HISTORY OF TUBERCULOSIS

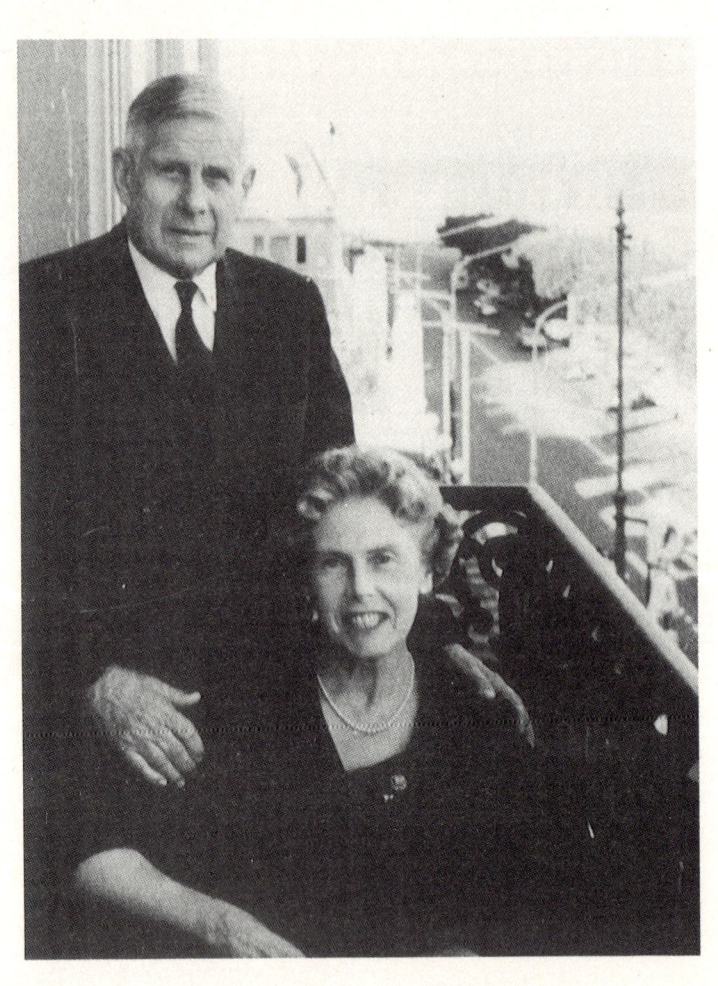

Sir Harry and Lady Wunderly, Geneva, 1964
(Photo by Mrs May Douglas, courtesy of Dr M.de L. Faunce)

Dedicated to to the memory of Sir Harry and Lady Wunderly
— tireless workers for the control of tuberculosis —

HISTORY OF TUBERCULOSIS IN AUSTRALIA NEW ZEALAND AND PAPUA NEW GUINEA

Edited by A.J. Proust

Brolga Press
Canberra

National Library of Australia card number
ISBN 1 875495 02 9

Cover design: Jocelyn Proust

Published by Brolga Press, 47 McCormack Street, Curtin, ACT 2605

Printed by Australian Print Group, Maryborough, Victoria

Contents

Illustrations

Contributing Authors*

ABRAHAMS, E.W. Formerly Director of Tuberculosis, Queensland.

BRAITHWAITE, Peter*. Formerly Surgical Staff Specialist Royal Hobart Hospital.

BRYDER, Linda. Lecturer, Department of History, Auckland University,

CARRUTHERS, K.J.M. Formerly Director, Tuberculosis and Chest Services, Western Australia.

CROTTY, J.M. Formerly Specialist Pathologist, Darwin Hospital.

DAWSON, David. Senior Scientist, Laboratory of Microbiology and Pathology, Queensland.

ENTICOTT, Thomas. Formerly Medical Superintendent, Coronation Hospital, Christchurch.

FAUNCE, Marcus de L. Consultant Physician, Royal Canberra Hospital.

GANDEVIA, Bryan. Formerly Associate Professor of Respiratory Medicine, Prince of Wales Hospital, Randwick.

GOLDSMITH, Lindsay. Formerly Research Officer, Commonwealth Department of Health.

GRIGG, Lindsay. Consultant Thoracic and Vascular Surgeon, Royal Canberra and Woden Valley Hospitals.

HARRIS, Keith W.H. Director of Tuberculosis, New South Wales.

HARVEY, H.P.B. Honorary Thoracic Physician, Royal Prince Alfred Hospital.

HIDDLESTONE, H. John. Formerly Director-General of Health, New Zealand.

JOSEPH, Maurice R. Formerly Consultant Physician Royal Prince Alfred Hospital.

KETTLE, Ellen. Formerly Senior Survey Sister, Northern Territory Medical Service.

LAYLAND, Robert. Formerly Minister (Energy) at Australian Delegation,OECD, Paris.

MACKAY, John B. Formerly Senior Chest Physician, Wellington Hospital Board, New Zealand.

MARSHMAN, Raymond S.A. Formerly Director of Tuberculosis, Victoria.

McLEOD, John A. Medical Superintendent, Princess Margaret Hospital, Christchurch, New Zealand.

McMANIS, A.G. Formerly Consultant Physician (Thoracic Medicine) St Vincents Hospital, Sydney.

MILLS, R.M. Formerly Staff Specialist (Thoracic Medicine) and VMO Royal Newcastle Hospital.

NICKS, Rowan. Formerly Staff Surgeon Green Lane Hospital, Auckland, Staff Surgeon Royal Prince Alfred Hospital, Sydney.

O'CONNELL, John Michael*. Formerly Consultant Physician, Bendigo Base Hospital, and Chest Clinic, Bendigo, Victoria.

O'KEEFE, Leslie John. Formerly Principal Medical Officer, Commonwealth Department of Health.

PAXON, T.G. Formerly Director of Tuberculosis, South Australia.

PROUST, A.J. Formerly Senior Specialist, Canberra Chest Clinic.

SEWARD, David N.L. Formerly Consultant Chest Physician, Geelong Chest Clinic and Geelong Hospital.

SLOAN, H. Retired Public Servant, Tuross, NSW.

* Those authors marked with an * are deceased.

STOREY, John. Retired Public Servant, Canberra, ACT.

THOMPSON, John E. Staff Specialist (Thoracic Medicine) Cairns Base Hospital, Cairns.

THOMPSON, Heath.Formerly Thoracic Surgeon, Princess Margaret Hospital, Christchurch, New Zealand.

THOMSON, Neil. Head, Aboriginal and Torres Strait Islander Health Unit, Australian Institute of Health.

THOMSON, Roma. Formerly Senior Medical Officer (Tuberculosis), New South Wales.

WEBB Adam. Formerly Specialist in Charge, Chest Clinic, Lower Hutt, New Zealand.

WELLS, Athol. Tutor in Respiratory Medicine, Green Lane Hospital, Auckland.

WIGLEY Stanley C. Formerly Senior Specialist (Tuberculosis) Port Moresby, Papua New Guinea.

WOODRUFF, Philip. Formerly Director of Tuberculosis, Director General of Public Health, South Australia.

The following contributed significant material, published and unpublished, on tuberculosis in Australia.

CAMPBELL, Alastair. Formerly Consultant (Chest Diseases), Repatriation General Hospital, Heidelberg, Victoria.

CUMPSTON, Alan. Formerly Specialist in Occupational Medicine. The Zinc Corporation, Broken Hill, NSW.

O'CARRIGAN, Catherine. Teacher and Medical Historian, St Vincents College, Potts Point, Sydney.

WILES, Angus. Medical Officer, Joint Coal Board, Newcastle and Sydney.

Acknowledgments

My thanks are due to all who have helped and encouraged me in so many ways, to those who contributed original articles or who forwarded published and unpublished material, photographs or references. Without their assistance there would have been no book.

I acknowledge with gratitude the assistance of librarians and their staffs, especially those at the Royal Canberra Hospital, ACT Health Commission, The Departments of Health and Veterans Affairs, The Australian War Memorial, the Australian and the various state archives. The Librarians of the History of Medicine Library, Royal Australasian College of Physicians and the staff of the National Library of Australia have been of great assistance for which I am grateful.

I spent many pleasant hours writing and reading about tuberculosis in the Library of the Royal College of Physicians, London.

I am greatly indebted to Brolga Press for professional and friendly assistance.

Finally, my thanks to my wife and family who will be relieved to see the book published at last; and to the secretarial help I received from several quarters.

Preface

The introduction of tuberculosis into Australia, New Zealand and Papua New Guinea was an important medical and social milestone. Not only did the disease devastate the indigenous peoples, hastening their subjugation by the European invaders but it also gravely afflicted the European settlers. But tuberculosis was far more than a killer disease. It became inextricably intertwined with the short-comings of the new society including poverty, illiteracy, urban overcrowding, the migration of the sick and socially disadvantaged, the Great War and unhealthy working environments.

An attempt has been made here to address these various factors and to record how the challenge to control tuberculosis has been met.

The contributors come from many disciplines and include former patients and interested members of the general public. The volume of material was overwhelming and ruthless editing was inevitable. All contributions in their original form will be catalogued and offered to the History of Medicine Library, Royal Australasian College of Physicians, Sydney.

This "History" is formally dedicated to Sir Harry and Lady Wunderly who formed a unique partnership for over 40 years in the effort to control tuberculosis both in Australia and in the region. It also honours those who wittingly or unwittingly heeded the call to join in the fight made by Lt Col Cotter Harvey under unusual conditions:*

"A final word to the younger members. Those of you who haven't made up your minds what to do afterwards, consider the possibilities of the tuberculosis service. I am sure it will offer great opportunities and scope for first class men, be they physicians or surgeons, bacteriologists or other specialists. From personal experience, I can assure you it is a fight well worthwhile joining. You will not attain to wealth in money, if that be your object, and you will have many disappointments. But you will obtain a wealth of knowledge of your fellow men and women, especially in their reactions to adversity that falls to the lot of few, rarely even to those in general practice.

Your triumphs, and they will be many, the gratitude of patients and their families—often life-long—will be to you adequate compensation, and indeed, rich reward."

A.J. Proust

Canberra, April 1991

---

* "The Changing Face of Tuberculosis" A Presidential Address to the Changi Medical Society by Lt Col Cotter Harvey on October 9th 1942.

CHAPTER 1

The Tubercle Bacillus and the Natural History of Tuberculosis

A.J. Proust

Mycobacteria belong to a family of bacteria one of which, *Mycobacterium tuberculosis*, is the common cause of tuberculosis in man. Mycobacteria have been described as straight or slightly curved rods which share a high lipid content and as a consequence are resistant to decolorisation by acids after staining by certain aniline dyes, hence the term acid-fast. They stain either uniformly or irregularly and may show beaded or banded forms. Traditionally the Ziehl-Neelsen method of staining has been used since the bacilli were discovered by Robert Koch in 1882; however newer fluorochrome procedures are now increasingly used, enabling the bacilli to be recognised more readily.

Mycobacteria share other properties besides acid fastness—all are obligate aerobes and they are more resistant than most bacteria to heat and other environmental influences. Mycobacteria are generally slow growers; *M. tuberculosis* grows best at 37° Celsius, the temperature of the human body while *M. avium* prefers 42°C and *M. leprae*, the cause of leprosy (Hansen's disease), grows best at 35°C.

Mycobacteria are ubiquitous in the environment and are commonly believed to be among the oldest bacteria on earth. Most of the enormous family of mycobacteria are free-living organisms found in soil, animal dung, in fresh and salt water, in mud and attached to algae and grasses. Some are pathogenic for animals including fish, reptiles, pigs and cattle. In all cases of mycobacterial disease in animals, the characteristic tuberculoid lesions similar to the lesions in humans with tuberculosis are found.

It has been suggested by Arnold Rich[1] that "it seems altogether likely that the pathogenic tubercle bacilli were derived, by gradual adaptation, from the free-living forms which are continually taken into the bodies of animals with their food and drink."

The Natural History of Tuberculosis

Dr F.M. Burnet delivered the second part of the *Edward Stirling Lectures on the Natural History of Tuberculosis* on August 28, 1947: *[2]

Clinically tuberculosis differs from most of the common epidemic diseases by its chronic character, and epidemiologically it has several important features of distinction: (1) the infecting organism (M.tuberculosis) varies little in virulence, (2) the commonest result of infection is a trivial pulmonary lesion which heals without serious sequelae and leaves an increased resistance to subsequent infection, (3) a proportion of infected individuals (determined more by genetic than by any other factors) develops more serious lesions from which tubercle bacilli are liberated into the environment. (4) It is from these individuals that infection of others occurs. Any attempt at prevention or elimination of tuberculosis must be based on these four principles.

Burnet then addressed the question of the factors responsible for the development of adult pulmonary tuberculosis, including the genetic constitution of the individual and the environmental conditions including climate, occupation and nutrition.

There is sufficient evidence to make it certain that there are significant racial differences in response to infection with tubercle bacilli. Non-European races, e.g. Maori in New Zealand and the Melanesian in Papua New Guinea were very susceptible to tuberculosis to which they had never been previously exposed prior to the European invasion. However, following exposure over 4 or more generations, these races have apparently lost their former hyper-susceptibility to tuberculosis.

Burnet discussed the influence of environmental factors in determining the occurrence and severity of pulmonary tuberculosis in the adult. Occupations associated with lung damage caused by the inhalation of silicious dust were of major importance, for example underground miners and quarry workers. He also mentioned occupations associated with undue intake of alcohol (barmen and brewery workers). He wrote that:

It has yet to be proved that minor nutritional deficiencies in normal populations have an influence at all comparable to that of genetic constitution... It is salutory to realise that so far (1947) it is almost impossible to find any real evidence that therapeutic measures have been responsible for any significant part of the diminishing general mortality rate from tuberculosis.

He admitted that this may change as improved methods of collapse therapy were more widely applied, especially to less advanced cases of tuberculosis.

Symptoms of Pulmonary Tuberculosis

The Third Edition of French's *Index of Differential Diagnosis of the Main Symptoms* (1919)[3] states:

Phthisis is by far the commonest cause of haemoptysis (spitting of blood). It may be the very first sign of the disease, it may be the last or it may occur at any intermediate stage. The amount of blood is variable... it may be only streaked or a pint or more may stream from the mouth. In advanced stages, the diagnosis is not difficult. There is a history of cough, loss of appetite and weight, night sweating and expectoration.

There follows a long list of physical signs which may be elicited and continues:

> On the other hand the examination may not reveal any physical signs. In some cases the mottled appearance seen with x-rays may assist the diagnosis... tubercle bacilli may be found in the sputum quite early.

In the ensuing 60 years there has been a significant change in the symptomatology of pulmonary tuberculosis due probably to the earlier diagnosis of the disease, ready availability of chest radiography and possibly due to increased resistance of the population to the disease.

Holmes and Faulks[4] studied the presentation of 100 consecutive proven cases of pulmonary tuberculosis in Melbourne in 1980-81; 55 of the patients complained of cough, 52 of weight loss, 43 of breathlessness, 23 of night sweats and only 10 of haemoptysis. Sixteen of the 100 patients were without symptoms. The diagnosis was suspected at the time of the first presentation in only 52; the diagnosis was delayed in 32 patients and was made in 16 patients only when a "routine" chest X-ray was taken.

Minor Epidemics of Tuberculosis[5]

A minor epidemic of tuberculosis in a small Australian country town in 1970 illustrated all the principal manifestations of tuberculosis, adult pulmonary tuberculosis, disseminated or miliary tuberculosis, progressive primary pulmonary tuberculosis and primary tuberculous infection[6].

The index case was an 11-year-old child who, after some months of ill health, suddenly became critically ill and died despite transfer to a metropolitan children's hospital. Autopsy revealed acute disseminated tuberculosis in both lungs, hilar glands, spleen and small intestine. The organism was proven to be *M. tuberculosis*.

Contact examinations revealed the source of infection was a grandparent with active infectious pulmonary tuberculosis who infected her daughter, son-in-law and three grandchildren (including the dead child). The other two grandchildren were found to have progressive primary pulmonary tuberculosis. Fourteen of the dead child's 69 classmates were found to have strongly positive tuberculin reactions and normal chest X-rays (primary tuberculous infection).

CHAPTER 2

Tuberculosis in Australia: Part I

A.J. Proust

Tuberculosis in Australia before Koch

Captain Cook recorded in his diary that a seaman on the *Endeavour*, Formby Sutherland, died of "consumption" and was buried at Botany Bay on 1 May 1770. He was the first of many thousands to die of tuberculosis in Australia over the next 200 years.

Gandevia and Cobley[1] have made a detailed study of the mortality at Sydney Cove during the first four years of European settlement. They faced many problems including incomplete records with only a minority of deaths being recorded in other than anecdotal fashion. No strictly medical records have survived.

They divided the period into three phases, the first following the arrival of the First Fleet, January 1788 to June 1790, next the Second Fleet, July 1790 to July 1791 and finally the Third Fleet, July 1791 to December 1792. There was a minor epidemic of mortality following the arrival of the First Fleet, March to June 1788. This was followed by an eighteen month period of negligible mortality. A major epidemic of mortality began immediately after the arrival of the first three ships of the Second Fleet on 26 and 28 June 1790.

> Of the 104 convict deaths in July and August 1790 at least 98 were from the Second Fleet... the sharp and progressive decline in weekly deaths after arrival suggests an epidemic occurring on, or determined by, the voyage rather than one having its origins on shore.

Similarly at least two-thirds of the total deaths between August 1791 and July 1792 were allocated to the ships of the Third Fleet. These two epidemics associated with the arrival of the Second and Third Fleet did not significantly affect the First Fleet convicts.

Gandevia and Cobley reported the probable causes of 23 deaths during the period 1788–1792. The three main causes appear to have been dysentery (between four and seven deaths), tuberculosis (between two and seven deaths), malnutrition and scurvy (between two and five deaths). Other causes included childbirth (three deaths) and one death (each) due to of smallpox, stroke, alcohol and snake bite. In addition E.M. O'Brien[2] records four convicts killed by Aborigines and five were executed.

Gandevia and Cobley in relation to tuberculosis wrote:

> Cases 14 to 20 involved a long lingering illness... in two of which a lay diagnosis of consumption was made. Phillip observes that about one third of the deceased convicts up to February 1790 died

from disorders of long standing and which it is more than probable would have carried them off sooner in England, a comment
probably based upon conversation with his surgeons and perhaps
most likely to be made in regard to consumption.

O'Brien gave a general picture of life at Sydney Cove and Parramatta
during this same period. In the early days of the settlement, weekly
rations consisted of 7 pounds of bread or flour, 7 pounds of beef or 4
pounds of pork, 3 pints of peas, 6 ounces of butter and half-a-pound of
rice.

However before the end of 1788 the spectre of famine threatened.

Crops failed, the transports returned to England and only the
current stores and uncertain future supplies from England stood
between them and famine.

The *Sirius* was dispatched to the Cape of Good Hope for supplies and
67 more convicts were sent to Norfolk Island. O'Brien noted that the
number under medical treatment rose to 76 convicts and 27 others while
51 were unable to work because of age and infirmity.

Early in 1789 a further 27 convicts were sent to Norfolk Island and in
May 1789 the *Sirius* returned with only 4 months food supply. In April
1790 rations were reduced to about one third of the original and the
physical condition of all was impaired and at least 2 deaths were recorded
as a direct result of famine.

Following the arrival of the Second Fleet the death rate rose sharply as
recorded by Gandevia and Cobley and the food ration was increased.
However by the end of 1791, O'Brien reports that the famine was worse
than ever.

At Parramatta 400 prisoners were prostrated by sickness, to this
number more than 100 others might be added who were so weak
that they could not be put to any kind or labour, not even to
pulling grass for thatching the huts.

In 1792 local crops improved and more land was cultivated and by
1793 when Governor Phillip returned to England the food supply appeared to be more assured.

By 1800 alcoholism was a medical problem but hospital admission
rates were surprisingly low. Sydney Hospital was occupied in 1817 and
acute infections (dysentery, respiratory, venereal and exanthemata) were
the commonest causes of admission. [3]

By 1810 food was cheap and plentiful in New South Wales as farming
flourished in the Hawkesbury and Camden districts. Housing was much
improved, there was less overcrowding and most convicts were self-sup-
porting or relatively free on tickets-of-leave or had been granted conditional pardons. A growing proportion of the population was
Australian-born. In some areas and occupations convicts worked long
hours under awful conditions; in the coalfields at Newcastle, underground

mining in 1804 was combined with lime burning. While the overall death rate was high no specific mention of consumption is made.

Royle made several references to consumption in Sydney in the early 1820s. A French surgeon on a visiting ship, *La Cocquille*, reported that dysentery and alcohol-related gastritis and hepatitis were common. "The rather sudden variations in temperature... have a sharp effect on pulmonary organs and from this arises these catarrhs, these inflammations of the lungs which develop more particularly in the winter months... also one notices quite a lot of consumption". He also reported that some Aboriginal women were consumptive.[4]

Thomas and Gandevia[5] quote Dr Peter Cunningham on phthisis in New South Wales in 1827:

> On reaching the age of puberty, phthisis is likely to supervene from the rapid sprouting out in the stature of our youths at this period, but the European phthisis is uniformly cured or at least relieved by a removal hither if early resorted to.

In 1829 the Royal College of Physicians sent a questionnaire about health matters to the authorities in Sydney and Drs Bowman and McLeod responded. They prefaced their reply with the statement that the colony had always been "remarkably healthy". Nutrition was more than adequate; however this was counterbalanced to some extent by widespread intemperance. Dysentery, especially during the summer, was common and caused over 50 per cent of deaths.

> Consumption of the lungs is much more frequent than from the mildness of the climate might be expected and more in advanced life suffer from this disease than in England. It is remarked in people who arrive in this colony labouring under this complaint, it runs a much more rapid course than it is observed to do in colder climates.[6]

Tuberculosis in Victoria about 1849 was described as follows:

> Consumption consigns many victims in Port Phillip to a premature grave. To imagine as many do that emigration to this colony tends either to prevent the development of this complaint or to arrest its progress is a fatal delusion... the most intense cold of England does not produce so baneful an influence on a habit predisposed to consumption as the sudden vicissitudes of the Australian climate.[7]

In August 1851 the fabulously rich alluvial gold fields of Ballarat were discovered and in the next ten years the population of Victoria rose from 97,489 to 539,764. Most in this enormous increase were aged in the 25- to 35-year age-group.

> In this period dysentery and acute forms of pulmonary tuberculosis broke out... tuberculosis was a common cause of death throughout these colonial times.... pulmonary tuberculosis was the most obvious... and was often not diagnosed until it was fairly advanced.[8]

The Long Sea Voyage and the Australian Climate

In England during the first half of the 19th century, there was a well-estab-lished theory that sea air and sea water in conjunction with a mild equable climate were of great therapeutic value in pulmonary phthisis. These could be combined by taking the long sea voyage via the Cape of Good Hope to Australia. By 1860, a growing number of English consumptives were making the round trip, particularly to Melbourne which was then the usual first land-fall. The Victorian goldrush undoubtedly lured many to take a one-way ticket and try their luck on the diggings.

The theory behind the belief was almost totally unsupported by any scientific evidence. It was known that pulmonary tuberculosis was com-mon in England which had a large and growing population densely packed in an industrial environment. There was anecdotal evidence that the disease was rare in certain countries such as Australia which had mild equable climates and the assumption was made that the disease was rare because of the climate. There were many factors which were overlooked; the great variations in the Australian climate, the conflicting reports on the prevalence of tuberculosis there and the vast differences in population density and social and environmental factors between the million or so people in Australia and the 20 million in England and Wales. Increasing affluence probably played a role as also did the negative attitude towards treatment by the medical profession. What had previously been the op-tion only of the wealthy became popular with the growing English middle and artisan classes and the stream of tuberculous round-trippers and migrants to Australia became around 1870 a veritable flood. Books and pamphlets were written on the advantages of the voyage to, and the climate of, Australia and scarcely a volume of the *Lancet* over the period 1860-90 is without articles or correspondence on the subject.

Dr S. Dougan Bird was a leading proponent of the advantages of the long sea voyage and the Australasian climates.[9] Samuel Dougan Bird (1832-1904) was born in Staffordshire and qualified after training at King's College Hospital in London. He was awarded the MD degree by St Andrew's University in 1859 and served as assistant to the resident physician at the Brompton Hospital for Consumptives in London. He contracted pulmonary tuberculosis shortly afterwards and with symp-toms of cough, haemoptysis, fever and weight loss, he decided to "seek the cure" by taking the long sea voyage to Melbourne in 1860. His condition improved and he returned only to suffer a relapse. He then decided to migrate to Melbourne and with his wife and infant son, arrived in 1862. His condition improved and he established a successful practice as a physician with appointments to the Benevolent Asylum, the Immigrant Aid Society and, in 1871, as the first physician to the Alfred Hospital. His concept of tuberculosis was of a constitutional or humoral disorder affecting the whole body with the principal location in the lungs being almost incidental. The disease in his opinion was due to a dyscrasia (general disorder) associated with urbanisation, industrialisation, poor physicial development, lowered moral standards, materialism and all the other shortcomings a modern industrial society imposed on a person's life style. His own experience convinced him that the sea voyage and the Melbourne climate had saved his life. In 1862 Bird claimed that pulmonary phthisis caused only about 8 per cent of deaths in Melbourne compared with 20 to 25 per cent of deaths in England. The clear inference was that pulmonary phthisis was much less common or less fatal in Melbourne than in England.

Dr Bird believed the treatment of tuberculosis required a complete change of life style:[9]

> the institution of such a hygiene and regimen as we know from physiology and experience to be the best suited to the preservation of health... it was vital to find a climate whose characteristics will have a powerful constitutional effect... an alternative effect so complete that it overturned the patient's constitutional history, changed its vital functions so that the humoral condition which allowed tubercle gain a foothold would be reversed.

This climatic change combined with a new regimen of hygiene would halt the progress of tubercle in the blood as well as its local manifestations in the lung. The long sea voyage and settlement in Australia filled all these criteria.

The sea voyage in ships "as comfortable as your own home" should be undertaken, leaving England in October or November. Bird provided figures showing that the risk of shipwreck was infinitesimal. The pitching and rolling of the ship leading to some seasickness was actually beneficial—the constitution improved and the circulation was tranquillised and the symptoms of pulmonary phthisis diminished. Landing in Melbourne the patient found the climate equable and mild, the temperature and humidity stable, the prevailing winds were from the south-west filling the atmosphere with iodine and ozone. Dr Bird was reflecting the views of other well qualified physicians in England and his book doubtless was read there and served to support these popular assumptions.

Dr. William Thomson was born in Glasgow in 1819 or 1820 and educated there and in Edinburgh and was later awarded his FRCS.[10] He migrated to Melbourne in 1855 and practised in Prahran and later South Melbourne. He became a colourful and controversial member of the medical community and the author of several books including *The Germ Theory of Phthisis* and several analyses of tuberculosis mortality in Victoria.[11]

Thomson trenchantly criticised Bird's views on the value of the long sea voyage, on the prevalence of tuberculosis in the colony and on the benefits of the climate for both the locally born and migrants with tuberculosis. He claimed, with some supporting evidence, that the long sea voyage was damaging and dangerous to the individual consumptive; some died during the voyage and many more died shortly after arrival. During the period 1871–74, 105 deaths occurred among passengers during the voyage to Melbourne, 50 of these due to consumption; Thomson thought the real figure was more likely 70.

He also maintained that phthisis was more acute in Victoria than in England. Those who arrived in the early stages of disease did better in Victoria than in England. Those who emigrated from England with advanced disease did poorly.

Thomson, in his various statistical studies, showed that among those who died of tuberculosis in Victoria during the period 1871–80, the proportion of locally born rose from 12 to 34 per cent. In the susceptible age-group of 15- to 25-years, 84 per cent of the deaths were among the locally born. This age group had grown disproportionately due to the high birth rate in the 1860's. As a result there was an increase in the mortality due to pulmonary tuberculosis in Victoria from 115 (1864-71) to 138 per 100,000 (1880).

Thomson also opposed Bird's theory that a constitutional or blood dyscrasia caused tuberculosis, which could be reversed by the long sea voyage and residence in an equable climate. In 1882, his book on the *Germ Theory of Phthisis* was published. Thomson maintained that climate played no part in the prevention or arrest of phthisis; the social environment did.[12]

> If the cause of the disease was not in the atmosphere above or in the soil underfoot, it may be in the air we breathe.

He summed up his theory:

> This transference of infecting particles (in the inspired air) is the mode of communicating phthisis most obvious with present means of judging. The virus conveyed from a diseased to a healthy lung sets up therein the irritation and inflammation peculiar to phthisis.

Thomson also conjectured that ingestion of the (as yet unproven) germ led to abdominal tuberculosis and that rupture of a tubercle into a blood vessel released the germs into the circulation, leading to what we now call miliary tuberculosis.

Thomson realised that the entry of large numbers of visiting and migrant consumptives into the relatively small population of Melbourne could affect the incidence and prevalence of the disease in the colony.

A select committee of the Victorian Medical Society was convened to report on the prevalence of phthisis in the colony and the effect of the migration of phthisical persons from abroad. It reported in 1877 that the locally born population was relatively immune to the disease and tuberculosis mortality amongst it was low. There was however a much higher tuberculosis mortality among "non-Victorians". Thomas and Gandevia[5], using Thomson's data, calculated that:

in Melbourne and suburbs about 1 per cent of all deaths from phthisis occurred in emigrants within a month of arrival, another 2 per cent within 6 months and a total of about 5 per cent within the first year. These figures relate to a five and a half year period 1865–70 when about 1850 of a total of 2143 deaths from phthisis occurred among emigrants; the population of Melbourne at this time was about 175,000.

A leading article in the journal *The Lancet* commented upon Thomson's published views. It observed that Thomson treated the subject of the prevalence of tuberculosis in Victoria in a "spirit other than a strictly scientific one". The article quoted Dr Thomson's claims that tuberculosis mortality in Melbourne was higher than in London for which he blamed not only the climate but the poor drainage of large areas near the city which was a quagmire receiving a large amount of town sewage.

The Lancet was of the view that the reputation of the Australian climate as curative of phthisis led to an influx of consumption, significant enough to be "part of the explanation of the slight decline in mortality from phthisis in England and the slight increase in Australia". The article called for caution in recommending the Melbourne climate for phthisical patients except for those in the earliest stages of the disease. It concluded that:

unless there is imported phthisis or there is something in the morale of the emigrants favouring phthisis, it would almost seem as if the climate of Melbourne favoured its production.

This, of course, was precisely Thomson's argument. Shortly before his death in May 1883 he became aware of Koch's discovery of the tubercle bacillus which he had anticipated in his book The *Germ Theory of Phthisis.*

Dr W. Lindseay Richardson in Ballarat

In the *Edinburgh Medical Journal* of March 1869 Dr Richardson[13], formerly physician to the Ballarat District Hospital, wrote about his observations of the prevalence of disease in Victoria in the early 1860s.

Of 12,286 deaths registered in Victoria during the year 1866, 756 were from phthisis, in common with other forms of tubercular disease. Tubercular pulmonary consumption presents frequently; it certainly has become more frequent within the memory of the writer. In former years popular opinion expressed itself that consumption did not occur in Australia. Experience has however shown that, while a change to Victoria from this country (the United Kingdom) is beneficial to the sufferer, scrofulous and tubercular ailments are developing there as elsewhere. In these cases a further removal to Queensland has, to my certain knowledge, stayed haemoptysis, arrested the process of wasting and brought about complete restoration to active life.

Based on an estimated Victorian population of 600,000 in 1866, the tuberculosis mortality was 125 per 100,000.

Dr Richardson then expounds on his own views of the benefits of the Victorian climate for sufferers from tuberculosis. There was a wide range of climates to choose from:

Melbourne and Geelong are equivalent to Naples; Echuca being that of Egypt while colder Ballarat suits some.

The possibility of outdoor exercise throughout the year was also beneficial.

(In Ballarat) we have repeatedly seen cases in which copious haemoptysis in some and the expectoration of cretaceous matter in others left no doubt as to the diagnosis, improve and resume work. There are many now hale and robust who tell with natural rejoicing, of a gloomy prognosis made by practitioners in this country (the UK).

That consumption was curable in Australia was no empty boast. The various Australian climates combined with outdoor living and physical exercise was the answer. Richardson mentions the widespread use of cod-liver oil in treatment.

Dugong oil was brought to the notice of the profession by Dr Hobbs of Moreton Bay as a substitute for cod-liver oil:

It was said to be more palatable and it was said to be easily obtainable as at first the Dugong frequent the Queensland coast in considerable numbers, I applied to Dr Hobbs for some of the oil but I was informed that the local demand was greater than the supply.

Tuberculosis in Tasmania 1863

In 1863 Dr E.S. Hall published a paper in the *Transactions of the Epidemiological Society of London* on the " Epidemic Diseases of Tasmania".[14] In 1861 the population was 89,977 (and of Hobart 24,773) in which:

The sexes on the whole nearly balanced but there was singular predominance of females over males at the ages 15 to 20 (years) owing doubtless to the rush of the latter to the Australian and Californian diggings.

Public registration of births, deaths and marriages had been enacted in 1838. Hall had for many years compiled a monthly *Health Report* in the Hobart district, using the nosology of the International Statistical Congress (1855). In addition medical practitioners had reported the causes of death of their patients to the Registrar-General.

Hall provides some epidemiological data on the epidemic diseases such as measles, scarlatina, diphtheria, typhoid (he devotes six pages to this) dysentery and phthisis. He estimates that phthisis is in second place as a cause of death (febrile convulsions is first) and the phthisical mortality rate was 188 per 100,000 in Hobart. He observes that 37 per cent of the population was born in Tasmania and only 15.7 per cent of the notified phthisical deaths were in this group. He does not indicate whether the majority of deaths were in those born overseas or in mainland Australia—probably the former, as intercolonial migration in the 1850s with regard to Tasmania would almost certainly have shown an excess of departures over arrivals.

Hall was convinced that wholesome food and the salubrious Tasmanian climate played major roles in the low tuberculosis mortality in the native born and in the healing of early cases in some English migrants.

Tuberculosis in Western Australia 1829 – 1955

From parish records (1829–41) and the records of the Registrar-General (1842–55) the causes of 1067 deaths (including two Aboriginals and eleven Asians) were investigated. In 862 deaths a cause of death was stated:[15]

Trauma, Violence	171
Pulmonary Disease	150
Fever (acute, chronic)	137
Diseases of Infancy	122
Nervous System Disease	81
Gastro-intestinal Disease	63
Cardiac and Renal Disease	47
Other	91

"Diseases of the lung were a frequent cause of death. Most important in this category were phthisis, consumption and haemoptysis, 74". One may conclude that tuberculosis was second to dysentery as a leading cause of death especially after 1850 when convicts were transported to Western Australia.

Tuberculosis in Australia 1850 – 1900

By 1850 the population had grown to just over 400,000. Almost half the population was Australian-born. The proportion of convicts in the population in 1850 was only 1.5 per cent. A steady stream of free and assisted migrants was coming from the United Kingdom. Only about a quarter of the population was concentrated in the principal towns (Sydney was the largest with 54,000, Melbourne and Hobart 23,000 each and Adelaide 15,000).

The goldrush of 1851 brought great demographic, political, economic and social changes to the whole of south-eastern Australia. It also directly and indirectly influenced the epidemiology of tuberculosis. These changes may best be traced in the publications of Lane Mullins and Trivett in New South Wales and of Thomson and Hayter in Victoria.

Dr George Lane Mullins

In 1898 Dr Lane Mullins published a booklet, *Tuberculosis and the Public Health*[16] in the introduction of which he stated that "in all the Australian colonies, tuberculosis stands at the head of the (medical) causes of death".

Lane Mullins was a physician at St Vincent's Hospital in Sydney and a member of the Legislative Council of the Parliament of New South Wales. He published the mortality rates due to phthisis, both pulmonary and non-pulmonary, in the years 1857 to 1896 based upon death certification. In a consolidated form the table traced the mortality rates of tuberculosis in New South Wales per 100,000 population:

	Male	Female
1857–64	88	84
1865–74	97	77
1875–84	114	94
1885–94	109	95
1895–96	92	66

The male mortality-rate peaked in the 1875 – 84 decade at a higher level than the female-rate which plateaued over a longer period at a lower level.

Lane Mullins thought the decline in the tuberculosis mortality was due in part to the Dairy Supervision Act of 1886 which reduced the risk of exposure to bovine tuberculosis through the milk supply in Sydney.

The magnitude of the problem of tuberculosis is shown in Lane Mullins's statistics. From 1857 to 1896 a total of 33,790 deaths due to all forms of tuberculosis were recorded in New South Wales (26,712 from pulmonary tuberculosis, 7,078 from non-pulmonary, principally abdominal and meningitic). Lane Mullins demonstrated the association between tuberculosis and urbanised overcrowding. In central Sydney, tuberculosis mortality was 196 per 100,000, falling to 116 in the outer suburbs and to 66 in rural areas of the state. He recommended that the Dairy Supervision Act be strengthened to ensure an even safer milk supply. He also advocated the compulsory notification of all forms of tuberculosis and the isolation of all sufferers from the disease in special institutions while still infectious; those who recovered could be released under the supervision of special dispensaries. Health education about tuberculosis should be promoted especially among the families and close contacts of consumptives. Central city slums should be replaced by well-drained and ventilated public housing.

He concluded:

> we spend immense sums of money in the prevention of infectious diseases yet we neglect the most deadly of all... we are bound to protect the health members of the community against tuberculosis —it is one of the most pressing questions in preventive medicine.

Mr J.B. Trivett

In 1909 J.B. Trivett, the Government statistician, published a booklet on tuberculosis mortality in New South Wales, (1876–1908). He emphasised the first step towards either prevention or cure of the disease could only be taken after a thorough examination of its epidemiology. Trivett proceeded to detail the age- and sex-specific tuberculosis mortality rates in metropolitan, rural and whole state populations, excess mortality due to tuberculosis, changes in mortality over the 33 years of the study, pulmonary compared with non-pulmonary and other data.[17] The preponderance of tuberculosis deaths in metropolitan areas was confirmed; however the metropolitan to country ratio of 100 to 42 (1876– 80) fell to 100 to 79 (1904–08) as the tuberculosis mortality fell more steeply in Sydney than in the country areas.

The maximum mortality rate was 161.1 per 100,000 in 1886; the male-rate was 181.7 and the female-rate was 136.6. The mortality rate fell dramatically within 10 years to 111.0 (119.9 in males, 100.9 in females) in 1896 and continued to fall much more slowly to 80.3 in 1908 when the male and female mortality-rates were equal.

The mortality rate in male infants aged 0–4 reached a peak of 618 per 100,000 in Sydney in 1885; the country male infant death rate in the same year was much lower at 220 per 100,000. These deaths were due principally to tuberculous meningitis and peritonitis and the rate fell dramatically after 1890, due to various Public Health Acts principally involving the milk supply.

The mortality due to tuberculosis was similar for both males and females in the 20–29 year age group. After that the male mortality rate was consistently higher than the female and it peaked in the 40–49 year age group at a level 50 per cent higher than the female rate. This bias towards a higher male tuberculosis mortality extended to the over 50 year age group and it became more evident after 1900.

Trivett concluded that the dramatic fall in infant tuberculosis mortality from 618 per 100,000 in 1885 to 59 in 1907 was:

> melancholy testament to the salvage of life which might have been effected in bygone years ... In 1881 one of the wisest and most valuable of all our laws (the Infectious Diseases Supervision Act) was passed. This created the Board of Health... From the time the Board brought the provisions of the law into full force we can trace a rapid reduction in the tubercular death rate.

The Dairies Supervision Act of 1886 reinforced this reduction by registering all dairyman and milk vendors and excluding those suffering from infectious diseases. Dairy premises had to be maintained in a sanitary state and the milk wholesome. The final advance was the Diseased Animals and Meat Act of 1892 which provided for animal and meat inspection at abattoirs and the condemnation and destruction of diseased animals and carcases.

Mr Henry Hayter

Henry Hayter was born and educated in England; he migrated to Victoria in 1852 and was appointed collector of statistics for the Western Province. He was appointed assistant Registrar-General in 1859 and in 1874 he became the first Victorian Statistician. During the next 21 years Hayter and T.A.Coghlan, New South Wales statistician, set standards unsurpassed in the world. Both received the highest international recognition for their work.

In his 1874 *Victorian Year Book*[18], Hayter reported 15,356 deaths from phthisis during the 21 years from 1853– 73. Phthisis (pulmonary tuberculosis) was the leading medical cause of death from disease during this period. Hayter estimated the average tuberculosis mortality in Victoria 1864–73 was about 120 per 100,000, about half that of the UK (250 per 100,000); however the tuberculosis mortality in Melbourne (225 per 100,000) was at least three times higher than in rural Victoria.

Hayter explained the difference in the Victorian tuberculosis mortality (140 per 100,000) in 1853 - 63 and the lower rate (120 per 100,000) in 1864 - 74 was due to the exodus of nearly 50,000 young males to other states following the winding down of the goldrush. This age-group (20 to 35 years) was most susceptible to phthisis and taking this change in the demographic profile into account, Hayter concluded "that the disease (phthisis) must be increasing". This is probably the first reference to the importance of the age-group profile of a population in relation to tuberculosis mortality.

In his *1875 Year Book*, Hayter recorded "Deaths from phthisis according to age, sex and period of residence in the colonies". Only 13.4 per cent of 588 deaths in 1876 were in the native-born. Among migrants, 89 per cent of those who died from phthisis had been resident in the colonies for 5 years or more. Hayter concluded that the "commonly held view" that tuberculosis was extremely rare in the Australian-born population was a fallacy and he referred to the work of Dr W. Thomson with approval. Hayter also noted that all deaths in the age group 15 years and less were in Australian-born while the migrant deaths were concentrated in the 30 to 35 year age-group.

Hayter refers to two female Aborigines dying of phthisis in 1876, and to eleven deaths from phthisis among Aborigines in Victoria in 1881. Hayter quoted H. Jennings, of the Victorian Board for the Protection of Aborigines to the effect that:

> lung disease (in Victoria) is the chief cause of death of aborigines who, once affected, seldom recover... from my experience among the blacks (in South Australia) I believe nine-tenths of them die of consumption.

In the 1877 *Year Book* Hayter reported that 48 per cent of 839 phthisical patients died within a year of the onset of their illness and a further 38 per cent within one to three years. From this Hayter concluded that 96 per cent of migrants who died of phthisis contracted the disease here. In successive *Year Books* Hayter pursued this topic; an increasing proportion of deaths due to phthisis were in the Australian born and that less than 7 per cent of phthisical deaths in migrants occurred in the first five years of residence in the colonies.

The Bendigo Epidemic
J. O'Connell and A.J. Proust

A rich alluvial goldfield was discovered in Victoria in October 1851 along a creek near Ravenswood sheep station between the Loddon and Campaspe rivers. The creek was later called after the Aboriginal Bendigo, a shepherd who accompanied the discoverer William Johnson. This was only one of a series of almost simultaneous major gold discoveries in Victoria leading to the great Victorian goldrush of 1851–60. The Victorian population grew five-fold during this period due to migration from other colonies and from overseas by British, Europeans, Chinese and Americans. It has been estimated that in 1857 alone, 40,000 Chinese entered Victoria. This mass migration undoubtedly brought tuberculosis with it.

The surface alluvial gold quickly petered out and shallow shafts were sunk by small groups of miners to extract gold from quartz reefs, using primitive crushing and washing methods. By the mid 1860s large companies were floated to sink deep mines and introduced new technologies, notably the machine rock drill (1870). This machine caused a marked worsening of the quartz dust hazard which was later recognised as a cause of "miners' lung" or silicosis. However, at that time, little action was taken in Australia or overseas to reduce the dust hazard. The association between silicosis and tuberculosis was also being recognised, the combined disease being called by various names, most commonly "miners' phthisis".

The first available data on tuberculosis mortality in Bendigo miners and also in the Bendigo and Victorian populations as a whole dates from 1870–72.[19]

The ratio of tuberculosis mortality in Bendigo compared with Victoria as a whole was 1.4 to 1 (1880–82) rising to 2.3 to 1 (1900–02). The only

conclusion which can be drawn from this data is that tuberculosis in
Bendigo miners became an occupational disease in the 1870s and they in
turn infected the non-mining Bendigo population.

Table 1.
Tuberculosis Mortality per 100,000 [a]

Year	Bendigo Miners (Miners' phthisis)	Year	Bendigo Pop. (Phthisis)	Vic. Pop. (Phthisis)
1875–79	485	1880–82	196	140
1890–94	846	1890–92	274	137
1900–04	1008	1900–02	267	117

[a] Data from Dr Summons report (1906)

In 1903, a series of articles in the *Bendigo Advertiser* entitled "Miners
Complaint, Bendigo's Dreadful Scourge" drew attention to this epidemic,
correctly linking the problem of quartz dust and tuberculosis among the
miners and the spread of contagion to the city's population. This conclusion owed a lot to Koch's discovery of the tubercle bacillus in 1882; the
writer of the articles was abreast and even ahead of the times as even in
1903 the implications of dust hazard and silicosis, silicosis and tuberculosis and transmission to the non-mining population were not generally
accepted. The articles suggested that the Bendigo District Friendly Society
might establish a fund to enable "victims of the disease to be properly
treated in the early stages of their illness".

In 1906, doubtless as a result of the efforts of the *Bendigo Advertiser*, Dr
Walter Summons was asked by the Bendigo Hospital Board and by the
trustees of the Edward Wilson estate:

> to make investigations into the incidence of miners phthisis and
> (the problems) of ventilation in Bendigo mines.

Dr Summons was a Melbourne graduate aged 26 when he began his
investigation. The investigation extended over six months and included
research into the clinical and pathological aspects of the disease, a review
of conditions underground and the domestic life of the miners. He reviewed the mortality data back to 1875, before which date machine rock
drills were not in common use. The machine drills increased the dust
undergound and the miners' mortality rate, especially the tuberculosis
rate. The number of miners employed over 1875–1905 varied between
2,850 and 3,990. Interestingly while Ballarat had a tuberculosis mortality
higher than that of Victoria and at times marginally higher than that of
Melbourne, only for a brief period (1894–96) was it as high as Bendigo's.

Dr Summons[20] compared respiratory (pneumonia, bronchitis and phthisis) mortality rates of adult males in Victoria, occupied (working) males in England and Wales and tin, coal and iron miners in England, with Bendigo miners. Only the tin miners of Cornwall had a comparable respiratory disease mortality with the Bendigo gold miners. There was obviously a very serious occupational health problem in Bendigo miners and a lesser but still serious public health problem in the Bendigo population. Bendigo itself was suffering the highest tuberculosis mortality in Australia just as Victoria and other states were recording falls of 50 per cent in their tuberculosis mortality rates.

Summons did not confine his research to mortality statistics. He examined many miners, their domestic living conditions, their medical records and autopsy material. By taking detailed medical and occupational histories, he was able to describe most accurately the course of chronic obstructive lung disease (COLD) from the stage of chronic bronchitis to emphysema ending usually with superimposed or associated tuberculosis or in heart failure. He noted that in some cases the chronic bronchitis did not always progress and improvement occasionally occurred if the miner changed to an above-ground occupation. No mention of cigarette smoking was made. No chest X-rays were available although three patients were fluoroscoped. Sputum was examined for acid-fast bacilli in some cases.

Summons was of the opinion that virtually all cases of severe silicosis proceded to tuberculosis before death. He found acid-fast bacilli in 47 per cent of miners with silicosis. He reported on 27 autopsies and all except one had pulmonary tuberculosis superimposed on silicosis and he found that the only exception was one man who died of acute pneumonia. The only solution was to prevent silicosis and tuberculosis. Silicosis should be prevented by dust suppression. Summons felt that the best method was to ensure the use of water jets with the rock drills and he found the unwillingness of individual miners to use a water jet with a rock drill " almost beyond comprehension". He also recommended enforcing the use of water sprays in blasting, shovelling and throwing rock and quartz down the chutes. The ventilation of the mines should also be improved. The use of masks was considered impractical as they were uncomfortable and were universally discarded. Summons also recommended methods to reduce transmission of tuberculosis infection. Invalid or special pensions should be paid to discourage tuberculous miners from working underground. In the community, tuberculous patients should be isolated in the special consumptive homes or special wards of the hospital. They should cover their cough and be taught the safe disposal of sputum.

There should be a special miners' medical officer, who should be able to reduce the incidence of tuberculosis, just as special mines safety officers reduced mine accident fatalities by 67 per cent during the period 1875-79 and 1905–06.

This document is remarkable for its observations on the natural history of COLD-silicosis and silico-tuberculosis and for the preventive measures for both diseases.

In 1909 tuberculosis was made a compulsory notifiable disease in Victoria. Attempts were made to obtain workers compensation for silico-tuberculosis (1910), to enforce dust suppression in the mines and to raise funds for a sanatorium. A local fund was set up and land was reserved at Spring Gully, 5 kilometres. from Bendigo for a sanatorium. The Government promised funds to equip three wards of a sanatorium to be named the King Edward VII Memorial Sanatorium. In 1911 Mrs George Lansell provided funds for a bacteriology laboratory at the Bendigo Hospital. Unfortunately matters ended there when the onset of he World War I set back the scheme for a sanatorium.

In 1920 the Federal Government in co-operation with the Victorian Government ordered an *Inquiry into the Prevalence of Tuberculosis at Bendigo*.[21] In the report Dr D.G. Robertson covered much the same ground as Dr Summons, and brought the epidemiological data up to date.

Table 2
Tuberculosis Mortality per 100,000 in Bendigo

Year	Bendigo Miners	Bendigo Pop.	Victorian pop.
1880–2	569	197	140
1903–5	1008	220	108
1913	942 [a]	200	75
1919	1406 [b]	147	74
Ratios			
1913	15.7	2.3	1

[a] 3156 miners; [b] 1138 miners

Dr Robertson recommended a 100-bed sanatorium and a tuberculosis dispensary staffed by a medical officer, nurse and radiographer. More generous assistance to tuberculous miners should be made available under the Workers Compensation Act. Advanced cases should be isolated and all contacts tuberculin tested and supervised. A laboratory service should be readily available to the dispensary, repeating the recommendations made by Summons 14 years previously. In these two reports one can see the genesis of the National Tuberculosis Campaign established 28 years later. As a direct result of the inquiry, and after considerable local agitation, a Commonwealth Health Laboratory was opened in Bendigo in 1922 which, combined with an X-ray unit in the Bendigo Hospital provided a tuberculosis and silicosis diagnostic service.

Bendigo continued to have a relatively high incidence of tuberculosis and in 1927 Dr J. Bell Ferguson, the first full-time Director of Tuberculosis, established there the first tuberculosis chest clinic outside Melbourne. In 1933 a 24-bed annexe for tuberculosis patients was built in the grounds of Bendigo Hospital.

Tuberculosis mortality in Bendigo fell from 241 per 100,000 in the decade 1891–1900 to 119 (1921–25) and more slowly to 93 (1938). These data were included in Dr F.R. Kerr's "A Hundred Years' Epidemic" in the *Health Bulletin* of the Victorian Department of Health[22]. In this article Dr Kerr concluded:

> It will be a sad day for Bendigo if gold mining is revived and if it is, it is essential that only fit men be employed (in the mines) and that they be X-rayed six monthly, that the tuberculous be excluded and that the disabled be compensated.

One can only speculate why the incidence in Bendigo was so much higher than in the rest of the state, including other gold mining towns.[23] It was probably due to the great depth of the mines with resultant ventilation problems and to the peculiar saddleback quartz formation in which the gold was located.[24] The last mine closed in 1954, however in 1987 mining is undergoing a resurgence, but the regulations, as suggested by Dr Kerr, are now in effect. One can only hope that Bendigo does not have another epidemic of tuberculosis.

Tuberculosis in the Mining Industry in Kalgoorlie and Broken Hill 1910 – 22

Almost certainly as a consequence of Summons' reports a Royal Commission chaired by Dr J.H.L. Cumpston was appointed to investigate the health of miners in Western Australia in 1910; it found that pulmonary tuberculosis was twice as prevalent among miners in Kalgoorlie compared with their non-mining counterparts.[25]

In 1916 the Broken Hill miners were granted a 44-hour working week largely because of their work-related risk of tuberculosis and other respiratory diseases.

In 1919 the Board of Trade carried out a survey of 3,967 Broken Hill miners.[26] The miners were given a physical examination together with a chest X-ray and, where indicated, sputum examination. The results may be summarised:

Completed examinations	3,967
Uncomplicated silicosis of the lungs	134
Silico-tuberculosis	59
Uncomplicated tuberculosis of the lungs	65

The overall prevalence of lung disease was 6.5 cases per 100 miners examined and of tuberculosis was 3.1 cases per 100. The prevalence of pulmonary tuberculosis was 20- to 30-times that found in male railway workers in New South Wales in 1924. Further surveys at Broken Hill in 1922 showed a much higher prevalence of tuberculosis (8 cases per 100) among 2,618 underground miners.

As a result mining practices were modified to reduce the dust hazard and pre-employment medical and radiographic examinations were introduced.

In its final report the Commission quoted Dr Gordon Smith, a member of the Technical Commission, to the effect that silicosis at Broken Hill differed from that seen in Bendigo and Kalgoorlie in that it affected the airways rather than the lung tissue and this resulted in a definite susceptibility to tuberculosis which was more likely to be a new infection rather than a reactivation of a primary childhood infection.

As a result of these seminal investigations in Bendigo, Kalgoorlie and Broken Hill the dust hazard in mines was reduced and medical services were established to undertake regular examinations of miners.

Tuberculosis in Coal Miners in New South Wales[*]

Black or bituminous coal was first discovered in 1795 at Coal River, later renamed Newcastle, about 160 kilometres north of Sydney. In 1797 George Bass discovered coal outcrops on the Illawarra coast, near present-day Wollongong, south of Sydney. In 1804 a permanent settlement was established at Newcastle and coal was exported to India soon afterwards. Coal mining around Wollongong began at Mt Keira in 1849 and the construction of the railway over the Blue Mountains to Lithgow in 1869 stimulated coal mining there so that by 1880 the Newcastle, Cessnock, Western (Lithgow) and Southern (Wollongong) districts of the Sydney coal basin were all in production. Production increased rapidly to 6.2 million tons in 1900 and doubled to 12.24 million tons in 1913. Coal was exported to other states and overseas as far away as South America. The New South Wales coalfields were by far the major producer until the Bowen Basin fields in Queensland were mined by the open-cut method on a large scale in the early 1960s. The work force in the New South Wales mines peaked at about 17,000 in the 1950s.

In 1946 the Joint Coal Board was established under joint Commonwealth and State legislation to carry out special administrative functions including the "promotion of the welfare of workers engaged in the coal

* In preparing this section the assistance of Dr A.N. Wiles, Medical Officer, Joint Coal Board, Sydney, is gratefully acknowledged.

industry in New South Wales". Hence coincidentally in the immediate post-war period in New South Wales there were two commonwealth-state programs—the Joint Coal Board's medical program to control pneumoconiosis and pulmonary tuberculosis among mineworkers and the National Tuberculosis Campaign, both established in 1948.

The Joint Coal Board's medical service was established by Dr W.E.George and Dr Gordon Smith. Dr George had for many years been a mines medical officer at Broken Hill and was a pioneer in the use of chest radiography to diagnose pneumoconiosis (and tuberculosis) in the underground miners of the enormous silver-lead-zinc Broken Hill lode. Dr Gordon Smith was a medical pioneer in occupational health, senior lecturer in that discipline at the University of Sydney and later a member of WHO expert committees on occupational health.

In 1949 just as the National Tuberculosis Control Campaign was getting started, Dr George approach Dr Marshall Andrew, State Director of Tuberculosis, with an offer to use the newly established chest clinics established by the Joint Coal Board as part of the state tuberculosis campaign. Dr George reasoned that pneumoconiosis and tuberculosis could not be separated and that the Joint Coal Board's medical officers had to have control of treatment, follow-up and compensation for tuberculosis in miners. The medical officers of the Joint Coal Board were well qualified and hence the Board's chest clinics at Wollongong, Lithgow and Cessnock were used for the whole community as well as coalminers.

Between 1948 and 1966, 96 miners were diagnosed as suffering from pulmonary tuberculosis in a mean work force of 15,000 men, an average annual incidence of 35 cases per 100,000. The average incidence of all forms of tuberculosis in the New South Wales population over the same period was 43.7 per 100,000; Southgate concluded that the incidence of tuberculosis among coal miners was actually less than among the male population of all ages in New South Wales during that period.[27]

It soon became apparent that pulmonary tuberculosis in coalminers in New South Wales was not a major occupational health hazard and:

> so effective was the ever-improving chemotherapy of tuberculosis that as of 1957 about 75 per cent of new cases could achieve long term arrest of activity. Having regard to these two developments a decision that was perhaps somewhat courageous for that time was taken within the Coal Board medical service... there were no longer any valid grounds for permanently removing tuberculous sufferers from the coal industry.

As a result of this enlightened policy, by 1966, all 85 miners who received compensation for pulmonary tuberculosis and had been withdrawn from the industry, were reviewed and over 40 returned to the coal industry at jobs other than at the coalface; 20 were retired either voluntarily or on medical grounds and 25 were declared unfit for work because of sequelae of tuberculosis or other disease and twelve of these died during 1948–66.[27] In addition to pulmonary tuberculosis 12 of the 77 miners withdrawn prior to December 31 1961 were in the early stages of pneumoconiosis. The number readmitted to the coal industry (40) would have been higher by 10 or even 20 had there not been a decline in the workforce of almost 30 per cent during the period 1948–66. Six of the 40 who returned to work had either early relapses (2) or later reactivations of their disease (4). Overall of the 96 miners with proven active pulmonary tuberculosis followed by Southgate, only five were treatment failures; one of these "failures" was an uncooperative patient and one was allergic to the whole range of anti-tuberculosis drugs. This low failure-rate and high rate of rehabilitation in the coal industry testify to the expertise of the medical service of the Joint Coal Board and the co-operation of management and unions in accepting medical rehabilitation advice which to them must have been revolutionary.

Southgate observed that no miner with a history of active pulmonary tuberculosis or with radiological signs of old inactive disease was observed during periodic follow-ups to develop progressive massive pulmonary fibrosis despite the fact that a proportion of the men in each group were observed to have mild degrees of pneumoconiosis.

Some Studies in Tuberculosis Morbidity during 1920 – 40

A mini-epidemic of 8 cases of tuberculosis in the Melbourne office of the Commonwealth Taxation Department in 1926–27 came to the attention of Dr J.H.L. Cumpston, Director-General of Health.[28] He ordered a retrospective examination of medical and sick leave records of 3,000 Commonwealth public servants in Melbourne over the years 1922–26. Forty three notified cases of tuberculosis were found, an incidence of about 280 cases per 100,000. Cumpston considered this was lower than in the population in general, however he ordered additional ventilation in commonwealth offices and he recommended that supervisors should refer all staff with poor health records to the commonwealth medical officer to exclude tuberculosis. All employees with active tuberculosis were to be granted six months paid sick-leave conditional upon entering a sanatorium for a minimum of three months. At the end of the six months leave, the employee was to be re-examined with three options in mind; return to full duties, return on light duties or retirement.

The 43 cases notified during the years 1922–26 were reviewed during the two years after the diagnosis was made; during this period 19 died, 10 were invalided out of the service and only 14 achieved stability of their disease likely to result in their return to work.

Surveys among state public servants were done in the 1920s. Victorian railway employees had significantly higher incidence rates (276 per 100,000) than their New South Wales colleagues (109 per 100,000). Among Victorian teachers, the rates were about 300 per 100,000 in female teachers compared with a rate of 250 in male teachers.

In Adelaide during the period 1939-40, Dr H.W. Wunderly surveyed 3,056 women in the 18- to 30-year age group. In his subsequent report to Dr Cumpston, Wunderly identified these women as "at risk of tuberculosis", presumably nurses and family contacts of active cases. Tuberculin testing revealed 1,110 (36 per cent) were positive reactors who were then subjected to chest radiography; 61 (5.5 per cent) showed active and suspected active pulmonary tuberculosis. This represented 2 per cent of the whole group.[29]

The Invalid Pension and Sickness Benefits in Australia prior to 1948

In the 19th century voluntary agencies raised funds to provide some temporary relief to families rendered destitute by the illness of their breadwinner. State governments increasingly supplemented the funds raised by well-established agencies such as the Benevolent Societies but even so the help extended to these families was minimal and unreliable.[30]

In 1907 the New South Wales Government introduced the invalid pension which in 1910 was superseded by Commonwealth legislation. To qualify for the invalid pension the applicant had to be certified as totally and permanently incapacitated. The consumptive qualified only in the last stages of the disease when all hope of a cure was gone. In addition the pension was lost or severely discounted if the consumptive was admitted to a sanatorium. Thus the invalid pension was unavailable to the consumptive in the early stages of the disease when sanatorium care may have brought about a cure. During the years 1911–15 about 10 per cent of invalid pensions were granted for advanced consumption.

Miners in Victoria with silicosis and tuberculosis were awarded a supplementary benefit in 1913. In New South Wales a Dust Diseases compensation scheme was enacted in 1920 and significant benefits under this scheme were granted to sufferers form silico-tuberculosis of the lungs. At about the same time in Western Australia consumptive underground miners were awarded a pension equivalent to half-pay until they could be found employment in a dust-free environment on the surface.

There was then a long pause before further social security or sickness benefits were introduced. The Great Depression of 1929–33 was certainly a factor in this lack of progress. Despite the exigencies of the Second World War the Labor government introduced child endowment (1941), widows' pensions (1942) and sickness benefits (1944), all of which were relevant to consumptives with families. The Tuberculosis Act of 1945 provided for a supplementary benefit which however was not successfully implemented. It was only with the passage of the 1948 Tuberculosis Act that a generous allowance was made available to breadwinners suffering from tuberculosis. This allowance was well in excess of the basic wage and was conditional on the consumptive agreeing to undergo treatment including hospitalisation if necessary.

Tuberculous Lesions at Autopsy in Adelaide 1925-40[*]

Professor Cleland reported the results of a personal search he had made over the period 1925–40 for evidence of tuberculosis, active or healed, in a series of 1,500 autopsies at the Royal Adelaide Hospital and the Mental Hospital, Parkside.

In 1014 of the 1500 autopsies (67.4 per cent) he found no evidence of tuberculosis on naked eye examination. He found doubtful evidence of tuberculosis in 80 cases (5.4 per cent) and in 406 cases (27.2 per cent) he found definite evidence of active or healed tuberculosis.

Of the 406 autopsies with definite evidence of tuberculosis, in 202 the tuberculosis was considered active; 136 were in the lungs, 48 were far advanced with cavitation, 31 were in thoracic or mesenteric lymph nodes, 33 were principally non-pulmonary and 2 were generalised. Of the 48 with far-advanced pulmonary tuberculosis, 9 also had tuberculous laryngitis and 24 had tuberculous ulcers in the intestines. There was evidence of tuberculous meningitis in 17 cases, most of which occurred in the 33 who were classified as non-pulmonary.

Of the 204 with inactive or "healed" tuberculous lesions, 107 were in thoracic lymph nodes, 26 in mesenteric lymph nodes, 45 in the lungs, 20 in the lungs and thoracic or mesenteric lymph nodes and 6 were in the spine, kidneys, hip joints and spleen.

He found that carcinoma was just as common in the autopsies of those with no evidence of tuberculosis as in those with tuberculosis. On the other hand he confirmed that rheumatic valvular heart lesions (mitral stenosis) was present in 26 of the 1,014 autopsies showing no evidence of tuberculosis compared with only 2 valvular heart lesions in 406 with evidence of tuberculosis.

---

[*] An abridged version of a paper by J.B. Cleland[31]. Copyright © 1942 the *Medical Journal of Australia*. Reprinted with permission.

CHAPTER 3

Tuberculosis in Australia: Part 2

The Goddard Papers[*]

R. Layland and A.J. Proust

Dr T.H. Goddard was a pioneer in tuberculosis control in Australia along with Sir Harry Wunderly, Dr W. Cotter Harvey and Dr D.R. Cowan. From 1920 to 1950 he was intimately involved in the effort to establish preventive and treatment facilities for the tuberculous in Tasmania and he was Tasmania's first Director of Tuberculosis from 1945 to 1950. He deposited his typewritten papers (the Goddard Papers) with the Tasmanian Archives to whom we are obliged for a photocopy of the 106 pages of foolscap (an estimated 25,000 words).

The Goddard Papers begin with the first moves to establish a sanatorium in Tasmania which resulted from the inspiration and enthusiasm of a small group of women led by Mrs Colonel Cox and Mrs Henry Dobson. They were concerned at the lack of treatment facilities for tuberculous patients and were enthusiastic about reports of the "open air" treatment of the disease. These women were also keen on health education as a preventive measure. They were confident that if they could establish the sanatorium and demonstrate its effectiveness then the state governnment would take it over and develop it further.

A public meeting was called, the response was positive and their concept of a sanatorium was endorsed. The appointed committee included Sir Gerald Strickland who was the Governor and Patron, the Hon. J.W. Evans (Premier), who was elected President and the Bishop of Tasmania, Rev. Dr Mercer, who was elected Vice President; the committee consisted of four doctors, six gentlemen and ten ladies.

The Tasmanian sanatorium was completed in 1905, and was operated by the committee of voluntary workers who organised fund-raising activities. The Association of Friendly Societies, the Australian Natives Association, trade unions and sporting organisations made regular donations. In 1916 the Tasmanian government built an administrative block, staff quarters and a separate unit for the treatment and isolation of advanced cases. The government increased its subsidy to £1,000 annually and in addition paid for the operational costs of the unit for advanced cases. The state later built other units and progressively increased its subsidy to £2,300

---

[*] The assistance of Mr Ian Pearce, Tasmanian State Archivist, is gratefully acknowledged.

(1922) and £3,000 (1937). In 1945 the state government took over the whole project.

Early Operation of the Sanatorium

The sanatorium was, even by the standards of the time, poorly equipped. There was no bacteriological laboratory and patients were taken to the Hobart Hospital nearby for X-rays. Dr Goddard related the method of diagnosis of tuberculosis:

> Strong reliance was placed on the medical history given by the patient, on his cough, his wasting and lassitude, his fever and night sweats. The stethoscope and sputum test (for tubercle bacilli) were the physician's two great aids in diagnosis.

The treatment was basically "open air therapy" combined with graduated exercise and good food especially milk and eggs. The chalets were spartan and provided little protection against cold winds and rain. Dr Goddard later recalled:

> (chalet treatment) was an altogether too rigorous a remedy to subject a tuberculosis sufferer to and yet it was the accepted treatment all over the world; the open air treatment, day and night, summer and winter.

Over the next decade more emphasis was put on complete bed rest. Dr Goddard again:

> The theory was that rest allowed the fatigued body to recover, it conserved strength while the disease was being arrested and till the fever had abated, it prevented additional wear and tear on the tissues.

In the late 1920s the sanatorium was given a portable X-ray machine by a patient of Dr Goddard who was grateful because he was told he did not have abdominal tuberculosis. The patient made the gift, observing, "he was only too happy to provide the apparatus at Dr Goddard's request although he (the donor) personally had not much faith in this X-ray business". The matron was trained as a radiographer and provided an excellent service for many years.

Some newer methods of treatment were used in the 1920s and 1930s. Little use was made of tuberculin therapy as it was by then largely discredited. The medical staff were involved in the nationwide trial of Dr Smalpage's serum and vaccine (about 1925) which ended in a unanimous opinion that the vaccine was useless. Mutton bird and cod-liver oils were used extensively as was creosote and Waterbury's compound. Dr Goddard recalled that one of his most poignant memories of those days was the ever-present smell of creosote at the bedside. Then the era of gold injections began (1925–35) and was followed by tonics of calcium salts. All were disappointing and for most of the period 1920–35, the sanatorium was noted for its comparative absence of drug treatment.

The rest treatment was applied more rigorously. The patient remained in bed, absolutely at rest, discouraged from talking or laughing. Meals were cut up for the patient and eaten in the supine position. After three months, under the most favourable conditions, the patient graduated to the use of the toilet and bathroom and if all went well, he could then have some meals in the dining room. Finally he would be allowed to walk in the grounds starting at ten minutes each day. The patient would then be classified as "quiescent" if he remained without symptoms or fever and the sputum was negative; "arrested" was achieved after two years of quiescence and "cure" was declared after a further three years of absence of symptoms and signs and of negative sputum tests.

Dr Goddard spoke highly of the nursing staff:

> Firstly I must speak of the Matron and nursing staff. Matron Luckie was a remarkably able woman... there were no resident medical officers in those days... she undertook the x-ray work when we obtained our first X-ray machine... Sister McKenna was an excellent assistant who, after seven years of devoted work at the Sanatorium took up duties as the first Sister in Charge of the new Chest Clinic in 1936, the first in Tasmania. I must refer to the work of the "nurses". They were not ATNA nurses but were generally women over 30 years of age who, without previous experience, volunteered to work at the Sanatorium. They were not afraid to come in the days when there was a distinct phobia against tuberculosis. I cannot speak too highly of their devotion. I do not (and this is significant) remember any of them developing tuberculosis and this was in the days when there was no routine staff x-rays, Mantoux testing or BCG vaccine. It was a tribute to the way they were instructed by the Matron and Sisters to look after themselves.

The nurses remained cheerful despite the inexorable progress of the disease in at least half of the patients. The symptoms of haemoptysis, malaise, fever and wasting rendered the atmosphere somewhat morbid especially when one after the other, patients succumbed to the disease. On the other hand, many of the cases were admitted in an early stage of the disease and restoration to good health could be promised.

Introduction of Artificial Pneumothorax

By 1935 artificial pneumothorax (APX) was the recognised standard treatment for selected cases of tuberculosis. Chest surgery was just coming into prominence overseas. In 1935 Dr Goddard, who had started APX treatment the previous year, went overseas to study the latest trends in treatment at the Brompton Hospital for Chest Diseases in London. He also visited Montana Sanatorium in Switzerland where Dr Hilary Roche was medical superintendent, and various other cities in Europe and the USA.

He returned full of enthusiasm for APX and determined "to apply it in earnest"; he was also keen to establish a chest clinic. He was soon doing a lot of APX treatments using the Maxwell apparatus he brought with him from overseas. The chief problem was the absence of a surgeon to cut pleural adhesions which prevented satisfactory collapse of the lung. Later, Dr J. Muir and Dr A. Pennington provided this service. Dr Goddard cited a family who owed much to APX:

> A young woman was admitted with advanced pulmonary tuberculosis and she died within three weeks. Her sister was then admitted and treated with APX first on one side and then the other. She became perfectly well. Then her two sisters were admitted, both had APX and both were cured. The husband of the second sister was admitted, treated with APX and returned to work. Then his sister came in, had APX and was cured.

This was a remarkable example of the infectious nature of tuberculosis and of the efficacy of APX. Dr Goddard continued to use it extensively up to the date of his retirement in 1950; in his last 12 months he instituted APX in 25 patients and performed 765 refills.

Chest Clinics

Dr Goddard had his mind set on the establishment of a chest clinic in Hobart even prior to his overseas visit in 1935. He sent Sister McKenna to Melbourne to work with Dr J. Bell Ferguson at his chest clinic. His overseas visit confirmed him in his determination to establish a clinic in line with the recommendation of the Federal Health Council, the forerunner of the National Health and Medical Research Council. The state government and the Hobart City Council co-operated and made a site available near the Royal Hobart Hospital. The clinic began operating in April 1937 and was followed by a similar clinic in the out-patients department of the Launceston General Hospital. Both chest clinics became part of the Tuberculosis Division of the State Department of Health in 1945. Chest clinics were seen by Goddard as:

> the first step in an organised campaign against tuberculosis. To these Clinics should be referred every case of tuberculosis, every member of the family concerned and every child noted by the School Medical Officers by reason of malnutrition. It is the coordination centre for all tuberculosis control activities.

Each new patient with suspected tuberculosis was handled as follows:

> A preliminary history is taken by the Sister with details of the home conditions, financial status and names and ages of every domestic contact. A full clinical examination is done by the physician and then x-rays and sputum examinations and other investigations such as blood sedimentation rates if necessary are arranged. Then the final diagnosis is made and if necessary admission is arranged to a suitable sanatorium.

Patients with early stages of the disease were usually admitted to the sanatorium for APX. Patients with far advanced disease had no hope of recovery and if there were children at home, admission would be arranged to isolate the patient and prevent the spread of the disease. Patients who were between these two extremes might be saved by bilateral APX.

Contacts of all patients were tuberculin tested and regularly followed up in the chest clinic. Dr Goddard noted that:

> Quite a lot of contacts under 14 years have, at the time of testing, proved to be already infected, the so-called (primary) childhood type of tuberculosis, which often tends to clear up, a different thing altogether from the consumption of young adults. A contact group in particular danger is that of young adults, especially females who have been infected when younger without necessarily developing the disease. They may later manifest disease either from within the body (endogenous disease from activation of a primary childhood focus) or from without (exogenous re-infection when resistance is lowered for some reason).

The chest clinic co-operated closely with the sanatorium in supervising discharged patients.

In Tasmania in 1941, 216 new cases of tuberculosis were notified, a rate of 90 per 100,000. About half (105) were admitted to the sanatorium; some were treated privately in nursing homes. The great majority of admissions to the sanatorium were referred by the chest clinics, although some were diagnosed by private practitioners or by the staff of the Royal Hobart or Launceston General Hospitals.

Some patients with chronic disease unsuitable for APX were discharged from the sanatorium with positive sputum. To reduce the chances of infecting others, these patients were educated in the necessary hygienic methods and supervised closely by the chest clinic.

In 1941 surgical treatment of pulmonary tuberculosis began at the Royal Hobart Hospital under Dr J. Muir, surgeon superintendent.

The Division of Tuberculosis

In 1945 the Tasmanian government established a Tuberculosis Division within the Public Health Service of the Department of Health. Dr Goddard was appointed Director of Tuberculosis and was directed to develop a campaign against tuberculosis. He gave up private practice and devoted his full effort to the task before him.[1]

The beds available for the treatment of tuberculosis were in the sanatorium at Newtown, Hobart, (72 beds), Ward 20 at Launceston General Hospital (20 beds) and some beds at the Repatriation General Hospital, Hobart. He had great plans including mass chest X-ray surveys, establishment and maintenance of a Central Register of all tuberculosis patients, provision of financial assistance to the family breadwinner who developed tuberculosis, to establish a chest surgical unit and provide rehabilitation and occupational therapy services. He also wanted to create an ongoing health educational program and to obtain the full co-operation of the medical profession (evidently some doctors were reluctant to notify cases of tuberculosis in case the patient would be lost to the practice or because the patient could not bear to be stigmatised as consumptive). Finally he had to solve the problem of a shortage of nurses which was so acute that half of the tuberculosis beds had to be closed down. Goddard solved this last problem by training returned servicemen as male nurses; this was an immediate success and all available beds were soon in use. He also appointed Dr. James Tremayne as resident medical officer at the sanatorium.

The Central Tuberculosis Register

Foremost in Dr Goddard's plans for the control of tuberculosis was an attempt to gauge the size of the problem. As a first step each case notified in the past five years was listed and an attempt made to record their present status, i.e. deceased or living and if living the status of their tuberculosis, i.e. active, quiescent, arrested. The Central Register was designed to record how the case was diagnosed, the X-ray report on diagnosis as well as the most recent report, results of sputum tests, treatment details and the present status of the patient. Dr Goddard standardised the definition of the extent of the disease.

Health Education

Dr Goddard felt it was essential to educate the public about tuberculosis and its mode of transmission. It was still commonly believed in 1945 that tuberculosis was an hereditary disease. He prepared a booklet setting out in simple language *What you should know about tuberculosis*.

One of the important items in Dr Goddard's tuberculosis control program was compulsory mass X-rays of the adult population. Mass miniature radiography commenced in Hobart on 1 February 1950.

Dr Thomas Goddard brought order into tuberculosis control in Tasmania in the short space of five years as the inaugural Director of Tuberculosis.

A Brief History of Tuberculosis in New South Wales
M.R. Joseph [2]

When I was a medical student (1929–35) tuberculosis was common and I well recall visits to Waterfall Sanatorium where we examined patients with advanced disease and elicited the classical signs of cavitation, consolidation, collapse, pneumothorax etc. There was also a government sanatorium at Thirlmere (Bodington) and a number of smaller private sanatoria dotted in the towns of the Blue Mountains. In Sydney, the major teaching hospitals had wards for tuberculosis and Randwick Chest Hospital provided especially for ex-servicemen with the disease. Smaller sanatoria operated at

Killara (Lourdes), Pennant Hills (Malahide, especially for advanced cases), Strathfield (the Eva Hordern Home for pregnant women with tuberculosis) and there were a few small private hospitals. In the post World War II period ex-servicemen with tuberculosis were treated initially at Concord Repatriation Hospital and then transferred to the Lady Davidson Home at Turramurra for prolonged convalescence. Dr William (later Sir William) Morrow was the consultant at Concord and in 1950 he invited me to join him.

The government sanatoria had full-time superintendents, e.g. Dr W.B. Fry at Waterfall and Dr Russ Godby at Bodington but a great deal of the treatment was controlled by visiting specialists, chief of whom were Drs Cotter Harvey, Bruce White and Gordon Bayliss. The linchpin of treatment was bed rest which was strictly enforced even to the extent, in advanced cases, of the patient being fed and sponged in bed. In some cavitatory cases the patient spent long hours in a plaster cast so postured that the cavity was in the most dependent position. Upgrading patients' activities was a painfully slow and gradual process and a sanatorium stay of two years was not by any means exceptional. At this time approximately one in every two newly diagnosed patients and two out of three of those with a positive sputum died.

Ancillary forms of treatment consisted of high calorie, high calcium diets, mutton bird oil and tuberculin which was favoured by Dr Fry. For cavitatory disease, some form of collapse therapy was used, artificial pneumothorax being the most popular. Some patients had bilateral APX's and all would have refills at weekly or fortnightly intervals depending upon the rate at which the air was absorbed. Large outpatient clinics existed for this purpose and in retrospect I am amazed at the amount of radiation we gave to our patients. They would be screened before and after each refill as well as having regular roentgenograms. In some cases the portion of the lung containing the cavity failed to collapse due to adhesions and a technique for dividing these was devised. It was termed "closed intrapleural pneumonolysis" and was performed with two thoracoscopes. Dr Gordon Bayliss was the chief exponent of this technique in Sydney. He taught me the method and published a monograph on the subject in 1945 incorporating his experience with 225 operations. Successful results were obtained in approximately 50 per cent of cases.

If the artificial pneumothorax failed a pneumoperitoneum was induced generally combined with a unilateral phrenic nerve crush to provide elevation of the diaphragm. The persistence of cavitation despite these measures generally meant that the patient was submitted to thoracoplasty. The surgeons whom I best remember performing these operations were M.P. Sussman who died recently at the age of 90, John McMahon, Harry Windsor and Ian Monk. About 1950 the use of extra-pleural pneumonolysis with the insertion of polythene sheets or lucite spheres to compress the cavitated lung enjoyed a brief popularity.

A *résumé* of the history of tuberculosis in New South Wales would be incomplete without acknowledgement of the important part played by the nursing sisters of the tuberculosis division of the Department of Health under the direction of the State Directors of Tuberculosis, first Andrew Marshall and later Keith Harris. They were responsible for running the clinics and for the follow-up of tuberculous contacts, In this field, Sister Betty O'Brien deserves special mention.

The Eva Hordern Hospital [3]

A.G. McManis

The Eva Hordern Hospital was opened by the Red Cross in 1945 as a convalescent home for ex-servicemen following treatment at Concord Hospital (Yaralla). In July 1948 it was converted to a hospital for pregnant women who had been found to have tuberculosis. At this time, it was the custom to X-ray all women who were found to be pregnant and a number of them were discovered as having tuberculosis. The demand for beds for tuberculosis was great at this time, and there were long waiting lists. Accordingly, it was considered desirable to have a special hospital for pregnant women with tuberculosis so that they could be admitted without delay. Dr Rhodes Hambridge, a trained chest physician, was brought out from England to organise this venture.

The Eva Hordern Hospital had been a private home with most extensive grounds. When it ceased to function, in 1956, it was sold to a developer who was able to erect fourteen large homes on the site. There was a cottage in the grounds in which Dr. Hambridge lived. Besides looking after the hospital, Dr Hambridge was head of the Red Cross services for tuberculosis. In addition to Eva Hordern, the Red Cross had two other hospitals for tuberculosis. These were Malahide which was for terminal cases, and Wentworth Falls-Bodington Sanatorium. At the latter, all routine treatment for tuberculosis, including surgery, was carried out.

At the beginning of 1951, Dr Hambridge returned to England, and Dr Russell Godby, who was then Superintendent of Bodington Sanatorium, became head of the Red Cross Tuberculosis Services and invited me to take over the care of Eva Hordern Hospital. I did this and lived in the cottage in the grounds. I remained in this position until it closed down in 1956.

The patients at Eva Hordern came from Crown Street Womens Hospital, Royal Hospital for Women, Paddington, the Royal North Shore Hospital, King George V Hospital and St. Margaret's Hospital. Resident medical officers from these hospitals visited the patients regularly during their pregnancy and when they came into labour, they were transferred to the appropriate hospital to have the baby and returned to Eva Hordern. They

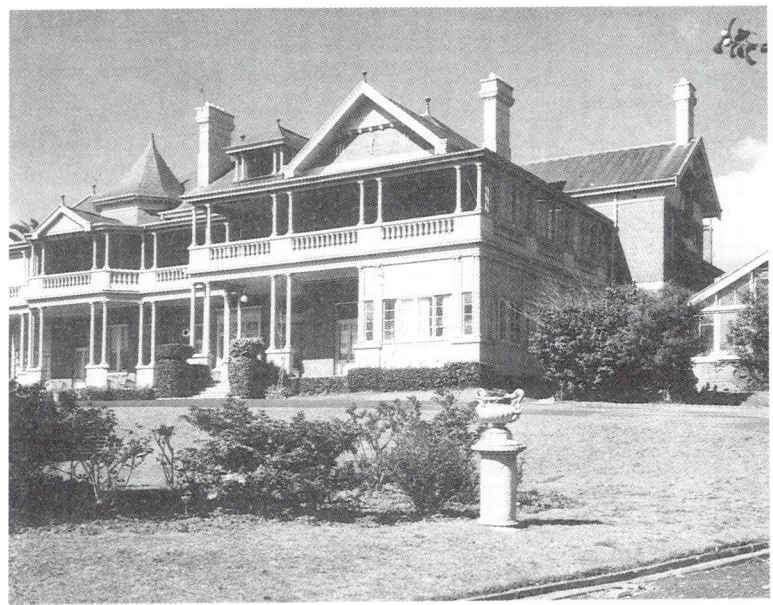

The Eva Hordern Home for Pregnant Women with Tuberculosis
(Photo courtesy of Dr A.G. McManis)

were separated from their babies, and various types of arrangements were made for the care of the offspring.

The treatment for the tuberculosis was modified during pregnancy only if surgery was needed. Surgery was extensively used in the treatment of tuberculosis at this time and, if performed in the middle trimester, was well tolerated.

All types of collapse therapy were also common then and were carried out without any problems. The chemotherapy of tuberculosis at this time was isoniazid, streptomycin and para-aminosalicylic acid. All these drugs were used and none of the babies had any ill effects from streptomycin.[3]

In addition to the in-patients at the Eva Hordern Hospital, there were three outpatient clinics conducted each week. Two were clinics for ex-patients and for contacts. The third clinic was a refill clinic for those patients with artificial pneumothoraces or pneumoperitoneum.

Tuberculosis in Newcastle and the lower Hunter
1953–1984

R.M. Mills

I obtained my membership of the Royal Australasian College of Physicians in 1950 and spent the next two years as the inaugural Fellow of the new Institute of Health at the Royal Alexandra Hospital for Children under Professor (later Sir Lorimer) Dods. My interest was tuberculosis in children.

In 1953 I was appointed staff physician to the Royal Newcastle Hospital with major responsibilities in chest diseases especially tuberculosis. Dr Ethel Byrne, the physician-in-charge of the unit welcomed me, allocating all new patients to my care. I quickly became part of a well-integrated tuberculosis service with a large chest clinic (and some acute beds) at the Royal Newcastle Hospital and 104 sanatorium beds at Rankin Park Hospital. This was ideal for a study of the epidemiology and long-term follow-up of tuberculosis in a defined community.

Dr Ethel Byrne was originally a pathologist in Newcastle in the 1920s but had slowly evolved into an infectious diseases physician with tuberculosis as a major responsibility. She was physician to the Infectious Diseases Hospital at Waratah where some tuberculosis patients were admitted and also conducted a chest clinic, initially in the city and in the 1930s at the Royal Newcastle Hospital. In 1929 Miss Thelma Bain a graduate nurse trained in public health was appointed to Dr Byrne's staff with responsibility for an area bounded on the north by Port Stephens, on the south by Gosford and on the west by Cessnock and Singleton.

Dr Byrne and Miss Bain were a remarkable pair. Each knew everybody of importance in Newcastle, managers and personnel officers of industry and commerce, trade union officials and other influential people as well as the scallywags and petty criminals about town—tuberculosis flourished as did petty crime in problem families aggravated by poverty. These women had prodigious memories for people and places. They could organise employment for ex-patients better than any government agency. They kept superb clinical and social records and their dedication to patients' welfare was outstanding.

Rankin Park Hospital

When Japan entered World War II, the Chairman of the Board of Royal Newcastle Hospital, Mr Archie Rankin, and the Medical Superintendent, Dr C.J. McCaffrey, were invited to Sydney by the Hospitals Commission. They were instructed to build urgently a temporary hospital in bushland more than three miles from the coast as the Royal Newcastle Hospital at Bar Beach was in obvious danger of sustaining damage from Japanese naval guns. Mr Rankin was quick to see the possibility that this new hospital might be converted to a chest hospital after the war. A site on the southwest outskirts of Newcastle, 110 hectares in area, was acquired, beyond the range of naval guns. Initially the new hospital was given top priority but by 1944 building languished and was completed only in 1946; it was called Rankin Park and subsequently taken over by the Royal Newcastle Hospital Board.

In 1955 I was privileged to participate in the planning of a large occupational therapy unit complete with a sheltered workshop in the basement and later a 12-bed male hostel for ambulant patients called Byrne House. This was designed for homeless and socially deprived males with chronic infectious pulmonary tuberculosis. They were given privileges and responsibilities and there was no problem with alcohol as they valued these privileges.

The occupational therapy unit played a vital role in the rehabilitation of the patient which began on the admission day when the occupational therapist was introduced. In 1956 a woodwork factory was established which was highly successful in winning large contracts in open competition. As a result over two-thirds of patients secured full-time employment on discharge. The remainder were able to continue in a "sheltered workshop" environment or were obliged to accept the invalid pension.

Treatment of Pulmonary Tuberculosis

No new cases were treated with artificial pneumothorax or pneumoperitoneum after 1955. Since 1951 no patient was referred for thoracoplasty and only one for pneumonectony despite pressure from those administering the tuberculosis allowance; closely supervised chemotherapy made surgery unnecessary in our closely followed up and supervised patients.

In 1966 I went on study leave to complete an analysis of the incidence and long-term outcome of tuberculosis in adults in the Newcastle region since 1950. I then went to Denver, Colorado to study the treatment of drug-resistant tuberculosis and acute respiratory care facilities.

On my return we obtained supplies of the new drug, rifampicin and along with ethambutol, pyrazinamide and capreomycin we had the drugs to treat drug-resistant disease.

It was only in 1984 that I presented to the Thoracic Society of Australia a review of 424 patients with proven pulmonary tuberculosis treated and followed up in the period 1966–80.

> With the exception of two patients who were moribund on admission and died from massive heamoptyses, all patients converted. Two patients relapsed, and refused to complete treatment and the other absconded. Resumption of treatment resulted in conversion in both cases. None of the other patients is known to have relapsed.

The dedication of the nursing sisters in this endeavour was remarkable. Treatment was on a fully supervised daily basis, at first for 18 months, more recently for 12 months. Co-operation from outside agencies was splendid; in one case an interstate lorry driver would have a schedule arranged, say chemotherapy at Kempsey, Brisbane and at Tamworth on the return journey. Many patients had chemotherapy supervised by nursing sisters at medical clinics in heavy industry plants. A number of housewives who were graduate nurses co-operated in supervising chemotherapy in outer suburbs.

Studies in Epidemiology*

By 1954 I had evolved an analytical card which enabled me to study the incidence and outcome of tuberculosis in Newcastle adults. This grew out of daily medical records I kept of each of the 720 men of F Force on the Thai-Burma railway in World War II.

Data on 2,012 Newcastle adults with active or inactive pulmonary tuberculosis from 1950 to 1965 were coded. A 7-year follow-up of 1,518 persons (1950–58) was completed by 1966. Less than 3 per cent were lost to follow-up.

The evidence showed the five mass X-ray surveys over nine years did not significantly reduce the incidence of new cases of tuberculosis. The obvious benefit of diagnosing previously unknown cases was offset by the incidence of new cases soon after the surveys, some of which caused local epidemics of tuberculosis infection and disease. Hence the basic tenet of compulsory chest X-ray surveys—to detect cases of pulmonary tuberculosis before they caused local epidemics of infection—was shown to be untenable.

In conclusion, I have given an intensely personal account of my experience with tuberculosis over nearly 30 years in Newcastle and the lower Hunter. It has been a team effort in which I have been privileged to participate.

The History of the Geelong Chest Clinic 1932-1983
David N.L. Seward

Among the early medical records containing a reference to tuberculosis in Australia is a pamphlet by Dr James Kilgour, a physician practising in Geelong. Entitled *Effect of the Climate of Australia upon the European Constitution in Health and Disease*. it was published in 1855. This pamphlet was the subject of a review in the first issue of the *Australian Medical Journal* in January, 1856. Referring to the effect of the Australian climate on consumptive patients, Dr Kilgour stated that "The *modus operandi*, or means, by which the climate operates favourably in such cases is probably by quickening the circulation of the blood, and thereby producing a higher and more equal temperature throughout the system, which in its turn, brings about an increased activity of the absorbents, and consequently, an improved nutrition of the body".

Dr Mingay Syder, MD, another physician practising in Geelong at "Celsus Cottage", Skene Street, Newtown,was an outspoken critic of

---

* Studies of infection by Dr Mills (as measured by a positive tuberculin test) are referred to in Dr Ken Carruthers' article on "Tuberculin as a Diagnostic and Epidemiological Tool" (Chapter 7).

Dr Kilgour. He had migrated to the colony from London in 1850 as a graduate of about thirty years standing. He published a pamphlet in refutation of Kilgour's pamphlet and also advertised the publication of a book entitled *A treatise on the causes and prevention of diseases, under the influence of the climate of Victoria*. He refers scathingly to Kilgour's publication— "I have searched from Alpha to Omega, and not one satisfactory word can I find as to the peculiarities of the climate of Australia". He ascribed the "fearful amount of disease and mortality" to factors other than climate and he stressed the need for healthy migrants in the following terms:

> This colony was not selected by its discoverers and first settlers, as a nursery for the idle, dissipated, scrofulous, phthisical... worn out constitutions; or for the "prostitutes", and other fungi, of Europe; and, until it has become what it is calculated for, a flourishing and highly civilised nation... invalids of any kind, had better not chance a change to this country.

Despite the controversy there is no doubt that the favourable reports about the climate attracted to the colony many patients suffering from tuberculosis and some with even advanced disease. Furthermore, some whole families who were thought to be pre-disposed to consumption joined the migration. The death rate was certainly formidable and although no early figures for Geelong have been found it is probable that these would have been similar to those for Melbourne.

To come nearer to the present time, but prior to the establishment of the chest clinic in Geelong, Dr George Cole, took an active interest in tuberculosis control. He commenced duty in Geelong as District Health Officer for the Western District in 1925. He was resident in Geelong and the Health Offices were in the Old Telegraph building situated next to the Post Office in Ryrie Street.

He refers to his early years in Geelong in an article published in the *Health Bulletin* in 1946 entitled "Tuberculosis in Country Towns and Shires". Despite his many other duties with diseases such as hydatid and diphtheria he was concerned with the problem of tuberculosis and the absence of a chest clinic in Geelong. During the years 1925–28, 118 cases of tuberculosis were reported from the country regions of the Western Health area, a yearly average of 29.5. From 1929–1932 he tried to visit every case reported and to persuade adults and child contacts to consult their doctor. This case-finding effort resulted in an increase of notifications from the same area to a yearly average of 39.4.

In 1927, Dr John Bell Ferguson was appointed as the first Director of Tuberculosis in Victoria. At that time, deaths in the state exceeded 900 a year for the population of 1,700,000 and only 512 beds were available. His appraisal of the situation led to a comprehensive tuberculosis scheme for Victoria and this included not only more sanatoria beds but the establishment of chest clinics in the provincial centres of Ballarat, Bendigo and Geelong. The Geelong chest clinic, established under the guidance of Dr George Cole (District Health Officer), was officially opened on 17 March, 1932. Dr Kenneth C. Purnell, Medical Officer of Health for the Municipality of Geelong refers to the clinic in his annual report for 1932:

> This institution, established at the beginning of the year, and controlled locally by the District Health Officer, has performed work of inestimable value in the detection, treatment and guidance of early cases of tuberculosis. Many doubtful cases of infection are seen and investigated in a stage early enough to permit successful treatment being undertaken—cases which, in the ordinary course of events would have drifted on until obvious symptoms prompted the seeking of advice at a stage when treatment would be of little avail.

For about the next fifteen years the work of the clinic concentrated on examination of contacts and the supervision of patients in the home and this was greatly facilitated by the appointment of a visiting Sister, Miss O.M. Gillies, who continued in this work till her retirement in 1947. In 1944 Dr Cole handed over the supervision of the chest clinic to Dr J.E. Piper, a general practitioner and also Medical Officer of Health in Geelong. He was appointed on a sessional basis, and carried on till 1947 when I was appointed as Medical Officer in charge, likewise on a sessional basis.

One notable step forward in case finding took place in the early years of World War II with the first trial of mass miniature radiography. In 1940 chest X-ray surveys with 35 mm. film had been instituted in Australia for service personnel and it had been found that about one in every 200 recruits had lesions suggestive of active tuberculosis. Dr Bell Ferguson instigated the extension of this method to civilians and several X-ray centres were established in Victoria. One of these was at the Town Hall at Newtown, Geelong, in 1943. These films were read by Dr A.R. Moreton, the only practising radiologist in Geelong who also held the appointment of radiologist to the chest clinic. Dr Bell Ferguson refers to this work in his annual report for 1944 – "An analysis of 2,000 films read by Dr Moreton shows that 1.8 per cent of those examined had tuberculosis: 0.85 per cent probably being active". In the following year 1,983 people were X-rayed but in subsequent years the numbers attending waned, presumably due to lack of publicity and the centre at Newtown closed in 1947.

Till the end of the 1940–50 decade there were difficulties because of inadequate bed facilities despite the increase in number of beds in sanatoria in Melbourne. There were long waiting lists and often a delay of six months before the admission of a patient. Local facilities for hospitalisation of patients were almost non- existent, at most a few balcony beds in the medical wards of the Geelong Hospital. Home conditions in the meantime were often appalling and under such circumstances spread of the disease to contacts continued to occur. In 1943 the Medical Officer of Health for Geelong gave prominence to some of the problems in his annual report.

> It is a calamity that some ward is not made available for the isolation and treatment of these patients in Geelong. There is one great innovation which I respectfully ask the Council to urge on the Government of the State, and that is to place any wage earner who has developed pulmonary tuberculosis on the basic wage if he has any dependents. For example, there is in our city now a man with pulmonary tuberculosis, and who has a wife and three very young children depending on him. He will not go into a Sanatorium because he is the sole support of his family. In the meantime he is undoubtedly infecting these young children, and young children are remarkably susceptible to infection by tuberculosis, as well as losing his chance of being cured of the disease. Also he is a danger to the men amongst whom he is working. From a monetary point of view the first expense would save a much greater one later on.

This situation was in no sense peculiar to Geelong and similar thoughts by physicians and lay people on a wide scale led in 1947 to Victorian state legislation for a tuberculosis allowance, and this legislation, of course, contributed towards the Commonwealth Tuberculosis Act of 1948. The great intensification of the anti-tuberculosis program which stemmed from this Commonwealth Tuberculosis Act marked the start of a new era which led to mass X-ray surveys, tuberculin testing in schools, increased bed facilities and, of course, greatly increased activity of the chest clinic. The scheme was administered through the existing Tuberculosis Branch of the State Health Service and under the control of the State Director of Tuberculosis, but with the Commonwealth providing the finance for capital expenditure for approved new hospitals, clinics, X-ray equipment, etc. The Commonwealth also supplied the finance for maintenance costs in excess of that spent by the state in the year 1947–48.

It was co-incidental that chemotherapy for tuberculosis emerged at about this time with the first cautious use of streptomycin at the end of the 1940s, and then PAS in 1950 followed by isoniazid in 1952. Another notable advance was the recognition of the value of BCG vaccination. The 1950s were exciting years with a great upsurge of case-finding and also witnessing the recovery of patients with advanced disease whose prognosis would have been very poor in previous decades.

Dr J. Bell Ferguson

Dr Bell Ferguson was appointed first full-time Director of Tuberculosis in Victoria on July 4 1927. He continued in office until 1950 and maintained his interest in tuberculosis until his death in 1971. He found on taking up office after an extensive assessment that tuberculosis control had been directed mainly at institutional care; the sanatoria were poorly equipped and staffed, there was little provision for domiciliary care, admission and discharge policies were rudimentary and newer forms of treatment (eg. artificial pneumothorax) were not encouraged. Bell Ferguson launched a co-ordinated attack on tuberculosis; all branches of the medical services (general practice, school medical, chest clinic, hospital and sanatorium) co-operated and Tuberculosis Nurses based in city and regional clinics assumed pivotal roles in assessing the home situation for possible domiciliary treatment; contact tracing and health and hygiene education were also important facets of their work.[4] The hospitals and sanatoria were upgraded and radiographic and bacteriological facilities installed. A system of state tuberculosis pensions was introduced in the 1940s to enable patients to undergo treatment without imposing economic hardship on their families.

His network of bureaux and chest clinics was the basis upon which was built Victoria's contribution to the National Tuberculosis Control Programme. He developed a fine team spirit in his staff and was ably assisted by Dr H.M. James and Sister Elizabeth O'Reilly.

Measuring the Impact of Tuberculosis on the South Australian Population in the 1950s

Philip Woodruff

Tuberculosis was present in the white population of South Australia from the earliest days of settlement. Harriet Gouger, wife of the first Colonial Secretary died of consumption within three months of the founding of the Colony in 1836. Three years later Colonel William Light, having surveyed and laid out Adelaide and a significant part of the surrounding countryside, became another notable victim of tuberculosis. In the succeeding 120 years great changes took place in the impact of the disease on the growing Australian community. The yardsticks for measuring this impact are mortality, morbidity, and rates of infection.

There had been a progressive decline in numbers of deaths from tuberculosis throughout the first half of the twentieth century, and this despite a continually growing population. Reasonably accurate age-specific death rates were available only in census years. In males in each successive census year there was not only a substantial decrease in crude death rates but also a distinct shift to the right, that is, to the older age groups. The result was that by 1954 it could be said that tuberculosis was no longer a major cause of death in young men, and its fatal impact had moved almost entirely into the period beyond middle age.

In females the high mortality in young women at the 1911 census was followed by a rapid decline in subsequent census years, but with no tendency for peak mortality to move to the higher age groups, so that by 1954 the disease was virtually no longer a fatal one for women at all. The significant change in mortality from non-respiratory tuberculosis in both sexes, in the same period, was a dramatic decrease in deaths from miliary and meningeal disease.

Morbidity information has always been more dificult to collect and examine than that of mortality. The National Campaign against tuberculosis made several significant alterations to this. First the special allowance for tuberculosis sufferers ensured not only the welfare of patients and their families, but also that virtually every known case would be notified to the health authority. Compulsory chest X- ray surveys, covering, as they did, the whole adult community, gave a remarkably complete picture of the radiological state of lungs throughout the population. In the five years from March 1952 to March 1957 almost 300,000 people in South Australia were examined; 2.8 per cent were reported as showing abnormalities probably of tuberculous origin. This included a large number of calcified primary complexes and many other quite inactive lesions. Considerable and successful efforts were made to ensure that all those needing investigation were fully investigated. In the event 262 new cases of active tuberculosis were notified. This represents a prevalence of previously unknown active tuberculosis of 0.089 per cent or one for every 1,124 persons examined.

Previously unrecognised tuberculosis was found to be twice as prevalent in males as in females. Taken over the whole age span, one man in 836 and one woman in 1,794 had active tuberculosis apparently without being aware of it. Almost 3,000 teenage males had to be examined to find each new case in this age group, but in men over 70 years old, one new case was found in every 256 examined. Although women were less often affected, this was not apparent in teenage girls who revealed one new case in every 1,751 examined. With a rising population during this period the actual case load of people requiring treatment remained remarkably constant year by year.

Of people who migrated to South Australia from overseas during the years 1952–57, 144 were found to have active tuberculosis. Migrants made up 11.4 per cent of new notifications of tuberculosis, nearly twice the proportion of migrants in the South Australian population (6.5 per cent).

In the Aboriginal population very few cases of tuberculosis were notified in the period 1952–54, partly because the main effort at case-finding in those years was in the metropolitan area of Adelaide. In 1955 and 1965 X-ray and tuberculin surveys took place in Aboriginal settlements at Point McLeay and Point Pearce, at Koonibba Mission on Eyre Peninsula and Gerard Mission on the River Murray, and in more remote areas such as Coober Pedy and Talawan Tank near the head of the Great Australian Bight, and at Ernabella Mission close to the north-west corner of the state. In the small groups involved, totalling some 2,000 people in all, six cases of active tuberculosis were found, five of them in persons living and working in a manner comparable with white Australians of low socio-economic standard, and only one in the approximately equal number living a semi-tribal lifestyle.

The third yardstick of the impact of tuberculosis on the community—infection rates—was studied using the Mantoux test employing old tuberculin 1:1000, or purified protein derivative (PPD) of equivalent concentration. In the five years 1952-1956, 47,000 were examined by this test, 11,763 national service trainees (males aged 18 years, or in a few cases 19 or 20 years), 16,005 primary school children of all ages in country districts and 19,544 seventh grade school children in the Adelaide metropolitan area. It soon became apparent that among the school children there were major differences in reactor rates between children born in Australia and those born elsewhere. In addition in both groups the reactor rate declined quite sharply in succeeding years.

Tuberculin Testing of Metropolitan Seventh Grade School Children

Year	Born in Australia			Born elsewhere		
	Number tested	Positive reactors	Percent positive	Number tested	Positive reactors	Percent positive
1952	3014	256	8.5	221	87	39.4
1953	3084	195	6.3	270	85	31.5
1954	3451	154	4.5	351	88	25.1
1955	3800	196	5.2	425	79	18.6
1956	4351	183	4.1	577	181	20.4

Australian born children aged 12 were then about five times less likely to have encountered tuberculous infection than were those born in other countries.

In 1958 certain conclusions were drawn from these examinations. It appeared that while environmental factors, and possibly changes in the host-parasite relationship had long been reducing the importance of tuberculosis as a cause of death, in the ten years to 1957 treatment seemed to have begun to make a significant contribution to lower mortality. X-ray surveys were making a significant and worthwhile contribution to the control program, and it was considered important that the survey of the whole state be completed as soon as possible, and then be repeated.

Tuberculin testing of school children year by year was clearly the best indicator of the decreasing threat of tuberculosis, and of the success of the national campaign. BCG vaccine given to children entering their "teens" was preventing primary tuberculosis of adolescent onset, and appeared likely to provide protection extending into early adult life.

Sir Darcy Cowan

M.de L. Faunce and A.J. Proust

Darcy Cowan was born in Adelaide in 1885, and was educated at Prince Alfred College and the University of Adelaide. He graduated MB BS in 1908. He excelled at sport, especially tennis, and remained an active and skilful player into his late middle age.

His interest in tuberculosis became a life-long crusade following a visit to the Chest Clinic in Edinburgh of Dr Robert Philip, the author of the "Edinburgh Plan" for the treatment and control of tuberculosis. He returned to Adelaide determined to achieve the highest level of medical care for tuberculosis sufferers at both the Chest Clinic and its associated tuberculosis ward, the Frome, in the Royal Adelaide Hospital. He served this hospital for many years as an honorary physician until his appointment as the first senior physician to the Adelaide Chest Clinic.

In many respects Darcy Cowan's career in Adelaide was remarkably parallel to that of the younger Cotter Harvey in Sydney. They were both superb chest physicians, well loved by their patients and admired by a generation of medical students and nurses. To the end of his professional life he maintained his faith in tuberculin therapy which he believed promoted healing in carefully selected cases.

Dr (later Sir Darcy) Cowan played a leading role in the formation of the National Association for the Prevention of Tuberculosis in Australia. He was the secretary of the provisional committee formed to draft the constitution for the association, which was adopted at the first formal meeting of the National Association in Adelaide in 1951. At that meeting office-bearers were confirmed and affiliation was granted with the International Union Against Tuberculosis (IUAT). He was also a foundation member of the Laennec Society, the forerunner of the Thoracic Society.

Dr Darcy Cowan played an important role, together with Dr Harry Wunderly and Dr Cotter Harvey, in securing the passage of the 1948 legislation, the Tuberculosis Act, which launched the National Tuberculosis Campaign. He did not hesitate to approach state and Commonwealth legislators: "official red tape, apathy and delay evoked (his) trenchant criticism in which he favoured the broadsword rather than the rapier".

The highly successful Bedford Industries, a rehabilitation centre, owed much to Darcy Cowan. Impressed with Papworth in England, Cowan was determined to establish a "sheltered workshop" where recovered tuberculosis patients could learn new skills and re-enter the workforce under medical supervision. In 1950 a new factory was built for this purpose in Adelaide and was named the "Cowan Building".

Frome ward was built in 1932 at the back of the original stone complex of the old Royal Adelaide Hospital for treatment of patients suffering from "open" or infectious pulmonary tuberculosis. It was badly needed and

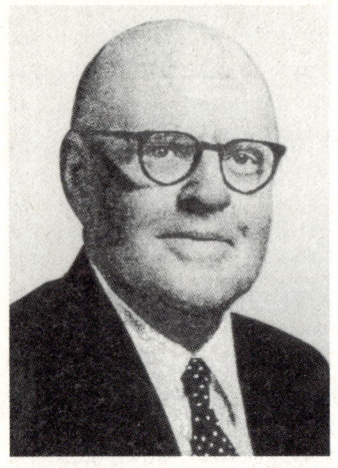

Sir Darcy Cowan.
(Photo courtesy of History of Medicine Library,
Royal Australasian College of Physicians)

when it opened on 16 September 1932 it filled with patients almost immediately. The Outpatient Chest Clinic was built soon afterwards and was
opened officially in July 1935.

The staff appointed to the new hospital department comprised Dr
D.R.W. Cowan as first physician, Dr H.W. Wunderly as Assistant Physician and Dr J.W. Rollison as clinical assistant. At that time Darcy Cowan
had been an honorary physician to the Royal Adelaide Hospital since 1924.
From this Royal Adelaide Hospital beginning, Cowan and Wunderly pursued their goal of a successful National Tuberculosis Campaign.

Tuberculosis Control in Queensland
The J.S. Elkington Oration, 1980 [*]

In the second half of the last century, tuberculosis, earlier in that century
described as the "Captain of the Men of Death", was very much the
equivalent of cancer in the popular mind today; a major cause of death, all
too frequently killing young people, infecting families by contact and
proximity to the point where it was regarded as hereditary.

The first of two great steps forward in its public health control was the
discovery by Koch of the acid-fast bacillus, now known as *M. tuberculosis*,
but for many years called Koch's bacillus, proving that the disease was an
infection, and therefore preventable; this occurred in 1882 when Elkington
was eleven years old. The other great discovery, the anti-tuberculosis

---

* E.W. Abrahams (Brisbane, Queensland) delivered the 1980 Elkington Oration, published in the
  Australian Health Surveyor 1981. 12(3), 51. This is an edited version (AJP).

activity of para-aminosalicylic acid and streptomycin, occurred in the late 1940s, the decade before his death in 1955. His working lifetime almost straddles the interval between these two dates. The discovery of Koch's bacillus produced an enormous explosion of hope and energy, directed to the care and prevention of tuberculosis; much of it, at a time when governments spent a minimum on health, by voluntary societies and private donations.

It is much to the credit of the political system of the time that Queensland was represented at the London conference on tuberculosis of 1901 by Dr Jeffries Turner. It was called to discuss the possibility that there were two types of Koch's bacilli—human and bovine, as well as the control of tuberculosis generally. Dr Turner reported to Dr Burnett Ham, the Commissioner for Public Health on his return to Queensland and completed his account of the conference by making the first of many recommendations to the politicians of the day on what should be done to control tuberculosis here. These were: voluntary notification, disinfection of premises, the establishment of sanatoria and of hospitals for the treatment and isolation of consumptives.

The next step forward occurred in 1911 with the first meeting of state senior medical officers to formulate Australian health policy. This was held in Melbourne, then the seat of Federal Government and there were representatives from all states except Queensland. One would dearly love to know why Elkington was absent—probably because he had just taken up duty as Commissioner of Health (January 1910) and there were many pressing problems. He was a federalist who subsequently accepted a commonwealth appointment—but he was new in his Queensland appointment and did not have time to attend. However he speedily implemented the recommendations of that conference.

In 1912, Elkington initiated a health survey of Torres Strait Islands (including phthisis, it uncovered only four cases) and all necessary powers for tuberculosis were covered in the Health Act of 1900–1911. (It is noteworthy that, in 1948–1950 when the present campaign on tuberculosis began, Queensland did not require new legislation, only regulations under its Health Act which dated back to this time.) By 1911 Queensland was reasonably well supplied with beds for the tuberculous, by the standards of the time. In other words there were beds provided in which the indigent tuberculous could die. Sanatoria, the creations of concerned persons, were established at Dalby, at South Brisbane (the "Dime" of recent memory—the Lady Diamentina Hospital for Chronic Diseases), at Westwood, near Rockhampton, and at Stanthorpe, this last for ex-servicemen.

The prevention of infection was another matter. In 1900 there were 234 deaths from tuberculosis— 102/100,000 of population. Perhaps this figure means more if I say that in 1977–1978 there were 197 cases notified, a rate of 9.2/100,000 and there were 19 deaths— 0.9/100,000. Notification figures fluctuated wildly in the early years of this century and were certainly inaccurate. They reflected the difficulty of collecting statistics at any time, particularly when the Commissioner for Public Health, Dr Burnett Ham, had just taken up duty.

A part-time tuberculosis medical officer was appointed, initially Dr Stewart and later, in the 1920s, Dr Jeffries Turner. His main duty appears to have been to recommend admission to one of the three sanatoria. A visiting nurse made home calls to advise on hygiene and prevention of infection and to arrange fumigation of the house or room into which the patient was often promptly returned. Sleepouts were strongly recommended and certainly at the Dime were in constant use. The sleepouts were really substantial tents: tiled roof, concrete floor, wooden uprights and canvas blinds which were rolled up in good weather but were very damp in cyclonic weather. Each sleepouts held four patients, and they were still in use in 1953 when Chermside Hospital was opened.

World War I provided its own tuberculosis casualties. A sanatorium was opened at Stanthorpe in about 1923 and Billy Hughes said that no ex-serviceman would lack care for tuberculosis and this produced the life-time pension for "war-caused" disease, equated with overseas service. This pension is only now being reviewed in the light of tuberculosis being a curable disease.

In 1927 the M.J. Holmes report was printed by the Commonwealth.[5] It reviewed tuberculosis facilities throughout the Commonwealth and found little to praise anywhere and damned Queensland with the phrase:

> No organised effort has been made to control tuberculosis in this State... The State Health Department takes no action on notification and action by the local authority is confined to disinfection of the premises after removal or death of a case. Patients on discharge from the sanatorium were lost sight of, there being no system in operation to keep them or their families under periodical supervision.

There were 67 recommendations appended to this report, commencing with a recommendation that all forms of the disease should be notifiable, not only pulmonary, and the 67th being a plea for research into infection of humans with bovine type organisms. It was an excellent comprehensive and eminently practical report, but the financial crisis of 1929 killed it absolutely stone-dead. The poverty of the depression years cannot be comprehended by anyone who did not experience it. Any progressive plan requiring increased government expenditure had no hope whatever of being implemented. Queensland was probably the hardest hit of the states and when appointments became vacant they were not filled, and the token service of part-time medical officer and visiting nurse stopped.

World War II made things even worse and disrupted administration, particularly in the far north, besides producing another crop of military tuberculous casualties. Groups of concerned persons throughout Australia, many of them medical and most of them either with personal or family experience of tuberculosis, became actively concerned and finally in 1948, following political pressure, the states and commonwealth came to an agreement that there would, at last, be concerted action to attack the problem. Most happily, this arrangement was instituted in the last year of the Chifley Labor Government, but most of the pressure group were not Labor supporters so that with change of government in 1949 impetus for the proposal was increased rather than lost—an unusual fate for an expensive innovation of an outgoing government. More happily still, overseas researchers were busy discovering anti-tuberculosis chemotherapy.

All states participated with varying degrees of enthusiasm. Queensland had to commence literally from square one with the appointment of a doctor and a visiting nurse—myself and Miss Blanche Craig with Miss Esme Wilson as typist and expert in Queensland Public Service ways. The only thing we had in abundance was patients.

The Commonwealth entry into the tuberculosis field could, with complete accuracy, be described as the moment of truth for Australia and tuberculosis. Many persons contributed to Commonwealth involvement. Perhaps Elkington himself was one—he clearly saw after only a few busy years as head of the Queensland Health Department, that definitive public health action was a national matter and transferred to a commonwealth appointment, junior to a young man whom he had himself recommended for the position of Commonwealth Director-General of Health, J.H.L. Cumpston.

Similarly, the group who persuaded the commonwealth to come to the party—D'Arcy Cowan, Alan Pennington, Cotter Harvey and last but by no means least, Harry Wunderly, had no doubts about it. At the end of the war, with tax-gathering power delegated to the Commonwealth, there was no point in trying to get money from the states. Senator McKenna's bill made funds available and Wunderly, as first Commonwealth Director of Tuberculosis with tireless energy saw that the states used the money in the way he believed it should be spent, and which was spelled out in his report on *Tuberculosis in Australia* in 1947. It was very similar in many ways to earlier reports. The difference was—it was implemented.

No discussion of this period is complete without a tribute to Harry Wunderly and his wife, Alice. They were a childless couple. If they had had children, it is unlikely that they would have abandoned their comfortable home and pleasant life-style in Adelaide to live for five years in a small hotel bedroom in the Hotel Canberra. While he travelled almost continuously from state to state, advising, cajoling, pin-pricking, lobbying politicians and public servants, she kept herself very fully informed on the political front, being almost a permanent fixture in the gallery of the House of Representatives.

With the change of government the fact that Wunderly and Menzies had been at school together in Melbourne was no small factor in the success of his plans which, almost at the drop of a hat, had to be modified to cope with the migrant intake from Europe in the late 1940s and 1950s which, at its maximum, was bringing 180,000 persons a year into this country. At one time, as well as everything else, Wunderly was consultant to a migrant sanatorium of some 200 beds at Bonegilla in Victoria and imported his successor as Director, Hilary Roche, to take over that clinical burden.

No project involving seven governments and seven departments of health could possibly survive without an expert on bureaucracy and "the system". Wunderly was ably supported in this field by Ted Dundas. Dundas, a product of Commonwealth Treasury, was seconded to Health in 1949 as Administrative Officer and briefed to keep the doctor "in hand" financially. Dundas caught the missionary zeal from Wunderly and in drive and enthusiasm excelled his leader. I well remember them, after a battle with Treasury when they "won" the Tuberculosis Allowance for tuberculosis sufferers, being as happy as two schoolboys in an ice-cream parlour.

There were 500 notifications in Queensland in 1950, which jumped to 943 in 1953 with the only case-finding measure being the offer of a tuberculosis allowance. To be paid the allowance, tuberculosis had to be notified. There was considerable concern about an alarming increase in tuberculosis in the Aboriginal and Islander population in the north. There were about 100 patients in the "Dime", renamed the South Brisbane Hospital, and about 80 on the balconies of the Royal Brisbane Hospital until 1953, when the first pre-fabricated units at Prince Charles Hospital came into use.

By 1959 we were able to commence mass miniature radiography on a compulsory basis. Before this could be done, thoracic beds had to be available—50 bed units at Cairns, Townsville, Rockhampton and Toowoomba, a 100 bed sanatorium on Thursday Island at the Weiban Hospital and 40 beds at Cherbourg for Aboriginal patients, and of course Prince Charles Hospital. Staff was difficult to recruit , particularly medical staff, and we were in the "import-a-doctor" business with medical officers from the United Kingdom and Africa.

With effective drugs available, and by this time knowledge of how to use them, our campaign really began. The next ten years saw the notification rate fall. Mean annual notifications for the 1950s was 739, for the 1960s was 629 and for the 1970s was 237. For the first time it fell below 200 in 1978–1979.

I could have called this "A Study in Public Health" but so far it has been merely historical. The public health lessons, however, seem clear to me.

1.Knowledge

Before Koch, no practical steps were possible because no-one knew what needed to be done. Koch identified the cause.

2. Awareness and public demand

This, in Australia, grew very slowly. Our tuberculosis incidence was lower than most parts of the world and as with motor vehicle accidents today, the "it won't happen to me" attitude prevailed. Education reduced public apathy.

3. Means

That is, money for mass radiography, beds, personnel and financial aid to patients—the Tuberculosis Allowance—was provided. By 1959 the effect of commonwealth money had made itself felt.

4. Persistence

And here, we must consider the future. The decline of tuberculosis in the western world has been going on for over 100 years. All we have done in the past 30 years is accelerate a declining trend. Will the decline continue if we now stop in our tracks?

We must now consider that refugees and migrants are coming to Australia from countries where tuberculosis is not effectively controlled—in some cases it is out of control. We must maintain medical and nursing expertise here in Australia. We must also maintain public awareness and avoid complacency about the possible threat posed by uncontrolled tuberculosis to the north.

Tuberculosis Control in Western Australia[*]

In 1829 the British decided to forestall the French and Captain James Stirling was sent to found the Swan River settlement. The early settlers battled with poor soil, drought, Aborigines and their own lack of farming skills in a generally hostile environment. Progress was slow and by 1840 the population had actually fallen to 1100; transportation of 10,000 convicts during the period 1850-68 gave some relief to chronic labour shortages but the population was still less than 30,000 by 1870. Joske and Joske have been able to trace phthisis mortality in Western Australia back to the earliest days of the settlement.[6]

Tuberculosis was mentioned as a cause of death by the Registrar of Deaths in 1848. He noted deaths from phthisis in recently arrived English migrants who sought a cure in the warm dry Mediterranean climate of the south-eastern region of Western Australia. Agriculture languished but the

---

[*] Prepared from material made available by Ms G. Oakley, Battye Library, State Library Service, Perth W.A. to whom the Editor is indebted. The authors include Dr F.G.B. Edwards and Ms L. Johnson.

wool industry flourished in this quiet backwater of Australia. All this changed quite dramatically between 1886 and 1892 when gold was discovered, initially in the Kimberley, and then at Coolgardie (the "Golden Mile"). Western Australian gold fields became major producer in world terms and by 1900 the State's population had trebled to 180,000. The gold seekers and gold miners came from the eastern states, mainly Victoria which at that time had the highest tuberculosis mortality in Australasia. Migrants also poured in from South Africa, Europe and California. Coolgardie and the adjacent towns of Kalgoorlie and Boulder had a population of 50,000 by 1905. By then the alluvial or surface gold was exhausted and deep shafts were sunk to extract the gold-bearing rock. Consequently the death rate from miners' phthisis soared. Tuberculosis was made a notifiable disease in 1902, a sanatorium was established at Coolgardie in 1906 and in 1909 Dr J.H.L. Cumpston was appointed Royal Commissioner to investigate the prevalence of miners' phthisis and other pulmonary disease, including tuberculosis, in the mining population. He was asked also to determine the nature of the pulmonary diseases associated with mining.[7]

Dr Cumpston reported that miners' phthisis was fibrosis of the lungs caused by the inhalation of quartz or silica dust and was far commoner in miners than in non-mining males of similar ages; tuberculosis of the lungs was an increasingly common complication of miners' phthisis or silicosis. He estimated that 24 per cent of the miners had silicosis and 3 per cent suffered from the complication of tuberculosis. Obviously Western Australia had serious industrial and public health problems and Cumpston recommended wide-ranging procedures to control them. Included among these were periodic health screening of underground miners, improved ventilation of mining shafts, some form of pension for disabled miners and facilities for the diagnosis and treatment of tuberculosis in miners and their families. It was no coincidence that at about this time Dr Walter Summons in Bendigo was making similar recommendations for the control of silicosis and tuberculosis in the gold mining population of that city. The Coolgardie sanatorium was extended and filled quickly with advanced consumptives. Water supply and hygiene were poor thus outweighing the perceived advantages of the hot dry climate. In 1915 the patients were transferred to the new Wooroloo sanatorium near Perth.

Wooroloo was a 200 bed sanatorium planned so that patients could be segregated according to the extent of their disease. Rehabilitation with graduated activities and part-time work in workshops and a farm were to be a features of treatment. Those who were permanently disabled could live in a farming village similar to Papworth in England.

Meanwhile the incidence of tuberculosis in Western Australia rose while in the eastern states it continued to fall. In Western Australia tuberculosis mortality peaked at 91.6 per 100,000 in 1919, 30 to 50 per cent higher than in other states.

Wooroloo was failing to meet the high expectations of its founders. Over half of the beds were hospice beds occupied by patients with end-stage tuberculosis; there were financial and staff problems leading to adverse criticism in the parliament and the press. Patients with early curable disease were reluctant to seek treatment there and the farm colony languished. The Medical Superintendent, Dr Mitchell, was obliged to assume the role of de facto State Director of Tuberculosis and divide his time between the sanatorium and Perth; he conducted regular chest clinics at Perth Hospital and directed the Visiting Nursing Service who followed up family contacts and supervised patients discharged from Wooroloo.

However, a Commonwealth Health Laboratory with X-ray facilities was established in Kalgoorlie in 1922, a mobile X-ray machine began screening miners for silicosis and tuberculosis and steps were taken to reduce the dust hazard in the mines. Also in the 1920s steps were taken to institute active treatment of tuberculosis at Wooroloo, initially with tuberculin therapy. An X-ray machine was installed in 1929 and artificial pneumothorax was followed some years later by thoracoplasty.

In 1940 Dr Mitchell retired and was succeeded as Medical Superintendent by Dr Linley Henzell. In 1947 Dr Henzell was formally appointed State Director of Tuberculosis.

The National Campaign in Western Australia

Alan King

Western Australia was lucky in having an experienced tuberculosis specialist in Dr Linley Henzell. He took over as Medical Superintendent of Wooroloo Sanatorium in 1941 and became the first Director of Tuberculosis Control in 1947 when I became his deputy. I remember assisting Dr Henzell at the Royal Perth Hospital chest clinic in 1947 which had over 100 sputum positive patients on its register in the first 3 months following its establishment. We gradually acquired about 80 beds for tuberculosis in the Royal Perth Hospital as Wooroloo was overflowing.

The Perth chest clinic moved to Murray Street in 1948. We built up case-finding by encouraging the general practitioners to send suspected tuberculosis patients to the chest clinic and by X-raying all in-patients and outpatients at all large public hospitals. Special surveys of mental hospitals, some industrial firms and close co-operation with the Kalgoorlie chest clinic increased notifications of tuberculosis cases.

The compulsory mass chest X-ray surveys were started in 1952 at Kalgoorlie so that we gained experience before commencing surveys in Perth. We had wonderful co-operation from the local authorities and community groups such as Red Cross, Country Womens Association and RSL. By 1960, 623,368 miniature chest X-rays had been taken leading to the diagnosis of 468 persons with infectious pulmonary tuberculosis (about 0.7 cases per thousand X-rays).

Prevention was based on isolating infectious cases until they were non-infectious. Contact-tracing identified those, especially children, who had been recently infected and the Morriston Preventorium was opened in 1950 to care for these and infants and young children of mothers with infectious tuberculosis. BCG vaccine was used for infants and children at risk. Later BCG was extended to nursing staff and finally was given to all 11 to12-year old schoolchildren with negative tuberculin (Mantoux) tests.

Medical care in the period 1945–50 was bed-rest and in some cases artificial pneumothorax. The gradual introduction of effective regimens of streptomycin, PAS and finally isoniazid led to a great increase in surgical intervention (e.g. lobectomy). Experience with, and confidence in, triple chemotherapy (the concurrent use of streptomycin, isoniazid and PAS) led to a decline in surgical intervention by the early 1960s. However the results of the surgical treatment of pulmonary tuberculosis in the Perth Chest Hospital were excellent; Mr Fred Clark was an ambidexterous surgeon of great ability, assisted in turn by Mr Archie Simpson and Mr Peter Gibson.

During my tenure of the office of Director of Tuberculosis in Western Australia the notification rate fell from 108 in 1950 to 53 per 100,000 in 1959. The mortality rate per 100,000 fell over the same period from 22.9 to 3.3. The battle against tuberculosis was being won.

The Community Health and Anti-Tuberculosis Association of New South Wales, a Great Voluntary Organisation

K.W.H. Harris and Roma Thomson

In the first decade of this century when the mortality rate for tuberculosis in New South Wales was about 66 per 100,000, a movement to provide some relief for the unfortunate victims of consumption was initiated by a small group of public-spirited citizens of Sydney. This group was led by Sir Phillip Sydney Jones, an eminent physician, and was assisted by a small grant from the New South Wales Government, a donation from the Walter and Eliza Hall Trust and subscriptions from a few private citizens who realised the great needs of impoverished consumptives and the grave dangers of the spread of infection in the community.

The National Association for the Prevention and Cure of Consumption was inaugurated on 29 June, 1910. From its very inception, the Association had three primary objectives:

- the compulsory notification of tuberculosis throughout the state,
- the establishment of tuberculosis dispensaries, and
- the education of the public in the causes and prevention of the disease.

It also advocated free bacteriological examination of sputum, a pure milk supply, the care of the families of breadwinners who were being treated in sanatoria and the transfer of convalescent patients from sanatoria to farm colonies.

On 25 September 1912, the Association established the first tuberculosis dispensary in Australia. This dispensary, situated in a small room off Hay Street in Sydney and manned by volunteers provided assistance to indigent persons suffering from consumption. Work continued at the dispensary until 1929 when, by voluntary public subscription, the Association established its first diagnostic clinic in Albion Street, Surry Hills, Sydney. This was the birthplace of our modern techniques of case-finding, contact-examination and patient follow-up and supervision. X-ray equipment was secured and operated by honorary radiographers. A bacteriological section was set up and honorary clinicians and radiologists were appointed. For a small fee, a person could be given an X-ray and a radiological report. The State Government provided a token but welcome subsidy. In 1930, the name of the Association was altered to the Anti-Tuberculosis Association of New South Wales.

In 1947, following the example of the armed services at the beginning of World War II, the Association acquired its first mobile X-ray unit. This was funded by voluntary subscription from residents in rural areas. The mobile unit was self-contained to provide accommodation for the staff, a 70 mm Phillips X-ray Survey Unit with a Fairchild Lens camera, (incidentally the first mobile 70 mm unit in Australia), processing equipment and an office fitted with a viewer for the medical officer-in-charge. This unit commenced service in the southern areas of New South Wales and was financed by a five shilling charge for each radiological examination; 50,000 radiographs a year was regarded as satisfactory.

The Unit remained on location until all film had been processed and then follow up X-rays were taken on full-size film of all people whose miniature rays were regarded as indicating possible radiological abnormalities. No further fees were charged for large X-rays or clinical examinations. A second mobile unit was put into service in 1948 to provide a diagnostic service to industry. This unit moved from factory to factory covering staff on a voluntary basis.

In 1952, the Association had gained considerable experience and prestige in mass radiography with mobile units and had developed a large out-patients clinic in Surry Hills. In one year alone, this clinic saw 32,918 people, 40,152 X-rays were taken and 74,216 attended for treatment.

By this time the Commonwealth Government, recognising the need for an Australia-wide campaign to eradicate tuberculosis brought down legislation ensuring adequate funding and arranged for the several state governments to act for them. Because of its experience and existing facilities, the Association was encouraged to expand. With this help a new clinic in Crown Street was officially opened on 25th March 1953.

Additional mobile X-ray units were designed and purchased using funds provided by the Commonwealth and in 1953 the first compulsory community mass-survey in New South Wales was undertaken. Ultimately the mobile unit force comprised eight mass miniature 70 mm mirror camera units housed in caravans covering Sydney every two years and the country areas north of Sydney every three years. Half a million X-rays were taken each year.

More cases discovered meant more medical examinations, more pathology tests, more contact-testing and domiciliary work. In addition to the diagnostic and medical facilities, the Association employed three nursing sisters, each with a car, for contact tracing and domiciliary care. In addition upwards of 1000 men and women voluntarily assisted the Association in a variety of ways, demonstrating the truly civic aspects of the Association.

In common with most anti-tuberculosis bodies, the Association conducted a Christmas Seals campaign each year. Seals not only produced income, but acted as a constant reminder of the Association and its campaign.

The Association had the distinction of being invited to assist in a number of assignments beyond NSW. At the Commonwealth Government's request a medical, technical and nursing team and portable equipment were sent to Nauru in 1956 and carried out a 100 per cent coverage of all residents. The statistical analysis of this survey clearly demonstrated the value of the assignment. In 1959 the Commonwealth Government again invited the Association to conduct a tuberculosis case-finding campaign among the residents of the Northern Territory. The Association's director of mass radiography surveys was twice chosen by the commonwealth as a tuberculosis expert in Colombo Plan tasks, in 1959, to Singapore and for twelve months in 1960–61 to British North Borneo. The Association also made available to the Commonwealth Government an expert medical team to demonstrate and teach tuberculosis control in Malaya (now Malaysia). Three members of the staff were seconded to Malaya under the aegis of the commonwealth for two year's service.

During 1972, re-organisation of some of the activities of the Association led to their transfer to the Health Commission of New South Wales and specificially to the chest clinics and the Division of Tuberculosis within the Health Commission. The activities of the Association's static clinic at its headquarters were very much modified and a great many patients transferred to other clinics and hospitals.

As the tuberculosis campaign began to wind-down in the mid–1970s the Association began to widen its activities in other community health fields. In 1975 the Association (now the Community Health and Anti-Tuberculosis Association) assumed responsibility for sheltered workshops previously conducted by the National Association for the Prevention of Tuberculosis in Australia (NAPTA). The Association also became involved in health-screening of industrial workers.

The Role of the Tuberculosis Nurse
A.J. Proust

The origin of the tuberculosis nurse may be traced to Dr George Philip of Edinburgh. In 1885 he proposed a new plan (later known world-wide as the Edinburgh plan) to control tuberculosis: "all preventive measures should be co-ordinated from a new type of dispensary specially devoted to this work with trained medical and nursing staff". Nursing was a relatively new profession in 1885 and it was significant that Dr Philip at the very outset of his plan specifically included a role for nursing staff.[8.]

At about the same time William Osler, foundation Professor of Medicine, Johns Hopkins Hospital and University, Baltimore, Maryland, USA, organised house visits to his domiciliary tuberculosis patients. The visits were undertaken by fourth-year medical students and nurses and his instructions as described by a Miss Dutcher, a medical student, and quoted by Harvey Cushing in *Life of Osler*:[9]

> Ie (Osler) was of the opinion that much could be done to prevent the spread of tuberculosis in Baltimore if the consumptive and his family knew more about the disease. He asked me to make a friendly visit... my duty should be to learn all I could about the patient, his family and his environment; to advise him about the nature of his disease, its mode and contagion and method of prevention; to teach him first of all to destroy his sputum because it contained the seed which caused the disease and was the only way of transmitting the disease to others; to give the reason why sunlight and fresh air were of preventive and curative value and to make any suggestions that would be of help in each home I went to.

Although this description of the role of the visitor to tuberculosis patients was made by a medical student it is an accurate description of the role of the tuberculosis nurse. Though the term "social worker" had not yet been coined, the work of the tuberculosis nurse encompassed some of the work later done by medical social workers.

Doubtless based upon the work of Dr Philip and Dr Osler, tuberculosis dispensaries were established in Sydney prior to World War I. Dr C.J. Cummins, Director-General of Health in New South Wales in the 1960s wrote *A History of Medical Administration in New South Wales 1788–1973*. It describes the functions of tuberculosis nurses as follows:

The first Director of Tuberculosis was Dr H.K. Denham who was succeeded by Dr H.G. Wallace. Dr Wallace was supported by a small staff of Tuberculosis Nurses who acted as health educators to the family where the tuberculosis patient had to be supported. They were partially trained as health and hygiene inspectors and so attempted to prevent the spread of the disease within the domestic household.

In Melbourne the first mention of tuberculosis nurses was made in "Notes on Tuberculosis in Victoria" (*Health Bulletin*, 12: 367, 1927). Dr J. Bell Ferguson launched a multi-pronged co-ordinated attack on tuberculosis in Victoria soon after he arrived to take up the post of the first full-time Director of Tuberculosis in Victoria (and in Australia) in 1927. A Central Tuberculosis Bureau was established in Melbourne with satellite chest clinics in major suburban and regional centres. Tuberculosis community nurses based in these clinics were of pivotal importance in assessing home conditions for possible domiciliary treatment; contact-tracing was also an important facet of their work. These nurses, also referred to as health visitors, were responsible for securing the co-operation of the patient treated at home and of the patient discharged from sanatorium or hospital.

At the Eleventh Australian Tuberculosis Clinical Conference held in Darwin in 1978, Sister Kay Barraclough presented a paper "Tuberculosis Nursing, a Brief Study of the Outpatient Nursing Sister's Role Past, Present and Future". She described her work over a period of more than twenty years in the chest clinics of the Blue Mountains region of the Department of Health, New South Wales.

The area was large and involved domiciliary, out-patient and epidemiological work. The population contained a relatively high percentage of geriatric and psychiatric patients; the region by virtue of its altitude and climate had traditionally attracted people with chronic chest diseases, including tuberculosis. In the past, several large and many small sanatoria had been established in the Blue Mountains but by the end of the 1950s, there were no hospital or sanatorium beds for tuberculosis patients in the area—all patients requiring hospitalisation were sent to Sydney.

In her everyday work, Sister Barraclough liaised closely with general practitioners and other health services personnel and she stressed that a good working relationship with these was essential. The recruitment of these nurses was usually from the nursing staff of hospitals which treated tuberculosis; most did some special training in tuberculosis. Their work however was different from hospital-based nursing staff and as they gained experience, they became a vital link in the overall tuberculosis control program. Their main role was to bridge the gap between the clinic physician and the patient. There was in the 1950s a large number of patients with active tuberculosis, many of whom were apparently healthy and discovered only on the compulsory mass X-ray program. The need to follow-up and supervise these patients and their contacts was of paramount importance. In addition to easing the patient-doctor relationship, the sister acted as the educator and confidant of frightened or confused patients and their families. In the early days of the program, she was a reassuring and easily contacted professional member of the chest clinic staff. Her nursing skills were used also in the early period for frequent surgical dressings of the patients who had undergone thoracoplasty or segmental resection. As this was phased out with the advances in chemotherapy, nursing skills were still of value in administering streptomycin, assessing possible adverse reactions to the anti-tuberculosis drugs and in checking that the drugs were taken regularly. Her role was then expanded to cover the field of contact examinations, follow up of unco-operative patients and the regular supervision of hospital staff and other high-risk groups. The load of clerical work increased as did her work as social worker and health educator.

In the 1970s two innovations further changed the nature of her work. Fully supervised intermittent chemotherapy became standard treatment in some regions, especially among refugee groups, and this became the top priority of clinic nurses in those regions. At about the same time the advent of the community health program heralded a major change in health care and was greeted initially with suspicion and even antagonism by clinic sisters; after all, they had been among the pioneers of community nursing and it appeared, on the surface, that their role was to be usurped by others who were newcomers in this field.

She was now obliged to be a member of a larger team, sometimes with other duties outside the tuberculosis field; there were qualified social workers and counsellors, other doctors and nurses in the specialities of psychiatry, child health and drug and alcohol dependency. The health bureaucracy multiplied. After a period of adjustment to the new team work the clinic sister found that the patient benefited from the expertise of other members of the team.

Sister Barraclough summed up the present position:

> This is where we come back into the reckoning; this is where the tuberculosis sister returns as the easily recognised person to whom the patient can refer. We see the patient at frequent regular intervals. We are there to allay fears, to explain and educate and to guarantee the patients co-operation in the treatment program until its conclusion... and the future, what does it hold for us, the nursing sisters in the field? I fear more forms, facts and figures and even less emphasis on our nursing skills. But because tuberculosis is not yet an eradicated disease in our community, the need for clinic sisters with expertise and specialist knowledge in tuberculosis will still be there.

At the same Eleventh Australian Clinical Tuberculosis Conference, Sister Sheila Summerton spoke on "The Role of the Nurse in Tuberculosis

Control in the Northern Territory".

The notification rate of tuberculosis in the Northern Territory during the period 1980–85 was five times higher than in the Australian population as a whole; BCG vaccination is more widely used in the Northern Territory than elsewhere in Australia. It is used also for its prophylactic value in leprosy which is endemic at a low level, especially in the Aboriginal population. All Aboriginal neonates born in hospital are given BCG as are children up to the age of 24 months in rural areas who have not previously been vaccinated. Over the age of 11 years Aboriginal children are revaccinated with BCG and again as young adults. At least three years must elapse between BCG vaccinations. Prior tuberculin skin tests are not routinely done.

The tuberculosis control nurse is closely involved with the Aboriginal population which comprises over 20 per cent of that of the Territory. Many of our concepts of health and disease are markedly different from those of Aboriginals. The causes of disease, the value of prophylactic vaccination and the need for long-term chemotherapy are three examples.

The transience of the population, excessive alcohol consumption and other social problems are other difficulties encountered frequently in the population, both white and Aboriginal. These interfere with the satisfactory completion of courses of chemotherapy and as a result almost all chemotherapy is wholly or partly supervised. Despite this, many patients fail to keep follow-up appointments.

Climatic conditions and the vast distances in the Territory compound the problems of the rural or "bush" nurses. The "wet" season frequently prevents visits to outlying areas, sometimes for many weeks. The tropical climate also is a cause of concern because drugs, BCG vaccine and tuberculin can all be affected and lose potency if storage conditions are poorly supervised.

In summary, the nurse in the Territory must be willing to learn and to adapt to the conditions there, to be patient, considerate and understanding and to show determination to teach the patient the significance of his illness and the need to complete the course of treatment.

Sister Barraclough and Sister Summerton, as summarised above, have described the roles they played in tuberculosis control in two different settings and in two different population groups. The central role which they played in the tuberculosis campaign has previously not been adequately acknowledged.

Chapter 4

Tuberculosis among Aborigines

Neil Thomson

One of the cardinal points in the epidemiology of tuberculosis [is] the terrible deadliness of the disease to newly exposed populations. We can hardly give adequate emphasis to the historical importance of this fact. Tuberculosis, so virulent and fatal in fresh soil, has been a major ally of the urbanised European and American white man in the conquest of new territory, the demoralisation and destruction of aboriginal people.[1]

Introduction

The impact of tuberculosis among Australia's indigenous peoples, the Australian Aborigines and the Torres Strait Islanders, was broadly consistent with that documented for indigenous people in other parts of the world. While probably not as important an "ally" as smallpox and some other infectious diseases in the "conquest" of Australia, tuberculosis eventually demonstrated its "terrible deadliness" for Aborigines in widely scattered parts of Australia. The spread of tuberculosis followed the non-Aboriginal occupation of the country, the disease appearing to have had its major impact *after* Aborigines had been virtually subjugated. This subjugation frequently resulted in extremely adverse environmental conditions, including substantial overcrowding in substandard dwellings, and significant malnutrition—fertile ground indeed for tuberculosis.

Even today, tuberculosis is much more frequent, and more severe, in Aboriginal than in non-Aboriginal Australians. The persistence of the disease among Aborigines is still related to poor housing and malnutrition, and is a clear indication of the extent of social inequality experienced by Aborigines, more than 200 years after the initial coming of the Europeans.

Before European settlement in 1788

Prior to the first European settlement in 1788, Aborigines had, over a period of at least 40,000 years, adapted successfully to a wide range of environmental conditions throughout Australia. It is likely that Aborigines in 1788 were physically, socially and emotionally healthier than most Europeans of that time. Evidence for this conclusion, and for the likely presence or absence of certain diseases comes from a combination of historical sources, palaeopathology studies and a knowledge of the nature of individual diseases in human populations.

Although it is probable that infant mortality was very high and life expectancy short by modern standards, those Aborigines who did survive infancy enjoyed an adequate diet and were probably free of many of the diseases which were common in Europe. It is almost certain that Aborigines did not suffer from smallpox, measles, influenza, other respiratory viruses, leprosy, tuberculosis, venereal syphilis, gonorrhea or dental caries. Yaws and endemic syphilis were present and it is probable that Aborigines suffered from hepatitis B and some intestinal parasites, and possibly even trachoma. Trauma is likely to have been a major cause of mortality, and arthritis, periodontal disease and tooth attrition are known to have occurred.

The impact of European occupation

European occupation of Australia had a catastrophic impact on Aboriginal health, resulting in widespread, though variable, population decline[2]. The most significant cause of depopulation, particularly in south-eastern Australia, but probably in many regions, was smallpox, with major epidemics beginning in 1789 and 1829–1831. Consistent with the mortality rate amongst previously unexposed peoples in the Americas, it was noted that about a half of the Aborigines in the neighbourhood of the first European settlement at Port Jackson had died from smallpox by 1790, and two early explorers in inland New South Wales noted the severe depopulation almost certainly resulting from the 1829–1831 epidemic.

Other infectious diseases certainly played a part in the depopulation, but their effects, at least until the second half of the 19th century, are less clear. In view of the pre-existence of yaws and endemic syphilis, some doubt exists about the extent of venereal syphilis. However, venereal diseases became widespread, at least in the south-east, and probably had a major effect on female fertility. Influenza, other respiratory viruses, pneumonia and measles became major causes of mortality, as did tuberculosis.[2]

Many of the Aborigines who escaped the scourge of smallpox and other diseases fell victim to the encroachment of European settlement on Aboriginal lands, directly through fighting or massacres, and indirectly through the disrupting effects of land dispossession on their economic and social organisation.

The combination of introduced diseases, conflict and dispossession from their lands had an enormous impact on Aboriginal populations. Recent research suggests that the Aboriginal population in 1788 was probably around 750,000,[3] much higher than the previously accepted estimate of 300,000. By 1933, when the total population was estimated at 81,000, Aboriginal numbers had declined to around 10 per cent of the likely 1788 figure.

The spread of tuberculosis, 1788–1900

By some reports, "consumption" accounted for up to half of the deaths of Londoners at the time the First Fleet sailed from Portsmouth.[1] Thus, with a likely high prevalence of tuberculosis among the first Europeans, it is probable that the disease was soon transmitted to Aborigines, at least those most closely affected by the initial settlements. However, there is no evidence of tuberculosis having had a major impact on Aborigines until around the 1840s,[2] when it appears that the disease became increasingly important. From around the middle of the 19th Century, tuberculosis probably became the leading cause of death among many Aboriginal groups, at least in the southern parts of Australia. The best documented spread of the disease among Aborigines comes from Victorian sources. Curr, in his four volume account of *The Australian Race* (1868), noted that when he first moved to Echuca in 1841 he could recollect not one case of consumption among Aborigines, but that cases began to be seen in the early 1850s. In 1860, a letter from William Thomas to the newly formed Board for the Protection of the Aborigines attributed "eight-tenths of the mortality" among the Aborigines of Victoria to intemperance, resulting in "pulmonary disorders, pleurisy, pneumonia, disorders of the chest, consumption, etc".[4]

William Thomas' description of the Aboriginal treatment of what was almost certainly tuberculosis shows that, by 1860, the Aborigines had already become accustomed to the symptoms and fatal nature of the disease:

> the blacks study much the colour of the spittle in those affected in the lungs, and know well its stages. When the patient begins to expectorate blood, much attention is paid to him; should this increase, which is generally the case, the [Aboriginal] doctors hold a consultation, and when once a consultation is held the doctors will not allow the patient to take any more medicine from the whites. The invalid is laid on his back and held firm by three or four blacks, whilst the native doctor keeps continually pressing with his feet, and even jumping on his belly.[4]

By 1879, concern was expressed about the "terrible death rate" among Aborigines in Victoria, death in the majority of cases being "the result of a disease of the lungs peculiar to the natives, which ends fatally in every case"[5]. Following an opinion from the colony's chief medical officer that the disease was due to the climate and inadequate diet, clothing and medical care, the Board for the Protection of the Aborigines requested an investigation of the causes of "tubercular phthisis" among Aborigines. Using information collected from both Victoria and Queensland, the investigator, William Thomson, concluded that climate had no bearing on the incidence of the disease and speculated that "contagion" could be the cause. Thomson "deplored the Board's failure to provide isolated quarters for the sick, suggesting that their infectious spittle impregnated cottages and could be 'breathed' by others" (quoted in Barwick[4]). The medical officers and the Board continued to ignore the theory of "contagion"—the sick were not isolated until the 1920s when the first station hospital was built.

Meanwhile, of the 736 deaths from known causes occurring to residents of the Victorian Aboriginal stations between 1876 and 1912, 39 per cent of the adult deaths were attributed to tuberculosis, as were 18–19 per cent of the juvenile deaths.[4] Elsewhere in the country, Aborigines also had a very high mortality rate from tuberculosis. In Western Australia in 1845, it was noted that there was an increase in the number of cases of tuberculosis, even though overall the number of deaths from influenza was higher.

By the second half of the 19th century, tuberculosis had also become a major cause of death for Aborigines in South Australia: "from 1864 to 1899, 13 per cent of all deaths at Point McLeay Aboriginal settlement in South Australia were attributed to pulmonary tuberculosis, and from 1880 to 1899, 28 per cent of all deaths at Point Pearce settlememt were attributed to the same cause".[6]

The continuing spread—into the 20th century

In contrast to Aborigines living in the southern areas of the country, for those living in more remote parts tuberculosis did not have a major impact until much later. For example, it was around the turn of the century before the death rate from tuberculosis began to cause concern on Aboriginal mission stations in north Queensland. Similarly, in the Northern Territory, tuberculosis did not have a significant impact on Aborigines until the non-Aboriginal population expanded in the latter years of the 19th century, at which time those Aborigines living in closest contact experienced a great deterioration in environmental conditions.

The discovery of gold some 200 kilometres south of Darwin, as well as the decision to link Australia to Great Britain by cable, triggered large scale non-Aboriginal immigration, particularly from the southern provinces of China, Hong Kong, Singapore and Macau. The introduction of tuberculosis to Northern Territory Aborigines was attributed largely to Chinese immigrants, among whom 27 per cent of the deaths occurring in 1913 were caused by the disease. At that time, it was noted that tuberculosis did not occur among Aborigines who had not had contact with "whites or Asiatics". In fact, it was noted by successive Colonial Surgeons over many years that the distribution of the disease was "strictly focal". However, for those Aborigines unfortunate enough to develop the disease, there was "a tendency to miliary infection with a rapid course to fatal termination".[7]

Some years later, Basedow[8] confirmed the focal nature of the spread of the disease:

> in all my wanderings among the primitive tribes of Central and Northern Australia during a period of over twenty years, I have never been able to find a single case of tuberculosis.

The mid–20th century

Although tuberculosis had spread to Aborigines in all parts of the country by the middle of the 20th century, its impact was still somewhat variable. In Aborigines living in areas long occupied by non-Aborigines, the disease was much more common and generally more severe than among non-Aborigines. In contrast, many Aborigines living in more remote parts of the country still experienced little or no disease. For example, Aboriginal children living in the Brisbane area were responsible for 8 out of 64 admissions to the Brisbane Children's Hospital for tuberculosis in the 10-year period 1939 to 1949. Although comprising "well below 1 per cent" of the total public hospital population of the area, Aboriginal children contributed 12.5 per cent of all cases of childhood tuberculosis, and "no less than 23.5 per cent of the more severe types".[9]

In contrast, a survey, in 1950, of 3209 Aborigines living in the remote Pilbara and Kimberley regions of Western Australia found evidence of only 15 cases of pulmonary tuberculosis, only two of which were described as "active" [10]. The overall prevalence of tuberculosis, less than 5 per thousand, was lower than that of the non-Aboriginal population. The low Mantoux conversion rates found among the remote-living Aborigines confirmed expectations that infrequent association with non- Aborigines, and the maintenance of less crowded living conditions, contributed to the lower prevalence of disease among Aborigines.

A similar survey of Aborigines living on settlements and missions in north Queensland[6] found an active case rate of 21 per 1000, and a reactor rate slightly higher than that reported for the Kimberley and Pilbara regions. The high active case-rate among Aboriginal nurses, midwives, and household servants of white Australians contributed to the impression that there was an increased racial susceptibility to tuberculosis among "full-blood" Aborigines.

For Queensland overall, between 1950 and 1972, there were 1089 new cases of tuberculosis reported among Aborigines, at an estimated average annual rate of 152 per 100,000 compared with a rate among "white Australian-born" of 32 per 100,000[11]. A detailed retrospective study of a sample of these cases found that tuberculosis among Aborigines was "more acute, more extensive and more frequently non-pulmonary" than among non-Aborigines. In particular, there was much more miliary and meningeal tuberculosis among Aborigines.

In 1964, reference to a mass X-ray survey of the southern half of the

Northern Territory reported that "less active tuberculosis had been confirmed in Aborigines than in other persons examined".12 In contrast, in the Darwin region of the Northern Territory, a radiological analysis of all cases of tuberculosis notified in the period 1969 to 1983 found that at least 229 (53 per cent) of the 434 cases occurred among Aborigines, comprising only about 20 per cent of the population.13 The manifestations of primary tuberculosis were seen in Aborigines and post-primary pulmonary disease was "more extensive and more often bilateral", and extra-pulmonary manifestations of the disease were much more frequent among Aborigines than among non-Aborigines.

In South Australia, 88 out of 573 Aborigines living in the north of the state were found to have a positive Mantoux reaction. Based on radiological investigation of these 88 Aborigines, the report concluded that:

> it is doubtful whether more than one or two of the natives tested are actually suffering from tuberculosis.[14]

For South Australia as a whole, including the densely settled southern areas, it was concluded that:

> the prevalence of tuberculosis among Aborigines was little or no greater than that in the general community.

In New South Wales, between 1958 and 1963, a series of surveys of the Mantoux reaction rates of more than 5000 Aborigines living on 45 Aboriginal communities found age-specific rates slightly less than those reported for the Kimberley and Pilbara regions, north Queensland and the Northern Territory.[6] For the early 1960s, it has been estimated that the new active case rate for New South Wales Aborigines was at least 1 per 1000 (the extent of the under-identification of Aborigines in tuberculosis notifications being uncertain), compared with slightly less than 0.4 per 1000 for other New South Wales residents.

In reviewing the various reactor-rates, Moodie[6] concluded that:

> the Aboriginal profiles are rather 'average' on world standards, being neither as steep as those for countries where tuberculosis has been a major health problem... or as gradual as in countries where tuberculosis has been well controlled.

Nature of the disease process

Once Aboriginal conditions had deteriorated sufficiently for tuberculosis to become established, the disease appears to have followed a particularly severe course. The rapidly fatal nature of the disease was noted for Aborigines in Victoria and South Australia in the second half of the 19th century, on mission stations in north Queensland around the turn of the century, and in the northern areas of the Northern Territory in the early 20th century.

Even in recent years, the disease has been reported as more severe and more acute for Aborigines, in Queensland and in the Darwin area of the Northern Territory, than for non-Aborigines.[11]

Particularly in the past, the greater severity of tuberculosis among Aborigines raised the possibility of an increased racial susceptibility to the disease. It would not be surprising if there were some genetic differences in susceptibility to the disease, based on the operation of selective survival among populations with long association with tuberculosis. However, it is most probable that the major reason for the higher incidence and greater severity of the disease among Aborigines, in both the past and present, is their socially disadvantaged position, involving substandard housing, overcrowding and, frequently, less than optimal nutrition.

Conclusions

The history of the impact of tuberculosis on Aborigines provides some valuable insights into their changing circumstances in a country in which they have lived for more than 40,000 years. The course of tuberculosis among Aborigines, a population with really no previous exposure to the disease, was perhaps somewhat less dramatic than may have been expected. While there is little doubt that some Aborigines in close contact with the first Europeans would have contracted the disease, tuberculosis did not make a major impact on Aborigines until well into the 19th century. At least from Victorian evidence, it was not until Aborigines had been virtually subjugated, and been subjected to European "protection" that the disease began to exact its fearful toll. A similar pattern is probably true for Aborigines in most other parts of Australia, be it on government reserves or missions. The key factors were almost certainly similar to those of importance in Europe in the 18th and 19th century: very adverse environmental conditions, including overcrowded, substandard housing, exacerbated by poor nutritional status.

The persistence today of much higher levels of tuberculosis among Aborigines than among other Australians no doubt reflects the continuing disadvantages experienced by many Aborigines. These social inequalities, seen in lower levels of education, employment and income, in inadequate housing for at least 30 per cent of Aborigines, and in malnutrition for many Aborigines, must be overcome if Aborigines are not to continue to bear a greater burden of tuberculosis than do other Australians. Of course, strategies to overcome these social inequalities must be accompanied by intensive efforts by health authorities to minimise the continuing impact of tuberculosis among Aborigines.

Tuberculous Lesions at Autopsy in Aborigines in the Northern Territory

J.M. Crotty

In a series of personally performed autopsies in Darwin between 1956 and 1964, the importance of mycobacterial disease in Aborigines in the Top End of the Northern Territory was strikingly shown. This series of 316 autopsies consisted of 137 under the age of 10 and 179 over that age. When traumatic deaths and deaths where the body was too decomposed for diagnosis were removed, 135 under the age of 10 and 148 over that age remained. These were the deaths diagnosed as being due to natural causes.

The only available records are summaries of the findings at each autopsy; detailed records were lost in the aftermath of the Darwin cyclone. During this time autopsies were obtained on over 80 per cent of Aborigines dying in the Darwin Hospital. Some coronial autopsies were also involved in the series.

The Aborigines concerned were of wholly Aboriginal descent and came under the care of the government department concerned with Aboriginal welfare, as did almost all "full-blood" Aborigines at this time. With very few exceptions these people came from the northernmost 40 per cent of the Northern Territory.

During the same period 273 autopsies were performed on the bodies of people who did not meet the definition of "full-blood" Aborigine. Of these 60 per cent died of natural causes. Of these 194 were over the age of 10 years. There were only three cases of tuberculosis in this group, all in middle aged or elderly men.

There were three major mycobacterial diseases occurring in the Aboriginal people at this time. These were due to *M. tuberculosis, M. leprae and M. ulcerans. M. ulcerans* did not contribute to death in any case in this series. However, it caused severe disease in people from one small area of the Northern Territory. Leprosy was present in 12 of the people in the series and in some it was in a reactive stage and must be regarded as contributing to the cause of death.

However, the major mycobacterial disease causing death was tuberculosis. There were 32 cases of tuberculosis in the series—17 male and 15 female. Over the age of 10 years 17 per cent of non-traumatic deaths in Aboriginal males and 20 per cent of non-traumatic deaths in Aboriginal females were due to tuberculosis.

Below the age of 10 years, causes of Aboriginal deaths were dominated by acute infections frequently associated with nutritional disease. Tuberculosis was rarely detected at autopsy in this age group (one case in 135). This may reflect the effectiveness of BCG, but it may also reflect distortion of the figures by the high death-rate from acute infection.

Accurate records of age were not always available so some were recorded simply as adult and some as aged. For younger people, accurate ages were available. In 21 of the 32 cases of tuberculosis, ages were available. If it is assumed, as is reasonable, that those listed as aged are over 50 and those listed as adults are under 50 a marked sex difference is obvious. Seventy-five per cent of male tuberculosis deaths occurred after age 50 years and 75 per cent of female deaths before that age.

Epidemics of a "flu-like" illness were important in these deaths. In a five year period I have records of four such epidemics of which three were proven to be influenza (two by virus isolation and one serologically). It is of interest that 60 per cent of tuberculosis deaths during this five year period occurred during these epidemics.

In all age groups tuberculosis was an aggressive disease. In those aged under 40 years (all except one were female) death was due to pulmonary disease alone or general disseminated disease.

In the group of seven made up of those aged 40–50 and those listed simply as adult, five were female. Four of these died primarily of tuberculosis; one of miliary spread from spinal tuberculosis, the others had pulmonary or disseminated disease. Three of the group died primarily of cardiac disease; one had associated pulmonary tuberculosis, one abdominal and one cervical glandular tuberculosis.

In the older age-group, pulmonary tuberculosis was a major cause of death. There were two cases of each of tuberculous pneumonia, disseminated tuberculosis in multiple sites and miliary tuberculosis. Three had pulmonary tuberculosis with tuberculous abscesses in distant organs. Five others had pulmonary tuberculosis as the major cause of death. In only two was the tuberculosis an incidental autopsy finding. The remaining case had massive effusions in serous cavities. The pattern of tuberculosis as a disease that kills, especially young women and old men, is aggressive in the lungs and is very often disseminated, is more familiar to earlier generations. What is missing from the pattern is the high incidence of childhood tuberculosis.

Tuberculosis in Indigenous Australians

E.W. Abrahams*

Much has been written about tuberculosis in various ethnic groups in the past but curiously little has been written in this field since the advent of effective drug treatment about 1950. Moreover, though differences in drug toxicity and the side effects of drugs have been associated with race, the possibility of variation in therapeutic effects in differing peoples has not been considered.

Cleland[15] in 1928 reported clinical and autopsy records from South Australia and commented that:

> these massive reactions cannot be considered as peculiar to the Australian native; on the other hand, the autopsy record would seem to show this massive type of reaction is more frequent in them.

---

* An abridged version of a paper published in the *Medical Journal of Australia* 2: 23, 1975..
Copyright © the *Medical Journal of Australia* 1975. Reproduced with permission.

The aim here is not to emphasise the differing incidence of the disease in Aboriginal and white populations or to discuss its aetiology but to describe the differing manifestations of the disease in individuals. These differences can be summarised briefly as follows: Aboriginals are likely to present with acute extensive pulmonary disease often with extrathoracic lymph node involvement at the same time. No Aboriginal patient showed calcified disease at the time of first diagnosis, though it developed during and after treatment, particularly in the lymph nodes. The pattern of long-standing disease of low-grade activity frequently seen in white patients ("chronic phthisis") did not occur. The response to treatment was equally satisfactory in both groups and radiological clearing to a complete or almost complete extent occurred more frequently in the Aboriginal group than in the white group.

In ordinary clinical experience, Aboriginal patients seem to have an excess of acute severe tuberculosis; this observation prompted the present investigation which was planned to compare the clinical features of the disease as seen in white Australians and in Aboriginals. The study is based on the use of matched pairs of patients.

A total of 229 pairs was studied. Clinical notes were obtained for evidence of bacteriological diagnosis and conversion and four X-ray films from each case were compared. These were taken at the commencement of treatment, three months later, a year after the beginning of treatment and as recently as possible. Based on the history of each illness, the radiological features of the X-ray films and the response to treatment, an attempt was made to infer the pathological features of the illness in each case.

There were almost twice as many cases of minimal disease in white patients as in Aboriginal patients. Pneumonic disease—that is, cases in which reversibility of the shadows leads one to assume that the lesion was largely cellular—is present in a marked preponderance of Aboriginal cases. Fibrocaseous disease on the other hand is markedly more common in white patients than in Aboriginal patients, but cases assessed as caseous are fairly evenly divided. White patients have disease confined to a single lobe much more frequently than Aboriginal patients.

Probably the most marked differences are seen in the amount of non-pulmonary disease occurring in the Aboriginal. Though the numbers are small, the difference is significant ($P < 0.001$); there is much more miliary and meningeal tuberculosis in the Aboriginal group. Marked differences are seen also in the extent of improvement with treatment in the two groups. Again the X-ray films of Aboriginal patients show improvement much more rapidly and more completely than those of white patients, evidence of a more cellular disease pattern with little fibrosis at the time of diagnosis. Though there was much more minimal disease in the white patients, the improvement in the Aboriginal group overall was better—that is, they have, with treatment, a more reversible type of disease pattern than the white group. There is little difference in either the extent, amount of calcification or of residual cavitation. However, in all white patients with significant calcification, it was shown to be present to some extent in initial films but in Aboriginals it developed during or after treatment. This suggests the disease in Aboriginals to be more active than in whites.

Tuberculosis in the Northern Territory
Ellen Kettle

No mention was made of 'consumption' or wasting diseases among the troops, prisoners or free settlers in the first three British settlements on the north coast of Australia during 1824–1849. Most deaths were due to malaria or scurvy. Although the Macassan seamen, collecting trepang, undoubtedly introduced malaria and yaws, there are no grounds for suspecting that they introduced tuberculosis to the Aborigines.

Permanent settlement on the Darwin site commenced on 5 February 1869 with the arrival of a party of very fit men from Adelaide to survey the new town. Dr Robert Peel accompanied the surveyors and a year later when settlement commenced he was replaced by Dr J. Stokes Millner. The Northern Territory was under the administration of South Australia until 1910 when it was taken over by the Commonwealth Government. Darwin (then Palmerston) was never without a doctor, but only once, in 1908, was a doctor permitted by the Government Resident, to leave Darwin to examine the health of Aborigines. On that occasion Dr C.L Strangman sailed along the Arnhem Land coast to Borroloola and back visiting the few existing settlements.

The famous Overland Telegraph line was constructed during 1871–72 and the first connection between Great Britain and Adelaide was achieved on 22 August 1872. Men had found gold south of Darwin and this news was blazed to the world. An uncontrolled gold rush followed in which men of many nations arrived by ship or travelled overland along the Gulf of Carpentaria where there was water for themselves and their horses. Within a couple of years there were over 3000 Chinese from Singapore and Hong Kong. Very few women came with any early arrivals so men of all races readily fraternised with the Aborigines.

A hospital with one ward was built in Darwin in 1873 and a second ward was added three years later to care for men with dysentery and malaria. It was staffed by a trained nurse-matron, and her husband was employed as a wardsman. In 1882 the husband of the second hospital matron, who had been working in the hospital, went to Adelaide for medical treatment and died from tuberculosis.

In 1913 Drs Anton Brienl and Mervyn Holmes carried out an extensive survey in the northern section of the Northern Territory.[16] They stated that "tuberculosis of the lungs exists sporadically amongst the natives..." They considered it had been introduced by the Chinese and were surprised that it was not more widespread. There had been many epidemics of malaria, whooping-cough and influenza which undoubtedly claimed the lives of any already sick.

Dr W. Bruce Kirkland presented a paper on health problems in the Northern Territory to the National Health and Medical Research Council, Adelaide, 24–25 May 1939. He made scant mention of tuberculosis except to say that it occurred among Aborigines and that some died within a few months. "In 1913, at least 30% of Chinese deaths were reported to be due to tuberculosis". He considered the situation had improved with the next generation living under better conditions.

Alice Springs was founded in 1873 with the establishment of a tele-graph repeater station. The first confirmed record of tuberculosis was that of the brother of the officer-in-charge of the Overland Telegraph Station. He came from Melbourne in 1901 because of his serious chest condition and six months later, following a severe coughing spasm, he died. As the telegraph station was a ration depot with a permanent camp of Aborigines there may have been some contact.

Dr Herbert Basedow, travelling by camel-drawn buggy, made a hasty survey of Hermannsburg Mission and several cattle stations in June 1920.[8] Many of his statements were sweeping rather than specific but he was convinced there was no tuberculosis there. In 1929 when both Professor J.B. Cleland and Dr C.E.A. Cook visited Hermannsburg, neither men-tioned any sign of tuberculosis. However, the Aborigines in Alice Springs may have had the disease and carried it to Hermannsburg.

Once the railway link reached Alice Springs in September 1929 many white men with tuberculosis came to Alice Springs hoping the dry climate would heal them. Once they took up residence in a guest house or hotel they remained there until they died. Dr W.B. Kirkland was appointed medical officer in 1930, and in 1931 he recommended that an Aboriginal in jail with tuberculosis be released in a bid to save his life. Over the next few years several Aborigines died and the diagnosis of tuberculosis was con-firmed by post-mortem.

The small Alice Springs Hospital with a separate unit for tuberculosis was opened in March 1939. There was an X-ray unit but with only one doctor in town, very little case finding was done prior to the take-over of the hospital by the army in June 1942.

During World War II, Major Raymond T. Binns recorded the number of Aborigines treated at Katherine during one year, when 21 were diagnosed by X-ray and sputum tests. He did not record their home areas. When this army hospital departed early in 1945 its records went too. The remaining patients were sent to Tennant Creek Hospital but no records remain.

Immediately post-war there were few medical officers prepared to work in the Northern Territory, the main reason being a lack of housing. In 1948 the Commonwealth Department of Health in Canberra set up a division of tuberculosis with Sir Harry Wunderly in charge. The commonwealth government undertook to finance the eradication of tuberculosis and Sir Harry Wunderly visited the six states to assess their needs. Each state was to have a director of tuberculosis to co-ordinate and direct the operation. The Northern Territory was omitted from the scheme; there was no special staff or extra finance.

In January 1951 Dr Richard Brock was appointed as the first Survey Medical Officer for Aboriginal health. Two more positions were created later and filled by Dr W.A. Langsford in 1953 and Dr John Hargrave in central Australia in 1956. All Aboriginal men, women and children received a full medical examination and individual medical records were established; these records were maintained by the Aerial Medical Service. Old tuberculin for Mantoux testing became available in the Northern Territory in June 1951 and was first used at Port Keats Mission by Dr Brock. Supplies of BCG vaccine became available in May 1952 and were first used at Millingimbi Mission, then Goulburn Island and Oenpelli before Dr Brock was sent to central Australia.

Dr Bertram Welton, an English doctor who had participated in the Normandy landing during World War II, was medical superintendent at Alice Springs Hospital from 1948–1956. Most of the time he was the only doctor in central Australia and was expected to look after community health as well as the hospital. He was most concerned about tuberculosis. In 1951 he taught Sister Saleen Lindner at Hermannsburg to do Mantoux tests. Those people who needed chest X-rays were taken to Alice Springs, a few at a time in the mission's truck. By 1952 there were 13 patients on domiciliary treatment with streptomycin, PAS (para-amino salicylic acid) and isoniazid (isonicotinic acid hydrazide) at Hermannsburg. The limited facility at Alice Springs Hospital was already overcrowded with patients from elsewhere.

Dr Brock and his wife Betty, a trained nurse, carried out a full medical survey at Yuendumu in June 1952. Sister Ellen Kettle was the trained nurse at Yuendumu. Mantoux tests on 260 people gave a positive reading of 34.2 per cent; 165 were given BCG vaccinations. All major central Australian centres were surveyed. Santa Teresa Mission, then at Arltunga, had seven people on treatment for tuberculosis in November 1952. Although only 55 per cent of the whole population had positive Mantoux reactions, 88 per cent of the young people between 16–20 years were positive reactors. Ten years earlier in September 1942 the Army had removed these people from Alice Springs to Arltunga. It was a barren area

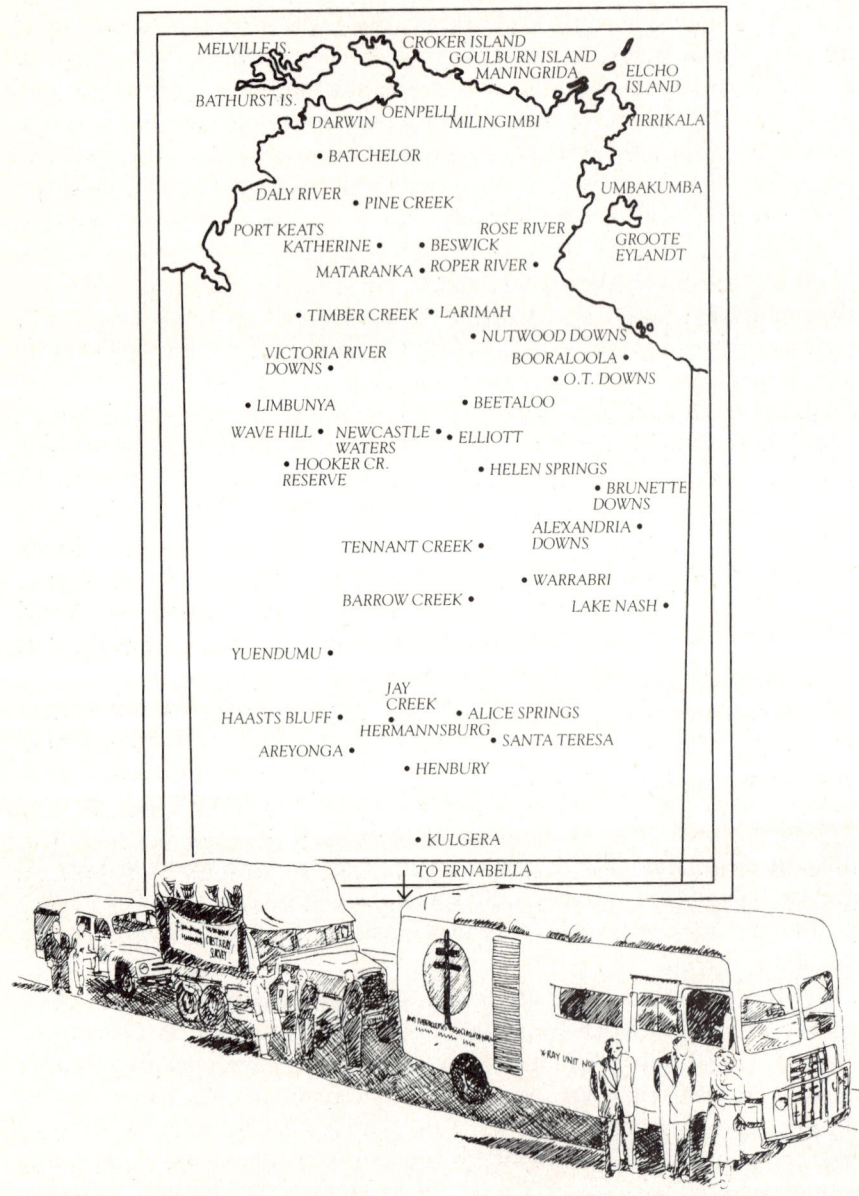

Settlements in the Northern Territory visited by the X-ray caravans of the
Anti-tuberculosis Association of New South Wales, 1959.
(Artwork: Jocelyn Proust)

and the mission was eventually shifted to better country south of Alice Springs.

Dr J.T. Rayment who replaced Dr Langsford in 1955 asked for a mobile X-ray unit suitable for transport by air. Sir Harry Wunderly helped in providing a SF 2 Watson Victor X-ray unit. It was first used on Channel Island to X-ray the leprosy patients. Port Keats Mission was the first large Aboriginal group X-rayed; all X-rays were sent by air to Sir Harry Wunderly in Canberra. Occasionally he came to Darwin to assess patients.

From the results of the Mantoux tests Sir Harry Wunderly gave priority to Milingimbi, Bathurst Island and Melville Island, all long-established missions and settlements. The RAAF flew Dr Rayment and his equipment to Milingimbi in a DC3 on 8 June 1955. The equipment was then recorded as weighing 907 kilos (2000 pounds). On his arrival he found six sick people in the hospital and sent them all to Darwin so Sister Jessie Smith, who knew the names of the people, would be available full-time to assist with the survey. Over the next sixteen days he examined 446, X-rayed 176 chests and gave BCG to 141. Many people with tuberculosis later received domiciliary treatment at Milingimbi.

Dr Rayment did medical surveys and X-rayed the people at Umbakumba and Angurugu on Groote Eylandt, Numbulwar on Rose River, Roper River Mission and Oenpelli. Elcho Island Mission proved a great disappointment as there was no adequate building in which to work and many films were spoiled by exposure to light. In total he X-rayed about 4000 Aborigines before his untimely death in late 1956.

Dr Hargrave examined 713 people on Bathurst Island betwen March-May 1957. He found 34 people with possible tuberculosis, 13 of whom later showed acid-fast-bacilli in their sputum. This number of people was too many for Darwin Hospital to handle so the Aerial Medical Service ferried them to Darwin for X-rays and then flew them home again to await the results. Sister Marita Scullion was the only trained nurse on Bathurst Island and the workload handled by her and other sisters later was very heavy.

By December 1957 Dr Hilary Roche in Canberra was exploring the possibility of having the Anti-Tuberculosis Association of New South Wales carry out a mass survey in the Northern Territory. The self-contained mobile X-ray unit came through South Australia and started X-raying at Ernabella Mission on 28 July 1959. As the films were developed Dr Leighton Anderson, the team leader, made the initial diagnosis. Sister Patricia Boland examined sputum for acid-fast bacilli from those suspected of having tuberculosis.

The "beef roads" that opened up the Northern Territory cattle country were still in the planning stages, but the X-ray team was well equipped with excellent vehicles and experienced no major hold-ups. The program was ambitious but they moved through the country amazingly quickly and surveyed a few other small population centres along the way. While half of the team spent four weeks in the Darwin area, the remainder were flown to the Aboriginal settlements and missions in a RAAF Dakota. On the missions top priority was given to the survey and staff were diverted to correctly and adequately identify illiterate Aborigines before they were X-rayed.

When Maningrida settlement was opened in May 1957 most of the population were still nomads. Dr John Hargrave, Sister Ellen Kettle and an Aboriginal medical assistant, Phillip Roberts, were flown to Maningrida in advance of the team to prepare the way. When the RAAF Dakota landed on 17 November the people came in hundreds including many not previously recorded. The radiographers could have worked faster but there were problems in getting people to take a deep breath and hold it. There was much nervous movement and laughter and many films had to be repeated.

In the final analysis 18,840 people had been X-rayed in the Northern Territory during the 1959 mass survey, comprising those of European descent (9,730) mixed race (1,038) and Aborigines (8,092). Eight Europeans and 13 Aborigines were diagnosed as active tuberculosis while 386 had other abnormalities warranting further investigation. The following year, as more people were followed through, a further 45 cases of pulmonary tuberculosis were notified. Dr L. Anderson visited Alice Springs, Tennant Creek, Katherine and Darwin during April 1960 to check the findings. Most of the 66 new patients received domiciliary treament as there were not sufficient hospital beds. The Aerial Medical Service greatly expanded its role to bring patients to Darwin for annual X-rays and review.

By 1965 a chest clinic was established at Darwin Hospital around which a tuberculous control programme was organized in the Northern Territory.

Tuberculosis in Far North Queensland

John E. Thompson

It was the foresight of Ellis Abrahams, as first Director of Tuberculosis for Queensland, that allowed tuberculosis services in far north Queensland to remain intact after 1978 when others outside the State have been largely dismantled. By appointing regional physicians, trained in thoracic medicine, he forsaw that as the incidence of tuberculosis declined the physician in Cairns would remain and deal with other chest diseases; asthma, lung cancer, emphysema for example. More importantly, this ensured that even when tuberculosis became a smaller part of the physician's duties, an adequate framework for tuberculosis control remained.

Originally there were two regional physicians for far north Queensland, in an area south to 16° latitude and north to easy wading distance of the Papuan coast. The physician on Thursday Island looked after a scattered tuberculosis empire that comprised not only the many Islands between Cape York and Niugini (formerly Papua New Guinea) but also large Aboriginal communities, then all Christian missions, lying on or near the east and west coasts of Cape York. Accessibility was a problem and at first slow boats provided the only communication. Many Cape York Aborigines first learnt to speak English fluently after spending a year or two in the Thursday Island sanatorium receiving triple therapy. Such a break of contact with one's family may have led to other less desirable sequelae but at least reactivation of tuberculosis occurred very rarely after such treatment. By the late 1960s the number of new cases had fallen and aircraft communication to remote communities by lumbering DC3 was a fact of life. They did not fly frequently enough and they needed constant repairs, but at least they got you there. The physician in Cairns then became responsible for the whole area. At this time mobile X-ray units from Cairns were able to visit most but not all settlements on Cape York. Even today, road transport is not an option unless the physician or chest clinic nurse has a four wheel drive vehicle, a "swag" and an extra week or two up their sleeves.

After 1987 daily plane services allowed more frequent visiting and follow up by tuberculin test and chest X-ray. The X-ray machine would be condemmed by modern standards but usually took a readable film. This is a tribute to the versatility of trained nurses, who staff these communities, and miraculously become, overnight, doctors. Telephones are still objects of great rarity. The Torres Strait Islanders are a people of a different culture, religion and language to the mainland Aborigines, and although scarcely affluent by Cairns standards, are seen to be glittering with wealth by their relatives in "sister" villages on the Papuan coast. With increasing numbers of Niuginians wanting to see this "El Dorado" for themselves, it is inevitable that the number of cases of active tuberculosis in the wards of Thursday Island Hospital has declined but little. Fortunately the organisms are not yet drug-resistant and short course chemotherapy ideally suits people who, after six months, may well wish, or have to, return to Niugini.

Around Cairns where most of the 170,000 population of this area live, tuberculosis surveillance goes on in school tuberculin surveys and BCG vaccination of high risk groups. The Aboriginal and Islander population makes up 15 per cent of the population and Aboriginal babies 20 per cent of all births.

The roads here no longer vary from dust bowls to waterways and to date the backpackers of many nations who flock here for the winter have not, like their Papuan counterparts, brought an influx of tubercle bacilli. I hope that we remain prepared.

CHAPTER 5

Tuberculosis in New Zealand

Linda Bryder

Tuberculosis arrived in New Zealand with the European, mainly British, settlers from the early nineteenth century. The death rate from all forms of tuberculosis in New Zealand in 1872, when national statistics were first collected, was 126 per 100,000 population. This was much lower than the equivalent rate in Britain of about 300 per 100,000, but a larger proportion of the New Zealand deaths were over the age of 25 which the Registrar - General thought "point(ed) unmistakably in the direction of a comparatively large number of adult persons arriving in New Zealand while suffering under that disease". He surmised that this group had come to the colony specifically for the therapeutic effect of the sea voyage and the New Zealand climate, although he admitted that no case histories had been kept as evidence to support this belief.[1]

Tuberculosis accounted for about ten per cent of all deaths in New Zealand in the late 19th century and was easily the major cause of death among the settlers, as shown in the table below.

Number of deaths (excluding Maori) from principal causes, 1899[a]

Tuberculosis (phthisis & other tubercular diseases)	795
Cancer	468
Accidents	462
Pneumonia	389
Bronchitis	369
Diarrhoeal diseases	298
Gastritis & enteritis	257
Diseases of the urinary system	255

[a] Source: *Statistics of the Colony of New Zealand 1899*, Registrar-General's Office, Wellington, 1900, p.40.

In the 19th century no specific health measures were directed against tuberculosis, but many of its victims found their way into the country's charitable institutions or became dependent on assistance from the Hospital and Charitable Aid Boards (set up in 1885). In the early 20th century an active anti-tuberculosis campaign was launched, which has continued to the present, although its strategies have changed markedly during this time. Different phases of the anti-tuberculosis campaign in New Zealand can be identified and these will be discussed in turn.

1. 1900 – 1913

Tuberculosis was already on the decline, at least in the European population of New Zealand, when the first active measures were taken to combat the disease. The last twenty years of the nineteenth century had seen a 29 per cent reduction in the death rate from tuberculosis among the settlers. In 1901 the Department of Public Health was set up, prompting the Chief Health Officer to the new Department, J.M.Mason, to state that "for the first time in the history of Great Britain and her colonies ... the physical welfare of the people (has) been elevated to a first place in the consideration of the Government".[2] While the immediate impetus for its inception was a plague scare, its energies were soon directed against tuberculosis. New Zealand was not alone in this new attention focused on tuberculosis. Anti-tuberculosis associations had been founded or were being founded in many Western countries around this time. Most significant for New Zealand was the establishment of a national association for the prevention of tuberculosis in Britain in 1898. Noting this and other such developments, the chairman of the New Zealand branch of the British Medical Association (BMA) advised in 1901; "we in New Zealand should not lag behind other countries in this matter, a matter deeply affecting the common weal of the people".[3]

Why did tuberculosis, endemic throughout the 19th century but largely neglected, suddenly claim so much attention in the early 20th century? New Zealand, like other countries, was influenced by the scientific advances relating to tuberculosis in the late 19th century, starting with Robert Koch's discovery in 1882 of the causal agent of tuberculosis, the tubercle bacillus. These advances precipitated a new confidence that tuberculosis was subject to medical control. At the political level tuberculosis was being identified as a national menace, detrimental to "national efficiency". The preoccupation with "national efficiency", defined as a concern for people's health as it affected economic and military strength, raised health problems to a new level of national consciousness in Western nations around the turn of the century.[4] Citing an American authority, Mason calculated that the 800 or so deaths from tuberculosis in New Zealand in 1903 cost the nation "the appalling sum of £304,000".[5]

The emphasis of the new anti-tuberculosis campaign launched by the Department of Public Health in New Zealand was on the institutional treatment of tuberculosis rather than on prevention. In this it followed the example of Britain. Mason's 1901 annual report noted that the Department had issued some leaflets and posters on tuberculosis but that "until some place has been erected where patients can be treated in accordance with the latest scientific manner, the best results cannot be hoped for".

In 1903 Te Waikato, the first sanatorium for the treatment of tuberculosis, was set up near Cambridge by the Department. It was intended to be an example to the hospital boards which normally ran hospital services. For a time this institution was the Department's pride and joy. Mason wrote in his 1903 report that "The Cambridge Sanatorium promises to be one of the finest institutions of that class in the world". The sanatorium was located in beautiful surroundings, 1,100 feet above sea level— "indeed it is hard to imagine more magnificent scenery— a factor not without its influence in the treatment", the Auckland Health Officer wrote.

The up-to-date "scientific" treatment practised at Te Waikato consisted of good food, fresh air, rest, and "graduated labour". The aim was to improve the patients' fitness and prevent them from becoming lifelong invalids as a result of a prolonged period of idleness in the sanatorium. In 1908 a tree-planting camp was erected for ex-patients from Te Waikato. Tree-planting was considered a suitable occupation for ex-patients as it involved fresh air and exercise. This "experiment" failed however, as not many ex-patients could be persuaded to take up the work and face the isolated existence which it entailed.[6]

The Department of Public Health launched a public campaign to raise money to build institutions and annexes at general hospitals for tuberculosis patients. Dr T.H.A. Valintine, who later became Chief Health officer and Inspector General of Hospitals in 1909, led a campaign to raise money for a small sanatorium near New Plymouth in 1904. In the same year Sybil Maude, a nurse who was responsible for starting the first district nursing service in New Zealand, raised money to erect a camp for poor tuberculosis patients near Christchurch. This was replaced in 1909 by Cashmere Hills Sanatorium, run by the North Canterbury Hospital Board. In Wellington, the Otaki Sanatorium was founded in 1906 and managed by the Wellington Hospital Board. From 1908 The Auckland Hospital Board accommodated tuberculosis patients at the Costley Home (now Green Lane Hospital). In 1910 the Otago Hospital Board also set up sanatorium, Pleasant Valley Sanatorium, near Dunedin.

Commenting on the anti-tuberculosis campaign in his annual report for 1910, Valintine expressed satisfaction with the situation for those in the early stage of tuberculosis, but regretted that there was little provision for those in the advanced stage of the disease. There was great reluctance on the part of hospital boards to admit advanced tuberculosis cases into their wards. The reluctance to admit tuberculosis cases was held responsible for a special public health threat as these people then remained in the general population, as Mason had noted in his 1904 report.

Compulsory notification of pulmonary tuberculosis was introduced to New Zealand in 1901. Notification held no immediate advantages for the patients themselves rather the reverse, now that tuberculosis was known to be an infectious disease. Patients were not anxious to advertise the fact that they had tuberculosis. Doctors sympathised with this, and some resented notification as an interference in their confidential relationship with patients. Few doctors carried out the notification regulations. Mason concluded in 1904 that "Notification in the strictest sense has proved a failure".

Another problem confronting New Zealand's anti-tuberculosis campaign in the early twentieth century was the tendency of physicians in Britain to dispatch tuberculosis patients to New Zealand for the therapeutic effects of the climate. Mason referred to this problem frequently in his annual reports. He claimed in 1903 that despite repeated warnings there was still a "steady influx" of such cases, and recommended a stricter insistence on the provisions of the Undesirable Immigrants Restriction Act. The problem was also discussed at a 1912 tuberculosis conference, where it caused friction. While some delegates called for stricter admission policies, others were in favour of admitting early cases of tuberculosis, arguing that, as British subjects, early cases of tuberculosis should not be "denied the advantages that were available to their more robust fellow-countrymen".

Thus the first decade of the twentieth century was the launching of a campaign against tuberculosis in New Zealand. The approach was very similar to that of Britain, with its emphasis on treatment in institutions and notification (although notification only became compulsory in Britain in 1912). Providing 260 beds for tuberculosis patients at the end of this period hardly constituted and effective preventive measure, given that there were probably about 8,000 cases in New Zealand at this time[7], and that the most advanced cases were least likely to gain admission to the sanatoria. Despite tuberculosis being rife among the Maori[8], the Department's anti-tuberculosis campaign was directed entirely to Europeans in the early twentieth century.

2. 1914 – 1939

The number of tuberculosis cases increased during the First World War, but this was believed to be the result of medical examinations of recruits, which led to the discovery of early cases, rather than an actual increase. The number of cases among ex-servicemen, however, was considered great enough to warrant the founding of a new government sanatorium specifically for ex-servicemen in 1918, Pukeora Sanatorium, near Wellington.

The period following the First World War was one of relative complacency in New Zealand in the fight against tuberculosis. The recorded death rates among Europeans continued to decline, and this was noted in the annual reports of the Director General of Health (the new name for the Chief Health Officer after 1920), together with the fact that New Zealand had one of the lowest rates in the world (when Maori deaths were

excluded from the computation, and they generally were). This complacency was reinforced by the conclusions of a committee of inquiry set up
in 1928 to consider the provision of accommodation for tuberculosis patients. This was a recipe for inaction, and accordingly the recommendations which the committee did make were not acted upon until much later.
These included the suggestions that a tuberculosis section under a director
be set up in the Health department, that hospital boards be encouraged to
establish tuberculosis dispensaries or chest clinics to diagnose and detect
early cases, that nurses be specially trained in domiciliary health visiting,
and that voluntary aid committees be set up to help rehabilitate tuberculosis patients.

There was little expansion in accommodation for tuberculosis patients
in the inter-war years. While there was little increase in the number of
beds, facilities within tuberculosis institutions were up-dated with the
advance of technology. Artificial pneumothorax was mentioned for the
first time in a medical superintendent's report in 1926, although there was
no reference to this or thoracic surgery in the report of the 1928 committee
of inquiry. A contributor to the *New Zealand Medical Journal (NZMJ)* noted
in 1929 that New Zealand lagged behind Canada and the USA in thoracic
surgery. He subsequently sent a questionnaire to all sanatoria, 25 hospitals
and 74 doctors, and found that thoracoplasty had been performed on 18
patients, and artificial pneumothorax on 256 patients.[9] Artificial pneumothorax was introduced in the Auckland Infirmary after Dr Chisholm McD-
owell was appointed visiting medical tuberculosis officer in 1933, taking
charge of all the tuberculosis cases.[10] In the 1930s a few articles appeared
in the *NZMJ* on thoracic surgery.[11]

In 1936 two dispensaries for the detection of early cases were set up in
the North Island. North Canterbury and Otago had dispensaries since
before the First World War, and this probably accounted for the greater
number of cases notified in the South Island. In 1930, for example, twice as
many cases of pulmonary tuberculosis in proportion to the population
were notified in the South Island as in the North Island. There is no reason
to believe that there were more cases in the South Island, the death rates
being practically equal, and so the difference really pointed to the futility
of using notification records as an indicator of the prevalence of tuberculosis in New Zealand.

The area in which there was most vitality in the anti-tuberculosis campaign in the inter-war years was in relation to school children. This seems
surprising at first since the death rates from tuberculosis among children
of school-age were relatively low. Yet it was argued in New Zealand and
elsewhere that if resistance to the disease were built up during these
"quiet" years, this might prevent the disease from developing in later life.

The School Medical Service had been set up in 1912, and was transferred from the education Department to the Health Department in 1920 (becoming the Division of School Hygiene). In 1926 Dr Mary Champtaloup conducted a survey of tuberculosis among 1,268 school children. The incidence was found to be considerably lower than in other countries. Yet this did not lead to complacency in relation to the school population. Rather, in the following years school nurses were instructed to keep an eye out for children who seemed likely victims of tuberculosis. The parents of such children were to be visited and given advice on precautions to be taken, and the children themselves were to be sent to convalescent homes or health camps.[12]

The first health camp in New Zealand for malnourished children predisposed to tuberculosis was held by Dr Elizabeth Gunn, School Medical Officer in Wanganui, in 1922. A voluntary organisation in Auckland called the Sunshine League set up a "Sunshine School" in 1929, with the co-operation of the Division of School Hygiene. Also in 1929, a campaign was started to raise money for health camps by the sale of Christmas card seals (an idea originating in Denmark in 1901 and practised in Britain and elsewhere). At the end of his first year as Director General of Health in 1930, Dr M.H. Watt reported on the success of the Christmas Seal campaign, which had raised £2,500. In the same year a permanent health camp was erected in Otaki. In 1926 the National Federation of Health Camps was formed to maintain a chain of permanent health camps throughout the country. Watt singled out the Children's Health Camp movement as the major advance, in his report on the progress of the anti-tuberculosis campaign in 1937, noting that some 2,500 delicate and undernourished children were treated in these camps during the year 1935.

Tuberculosis patients were not singled out for special treatment when social security was introduced by the first Labour Government in 1938, although like other invalids they profited from the new welfare benefits. Only much later, in 1955, when a degree of selectivity had been introduced into social welfare, were tuberculosis sufferers identified as in need of an additional benefit by the Social Security Department. The Labour Government's housing scheme was also thought to assist in the anti-tuberculosis campaign, with about 29,000 new State houses having been erected by 1949. Priority for relocation in these State houses was given to "tuberculosis households" in sub-standard accommodation.[13]

The provision of free milk in schools from 1937 was considered a valuable preventive measure. Additional milk was only of value if it was guaranteed to be free of tubercle bacilli, which sometimes caused tuberculosis in children. Pasteurisation was the surest way of ensuring that the milk was safe. This procedure had been objected to in the earlier 20th century on the grounds that it destroyed the nutritional value and taste of milk and also encouraged sloppiness among producers. However, by 1937 the medical profession lent its full support to pasteurisation of milk. Pasteurisation was still not universal however; by 1944, in Auckland only 70 per cent of milk delivered retail was pasteurised; in Wellington the figure was 77 per cent, in Christchurch 15 per cent and in Dunedin 31 per cent. Complete statistics of tuberculous disease of livestock had never been compiled in New Zealand.[14] Some estimates placed the proportion of cows with tuberculosis at ten per cent, but the 1928 committee of inquiry had stated that "repeated tests throughout the Dominion have shown that tuberculous infection of milk is exceedingly rare". The extent to which infected milk contributed to the incidence of tuberculosis in New Zealand remains unknown, and little action was taken before 1944.

The 1928 committee of inquiry noted that "little accurate information is available as regards the incidence of the disease in Maoris, and not much appears to be done to combat the disease among this section of the population". The committee recommended that more definite information be obtained in regard to the extent of tuberculosis amongst Maori, and that more active measures be taken for the control of the disease in Maori districts. The first systematic study of tuberculosis in a Maori community was undertaken on the East Cape in 1933 by Dr H.R. Turbott, at the time health officer for Gisborne.[15]

3. 1940 – 1970

The 1940s and 1950s was an extremely active time in the campaign against tuberculosis. This was a period in which medical intervention showed real influence on the disease for the first time. Innovations in this period included mass miniature radiography to detect early cases (first introduced in 1941), BCG vaccination (not generally available until around 1950), thoracic surgery, and, after 1950, effective chemotherapy (streptomycin and related drugs). In this period it was confidently predicted that medical technology would totally eliminate tuberculosis within a generation.[16]

In 1943 a Division of Tuberculosis was set up in the Department of Health, as had been recommended by the 1928 committee of inquiry, and Dr C.A. Taylor was appointed as Director. All forms of tuberculosis were made notifiable in 1940, and a National Tuberculosis Register was set up to classify cases in a standardised manner. By 1943 there were 6,772 cases (including Maori) on the register, and by 1958, 13,341.

District nurses were employed to look out for early cases of tuberculosis and instruct households (specifically mothers) in prevention and home treatment. In order to place the responsibility in the hands of district nurses the 1940 Health Amendment Act had taken pulmonary tuberculosis out of the list of infectious diseases which, under the 1920 Health Act, were to be notified to the local authority and followed up by sanitary inspectors. Instead, tuberculosis (all forms) was declared by an Order of Council to be a notifiable disease, to be notified to health officers and followed up by district nurses. It was believed that the search for new cases and the supervision of patients living in their own homes would be much more effectively undertaken by (female) district nurses than by (male) sanitary inspectors. One of the objections to notification was apparently the resentment caused by the visits of the sanitary inspectors, and it was hoped that district nurses would cause less resentment. By 1948, 8,101 outpatients and 23,104 contacts were being supervised by 221 district nurses in the employment of the Health Department or hospital boards. These nurses were responsible for identifying 314 new cases of tuberculosis that year. In 1953, over 11,000 "tuberculous households", containing more than 30,000 people, were under the supervision of district nurses.

Mass miniature radiography (MMR) was introduced in 1941 to detect early cases of tuberculosis. MMR, capable of taking 100 1 inch chest photographs per hour, had been developed in the decade before the Second World War and was first used in Britain in 1940. In 1941, 2,204 factory and office workers and secondary school pupils in Wellington were examined, and an active tuberculosis case rate of 0.6 per cent discovered.[17] MMR expanded as more equipment and trained staff became available. By 1954, there were approximately 95,000 miniature X-rays taken each year, and by 1957, with nine units operating throughout the country, there were almost 250,000 examinations. In the 1950s one to two new cases of active tuberculosis were found per thousand miniature X-rays.[18]

One of Dr Taylor's first priorities as Director of the Tuberculosis Division was the organisation of conferences to stimulate hospital boards to appoint tuberculosis officers, institute chest clinics and improve facilities for tuberculosis cases, including facilities for thoracic surgery and occupational therapy. He also campaigned for the formation of voluntary societies to help with social problems and rehabilitation of tuberculosis patients. The first such organisation was set up in Auckland in 1944, and by 1949 tuberculosis associations had been established in various provinces, guided by the newly formed New Zealand Federation of Tuberculosis Associations. In the 1950s the Director referred in his annual reports to the valuable work being done by these associations. Their activities also included the financing of a visit in 1962 by J.W. Crofton, Professor of Chest Diseases at Edinburgh University, as guest speaker at a course in Wellington on chest diseases.

In 1948 a Tuberculosis Act was passed. This was largely a consolidating measure. It included provision for the establishment of clinical, X-ray and laboratory services by hospital boards, as well as a more systematic notification of cases and compensation for certain employees in hospitals and Department of Health nursing services who contracted tuberculosis at work.

The following year regulations were added to the Tuberculosis Act to guide a national scheme of voluntary BCG vaccination against tuberculosis. BCG had been discovered in France in 1921 but little used outside France and Scandinavia before 1945.[19] Britain introduced BCG vaccination in 1949. Some countries, such as the USA, continued to oppose BCG as a public health measure against tuberculosis, but after World War II the World Health Organization pronounced strongly in favour of this vaccine as a tuberculosis preventive measure and this may have influenced New Zealand in its decision to adopt BCG. A start was made in New Zealand in 1948 when vaccination was offered to nurses in two provincial hospitals.[20] This program was extended throughout the country by 1950, with supplies coming from the Commonwealth Serum Laboratories in Australia. It was reported enthusiastically in 1949 that "This may well be an important step towards the ultimate goal of complete control of tuberculosis in this country".[21] The scheme was extended to school children, and a pilot scheme, under which about 80 per cent of the parents agreed to have their children vaccinated, was launched in several post-primary schools in the Wellington Health District in 1951. In 1952 approximately 12,000 vaccinations were performed; by 1955 about 25,000 were administered annually, and by 1960 over 35,000.

In 1951 compulsory tuberculin-testing of all dairy herds was instituted, together with the eradication of positive reactors (realising the 1944 Milk Act). Pasteurisation of milk was also extended, by still did not reach remoter areas. Rural areas continued to rely on voluntary tuberculin-testing of cattle to eliminate tuberculosis from milk supplies.[22]

Thoracic surgery took off in the 1950s. In 1955, J.M. Wogan, the Director of the Division of Tuberculosis, referred to the recent rapid growth of regional thoracic surgery services.[23] Thoracic surgery units had been set up in Auckland, Wellington, Christchurch and Dunedin. However, by the 1960s chemotherapy had made surgery almost redundant in the treatment of tuberculosis. In 1947 the editor of the *NZMJ* announced that the Department of Health had begun to distribute streptomycin, "a potential agent in the treatment of tuberculosis", in New Zealand hospitals. By 1957 streptomycin had been combined with other effective drugs (para-aminosalicylic acid, or PAS, and isoniazid). In the same year it was recorded that the shorter stay of patients in institutions, made possible by modern treatment, meant that some sanatorium accommodation could be diverted to other uses. One sanatorium, Pukeora, was closed altogether. In 1958, it was announced in the Department's annual report that "waiting lists for sanatoria and hospital beds throughout the country have disappeared and, indeed, surplus accommodation is available in most institutions." In 1960 when there were still 839 beds for tuberculosis in general hospitals, as well as 404 beds in four sanatoria, the overall bed-occupancy rate was less than 50 per cent. By 1965 the only sanatorium still operating was Gonville Sanatorium for Maori children with tuberculosis, administered by the Wanganui Hospital Board.

4. 1970 – present

In 1979, the Director General of Health pointed out in his departmental report that tuberculosis had been a declining problem since the early 1970s and was becoming a disease of the "aging New Zealand male", but that an undue proportion of the cases was also occurring in the immigrant Polynesian population of all ages. In 1969, 44 per cent of all notifications in New Zealand were among Polynesians, an ethnic group comprising only 9 per cent of the population.[24] In 1973 the first rise in notifications in twenty years was recorded, 688 compared with 552 in 1971. (This was still far below the figure for 1952, for example, which had been 1,705).

Dr J.F. Ryan, tuberculosis officer to the Auckland Hospital Board, asserted in 1972 that "The arrival of active cases of tuberculosis from overseas constitutes the public health hazard and represents a financial burden to the New Zealand tax payer". He instanced the 2000 or so Samoans who entered each year on a temporary work permit without any medical examination or chest X-ray, many of whom out-stayed the limit of their temporary permits. In his opinion, "it is from this group of people that our major problems arise as regards the control of tuberculosis in the community". He added that most of them could not pay for treatment. Ryan recommended that Pacific Islanders entering New Zealand be thoroughly checked either before leaving the Islands or on arrival in New Zealand. This recommendation was endorsed by the Thoracic Society.[25] However, Dr J.B. Mackay of Wellington pointed out that the majority of Pacific Islanders contracted tuberculosis once in New Zealand. He thought the solution was to offer BCG vaccination to all Polynesian children soon after birth and again at the age of five years when they entered primary school.[26]

In 1976 a program began by agreement with the governments of Western Samoa, Tonga, Fiji and the Cook Islands that all visitors or workers who proposed to stay in New Zealand for over two months should receive a chest X-ray.

The decline of tuberculosis

In 19th-century New Zealand deaths from tuberculosis outnumbered those from cancer, cardiovascular disease and cerebrovascular disease combined. By the 1960s tuberculosis deaths represented less than one-hundredth of the combined total of those diseases. In 1960 the Registrar-General showed a neat inverse relationship between tuberculosis and cancer in New Zealand. As tuberculosis declined, cancer increased. He explained this in the following terms: "The fall in the tuberculosis rate may be said to reflect the achievements of the public health service, whilst the rise in the cancer rate portrays in general the increasing age of the population". However the role of the public health service in the decline of tuberculosis has more recently be questioned in Britain by Thomas McKeown[27], and must equally be questioned in New Zealand.

Tuberculosis had been steadily declining since the late 19th century and effective anti-tuberculosis measures were not introduced before the late 1940s. Indeed some have argued that even after these measures were introduced, other factors such as housing improvements were of far greater importance in the decline of tuberculosis.[28] J.J. Collins carried out a study of the contribution of post-1947 developments to the decline of respiratory tuberculosis in England and Wales, Italy, and New Zealand by analysing death rates of birth cohorts. He concluded that medical factors played some part in the decline in England and Wales and in Italy, but that in New Zealand they barely affected mortality levels from respiratory tuberculosis. He reached this conclusion by estimating how many deaths would have occurred had the pre-1947 trends continued and found that in New Zealand the predicted coincided with the actual trend.[29]

Some commentators suggested that the favourable climate of New Zealand affected the incidence of tuberculosis. However, the rates were more or less equal throughout the century for the various provinces of New Zealand, where the rainfall, wind factor, and hours of sunshine differed dramatically. This suggests that climate had minimal influence on the course of the disease.

It appears in the final analysis that the low rate of tuberculosis in New Zealand (among European New Zealanders) compared to most other countries, and the decline of tuberculosis in the 20th century, lay in the favourable social and economic conditions of the country.[30] Infant mortality was also relatively low, and like tuberculosis, was often thought of as a "social barometer". By the 1980s tuberculosis in New Zealand was identified primarily as a problem of the Maori and Polynesians. In 1983, the incidence among Pacific Islanders and Maori was 9 and 4 times that of the rest of the New Zealand population respectively.

The Development of Tuberculosis Services in Canterbury

T.O. Enticott, J.A. McLeod and H.T. Thompson

The role of surgery in the treatment of tuberculosis is emphasised in this brief outline of the control of the disease in Canterbury during the first 60 years of this century.

The need for the isolation and care of cases of pulmonary tuberculosis in Christchurch led, in 1898, to the setting up of a tent camp on the sand dunes of New Brighton, a seaside suburb. Eight years later, as a result of public concern, the need for a more permanent institution was recognised and 10 acres of land were obtained on the Cashmere Hills four miles south of the city. In 1910 the Cashmere sanatorium was opened under the control of the North Canterbury Hospital Board with Dr G. Blackmore as Superintendent. There were 31 beds in open chalet-type shelters. Patients were ambulant on a strictly regulated regime of exercise and generous diet. Coronation Hospital, built on a six-acre block of land below the original sanatorium was opened in 1914. With 34 beds it was intended for the isolation and bed treatment of advanced and dying cases. By 1930 when Dr I.C. McIntyre succeeded Dr Blackmore the complex had grown to the extent that there were 102 beds in Coronation Hospital and 104, including a children's block of eight beds, in the sanatorium.

In 1919 a 70-bed military sanatorium on land (54 acres) above the original sanatorium was opened under the control of the Defence Department. In 1924 it was taken over by the North Canterbury Hospital Board. Having fallen into disrepair it was closed in the mid-thirties only to be rebuilt in 1942 in response to the needs of servicemen returning from World War II. From 1916 other hospital boards in the northern half of the South Island had rights to beds in the sanatorium. In 1930 Dr McIntyre began a three-monthly consultative service to clinics in these places.

In 1923 an institution unique at that time, the Fresh Air Home for Children, with 32 beds was opened near the upper sanatorium. The home cared for the children of sanatorium patients, especially the poor and underpriviledged. A regime of good food and healthy living was thought to confer resistance to tuberculosis. A model open-air school was a feature of this institution. The home continued to function for about 45 years, eventually to be taken over as an orphanage.

Under Dr McIntyre's influence the treatment of pulmonary tuberculosis became more active. He was joined in 1946 by Dr T.O. Enticott and in 1953 by Dr J.A. McLeod. Patients were initially admitted to Coronation Hospital and graduated from bed rest to controlled activity at the upper sanatorium and then to open shelters at the middle sanatorium eventually to return home. At least this was the general plan, not always realised as relapses occurred. Collapse therapy with artificial pneumothorax and pneumoperitoneum with phrenic crush was widely used and had its heyday in the 1940s. Streptomycin was introduced in 1948 and PAS in 1949 followed by isoniazid in 1952. There was a low incidence of atypical tuberculosis strains and a very low incidence of primary or secondary drug resistance which says a good deal for the efficient control of chemotherapy in Canterbury. Successful chemotherapy set the stage for a decade of surgical treatment.

Although a few three-stage thoracoplasties had been carried out in preceding years, it was not until 1955 after the appointment of H.T. Thomson as full-time thoracic surgeon that the surgical treatment of pulmonary tuberculosis came into its own in Canterbury. Until 1960 most operations were carried out at Coronation Hospital. The operating theatre was a small room where, in earlier days, artificial pneumothoraces had been induced and refilled. This rather primitive arrangement was presided over by a theatre sister, helped by a nurse aide. Any architectural deficiencies were more than compensated for by the skill and efficiency of this small team. At a time when resistant staphylococcal infection was epidemic in New Zealand hospitals, Coronation Hospital was relatively free from problems of infection. That the results of surgery were excellent was in no small measure due to the high standard not only of the theatre staff but also of the pre- and post-operative care of the patients.

By 1958 the backlog of patients with long-standing fibrocaseous disease had largely been overcome and the number of cases presenting for surgery fell dramatically. For the first time in many years there were empty beds in the sanatorium.

In 1960 Coronation Hospital ceased to function as a tuberculosis hospital and was converted to house long-stay geriatric patients. Surgery was transferred to the thoracic surgery department of the recently opened Princess Margaret Hospital. By 1965 the number of cases of pulmonary tuberculosis presenting for surgery had fallen to less than ten per year.

In the ten years from 1955 to the end of 1964, 410 patients had had resections for pulmonary tuberculosis. In this number there were 33 pneumonectomies and 355 patients had conservative resections, of whom 228 had segmented resections and 127 had lobectomies. Twenty-three patients in the conservative group had bilateral resections. All the pneumonectomy patients had corrective thoracoplasties. In this latter group the thoracoplasty was a limited osteoplastic operation of the Bjork type, normally carried out at the time of the resection. It was believed that the corrective thoracoplasty prevented over expansion of the remaining lung tissue and made the flare-up of any residual tuberculous disease less likely. Be that as it may, none of the patients in this group suffered any significant flare-up of their disease post-operatively and none developed empyemata, tuberculous or pyogenic. In addition to pulmonary resections 22 patients underwent pleurectomy for tuberculous empyemata.

There were for post-operative deaths, two in the pneumonectomy group and two in the conservative resections. In 433 operations this was well under 1 per cent.

Some Aspects of Tuberculosis in New Zealand and Western Samoa 1942-1985

J.B. MacKay

In 1942, while a sixth year medical student, I spent three months as acting house physician in the tuberculosis wards of Wellington Hospital. Six weeks later I developed erythema nodosum and after a further six months, pleurisy. A year later I had an abnormal chest X-ray and went on extended sick leave. I returned to work in a protected environment as the only resident doctor in a long-stay hospital in the country. Two years later, a cavity developed at the left apex—my sputum was bloodstained and contained *M. tuberculosis* and I was admitted to Cashmere Sanatorium in Christchurch.

Treatment in the sanatorium consisted of prolonged bed rest and subsequent graduated exercise, good food and fresh air. Considerable emphasis was placed on the latter, so one lived in a "shack" with folding walls, one of which had always to be open even in the most inclement weather. After three months of this regime, a left artificial pneumothorax was successfully induced. Life was rigidly controlled by rules and regulations which I found irksome and I earned the displeasure of the medical superintendent, Ian McIntyre, by walking over the nearby hills rather than doing the set daily walks up and down the sanatorium road.

Following discharge from the hospital after six months, I started to look for a job and was accepted as a resident physician at the mental hospital in Nelson; a hospital at which my grandfather had been medical superintendent over forty years previously. Coincidentaly he had been advised to come to New Zealand to recover from pulmonary tuberculosis.

As I was now married and had one child, the provision of a house with the job was the main attraction. However, before I could take up the post, my sputum again became positive for *M. tuberculosis.* Somewhat depressed at this stage, I was offered a job by Gilbert McLean, as a registrar in the chest department of Wellington Hospital for 1947. I enjoyed the work, and continued in the department until I retired in 1985, having spent the last 28 years as physician in charge. My pneumothorax was continued for five years and after it was abandoned I felt free to go overseas for postgraduate study.

My story was a not uncommon one at the time, although for many patients, the outcome was less satisfactory. During my stint as a house physician in the tuberculosis wards of Wellington Hospital I noticed that only a few patients were discharged during the three months I was there; some went on to sanatoria, a number died, and others continued in the ward, some having been in-patients for one or more years. I was somewhat alarmed on entry to the sanatorium to read in an article in the *British*

Medical Journal, that 50 per cent of newly diagnosed patients with tuberculosis were dead within five years—a fact which was supported by the eventual death from tuberculosis of many of my fellow patients in the sanatorium. Alcohol was a prominent factor in the development of tuberculosis in many patients.

During the 1940s artificial pneumothorax was the most effective treatment for pulmonary tuberculosis, and with the addition of adhesion resection was, in many cases, life saving. The patients were aware of the efficacy of artificial pneumothorax, and were often in tears when attempted induction failed. One religious registrar always carried a bible in in the pocket of his white, and after a failed pneumothorax brought it out as the next most effective treatment. Although surgical intervention was practised on some patients, the results were not encouraging. I surveyed all the cases where thoracoplasty had been undertaken, but cures were so few that I never published the results. Resection prior to the advent of effective chemotherapy was disastrous. Pneumoperitoneum and phrenic crush seemed to benefit some patients.

We began to use streptomycin in 1947, following its discovery by Waksman in 1944. Initially we were impressed with the improvement in sick patients only to be disappointed after one or two months of treatment. We were to learn that resistant organisms developed rapidly, and were soon the dominant organisms seen in cultures. It was not until other anti-tuberculosis drugs were developed that it was shown that two or more drugs given together would prevent the development of resistant organisms. About this time two trained thoracic surgeons, Jim Baird and Tim Savage, were appointed to the staff, and with the use of anti-tuberculosis drugs, resections were carried out in increasing numbers and with excellent results. I can recall one sad episode associated with chemotherapy. A young man of unconventional religious beliefs was opposed to taking any drugs. The medical and nursing staff spent considerable effort in persuading him to change his opinion. Shortly after he started treatment he was found hanging from a tree behind the hospital.

Tuberculous meningitis was a dreaded complication and invariably proved fatal prior to the advent of effective anti-tuberculosis drugs. In 1967 I collected the cases of tuberculous meningitis occurring in the Wellington Hospital Board area from 1941–65 inclusive. There were 132 patients, one third were under ten years, half were under the age of 20 and three quarters were under thirty. Fifty per cent of the patients were Maori. The incidence fell from 10.4 cases a year in the first five-year period to 2.2 in the last. BCG vaccination was introduced into the area in 1951 and it is significant that none of the patients who developed tuberculous meningitis were known to have had BCG vaccination. Mortality was 100 per cent between 1941 and 1947; 82 per cent between 1947 and 1952, and 26 per cent from 1953-1965 when isoniazid became available. In the first group all patients were dead within three weeks of admission to hospital and 40 per cent died within eight days of admission. The urgency of instituting treatment became apparent if cerebral infarction due to arteritis was to be avoided. The first patient to survive at Wellington Hospital was a 21 year old woman admitted in October 1947. She was treated with streptomycin alone, administered by intramuscular injection daily for six months and intrathecal streptomycin daily for the first two months. Subsequently an 18 year old Maori boy, treated with large doses of streptomycin intramuscularly and daily intrathecal injections for six weeks survived, although he became quite deaf. The treatment with daily lumbar punctures, for long periods, was stressful for both patient and doctor. When isoniazid became available and corticosteroids were used, intrathecal injections were no longer necessary. I was most impressed with the value of corticosteroids and although there was some controversy regarding their use, gave them to all patients. I felt that corticosteroids were effective in preventing arteritis of the cerebral vessels thus preventing cerebral infarcts and also in preventing spinal block. Of the last ten patients I treated the only one who died had the dose of corticosteroids reduced early because of apparent good progress. He subsequently died in spite of the dose being increased again. At post mortem examination widespread arteritis of the cerebral vessels was seen, producing multiple cerebral infarction.

In the early 1970s concern was expressed by chest physicians, hospital authorities and the press at the increasing numbers of Pacific Islanders in New Zealand suffering from tuberculosis. In 1974 there were 615 cases of tuberculosis notified in New Zealand, an incidence of 20 per 100,000. Although Island Polynesians made up only 2 per cent of the population they were responsible for 20 per cent of the cases; a third had been in New Zealand for less than one year, the probability being that they entered New Zealand with tuberculosis. The incidence of tuberculosis in Island Polynesians in New Zealand was 20 times that of the European.

The problem was highlighted by an outbreak of tuberculosis that occurred in Porirua College. A 16-year-old fifth form school boy was admitted to hospital with sputum positive pulmonary tuberculosis. He had been in New Zealand for 15 months and had had a cough for most of this period, and some blood-staining of his sputum more recently. The organisms from his sputum were resistant to streptomycin and isoniazid. Soon afterwards two Samoan boys from the same fifth form were admitted suffering from tuberculous meningitis. It was assumed that their organisms were resistant to streptomycin and isoniazid, and this proved to be the case. It was fortunate that the sensitivity tests of the organisms from the original patient were available when these two patients were admitted, because if we had used conventional treatment they would probably not have survived. Both did well, but one, about twelve months later on, fell from a second floor verandah and died of head injuries. His mother concluded that this was his destiny and that we had only delayed the inevitable by curing his meningitis. A further seven sputum-positive cases of pulmonary tuberculosis, all with resistant organisms, were discovered at the college by examination of 430 contacts. The thought of resistant organisms being disseminated in the community later on, prompted us to treat 29 fifth-formers who had a high degree of tuberculin sensitivity; a total of 38 patients were treated therefore as a result of one Samoan boy entering New Zealand with active tuberculosis. In an endeavour to discover the incidence of drug resistance in New Zealand, I wrote to all the laboratories where sensitivity tests were undertaken. Fifty seven patients were noted as having drug resistant organisms between 1975 and 1977. During this period 1,880 patients were notified as suffering from tuberculosis, 14 of the 57 patients patients with resistant organisms were Samoan and 12 of these had organisms resistant to isoniazid and streptomycin, whereas only one European had a similar pattern of resistance.

At a meeting of the advisory committee on tuberculosis to the Department of Health in 1975, it was recommended that a chest physician visit the Pacific Islands, and I was asked to undertake a four-week assignment to Western Samoa in March 1976—the first of seven official visits I made over the next ten years. Other chest physicians visited Tonga, Niue and the Cook Islands. I found a high prevalence of tuberculosis, a 50 per cent relapse rate, an appreciable mortality and I suspected considerable drug resistance. Sputum cultures for *M. Tuberculosis* were not done as a routine and no sensitivity tests were undertaken. I arranged for mass miniature radiography of the adult population. The population of Western Samoa was 160,000, 50 per cent of whom would be under the age of 15 years. The X-ray unit was taken out to the villages, often over poor roads, and some 60,000 Samoans were X-rayed during the next two years. The miniature films were sent to New Zealand for me to read. Approximately 3 per cent were recalled for a large film. The main reasons for recall were tuberculosis, bronchiectasis and cardiac abnormalities. I estimated the prevalence of tuberculosis to be 345 per 100,000 and bronchiectasis as 600 per 100,000; the latter figure was startling but was supported by the number of patients with bronchiectasis in the wards and in the out-patient clinics.

Arrangements were made for sensitivity testing of cultures of *M. Tuberculosis* to be undertaken in Wellington. On my first visit I returned with all the cultures packed in my baggage, and had some trouble getting them through Customs. In the first three years 188 cultures were tested; 50 per cent were resistant to one or more drugs. Half of these were resistant to both streptomycin and isoniazid. It was alarming to find a few patients with organisms resistant to rifampicin as well. Rifampicin was not available in Western Samoa but was being used in American Samoa. Treatment at that time was either streptomycin and isoniazid three times a week or daily isoniazid and thiacetazone. The main factor in the development of resistant organisms was irregular drug taking by out-patients. Samoans found it difficult to understand that it was necessary to continue to take treatment when they felt well, particularly if the drugs had unpleasant side effects.

John Alama, a Samoan graduate from the Fijian Medical School, was at that time a physician with an interest in chest diseases at the National Hospital in Apia. I arranged for him to spend six months as my registrar in Wellington Hospital—a friendship that has continued over the years.

The number of Samoans suffering from tuberculosis in New Zealand declined by 56 per cent between 1976 and 1983, in spite of a steady increase in the number of Samoans coming to New Zealand. The number of Polynesians discovered to have tuberculosis within one year of arriving in New Zealand, dropped markedly from 34 in 1974 to 13 in 1977. It is rewarding to have observed, and to have had some hand in, the steady reduction of the morbidity and mortality of tuberculosis in the Polynesian population of New Zealand. In 1947, when I joined the Wellington Chest Department, there were 180 beds in the hospital for the treatment of tuberculosis, and as well use was made of three sanatoria; Cashmere, Otaki and Pukeora, but still the number of beds was inadequate. Thirty eight years later, when I retired from the hospital, only an occasional patient with tuberculosis was in the chest ward at any one time. From a peak of 117/100,000 in 1943 the yearly rate of new cases notified in New Zealand had fallen to 9 per 100,000 in 1986.

Dr John Hiddlestone

John Hiddlestone was attracted to postgraduate work in Edinburgh by a seminar conducted by Professor Derek Dunlop on a visit to New Zealand in 1951. In Edinburgh he met John Crofton who pointed him towards a career in chest medicine; he worked for Norman Horne and Ian Grant at City Hospital where Crofton's professorial unit had 90 beds and large outpatient clinics; up to 50 patients received their "refills" at a single pneumothorax session. Each week Crofton led a group discussion on research projects and one whole morning was spent discussing the MRC Chemotherapy Trial to which the unit was the largest single contributor. At the same time all were encouraged to maintain their expertise in general medicine. Hiddlestone worked on a research project (glucose levels and glycolysis in pleural fluids in various diseases) which earned him his MD. This research suggested that the pleural fluid glucose level reflected pleural permeability and was part of the Donnan's equilibrium.

After further work in Brompton Hospital in London and Sully Hospital in Wales (where he became interested in the role of fungal allergy in asthma) he returned to New Zealand in 1955 to become chest physician at Nelson Hospital. With Rodney Francis (Napier) Alec Priest (Wanganui) Donald Malcolm and later Murray Kirk (Palmerston North), Hiddlestone met with Jim Baird and Tim Savage (thoracic surgeons) and John Mackay and Adrian Webb (thoracic physicians) in Wellington once each month. In turn each presented a major paper for discussion. Tuberculosis control in Nelson was based on case-finding using MMR, BCG vaccination of neonates and children, modern supervised chemotherapy and freely available thoracic surgery.

Hiddlestone's late career took him into medical administration as happened also to Halfder Mahler who became Director General of WHO and Gwyn Howells, Director General of Health in Australia.

Dr Adrian Webb

Adrian Webb wrote that in July 1939 while a houseman at Napier Hospital he developed a massive left pleural effusion; a replacement pneumothorax produced a frightening air embolus and later an empyema. He just avoided a thoracoplasty and was able to return to work only after 20 months. He resumed work at Wapeta Sanatorium 1941–45 and Cashmere Sanatorium 1945–47. In 1947 he reviewed 109 cases of artificial pneumothoraces (personally induced) and only 11 were free of complications. In 1947 he was appointed Tuberculosis Medical Officer for North Auckland, a region of poor roads, primitive hospital facilities, very few tuberculosis beds and whole Maori families dying of tuberculosis. In 1960 he was succeeded by Jim Ryan after his appointment as Senior Chest Physician to the Hutt Hospital. In the same year he was invited by WHO to establish a Tuberculosis Control Program in Sarawak over 3 years, a most satisfying task. Returning to Hutt, he resumed his active chest clinic practice in tuberculosis, asthma and occupational lung disease until his retirement.

Tuberculosis in New Zealand Maoris
Athol Wells

The first Maori migrations of the 9th century preceded European colonisation by over one thousand years. There is no evidence of tuberculosis in New Zealand during this period. Early European writers are unanimous in their description of the nobility and vigour of the Maori, a vigour that expressed itself, from time to time, in resistance to British dominion. It is among the ironies of the age that their final submission owed less to colonial coercion than to the various diseases introduced by the early European settlers.

The first known case of tuberculosis developed in the second Maori to visit England, Matara, who died of "phthisis" in 1807, shortly after returning from London. The Maori chief Ruatara, who was abducted to England in 1809, died five years later, most probably from tuberculosis. Infection spread rapidly from the whaling and trading stations of the early 19th century with disastrous effect. In 1827, Augustus Earle, draughtsman to *The Beagle*, was "very much astonished and shocked at seeing several beautiful young women, whom I left only a few months back in perfect health and strength, now reduced to mere living 'skeletons' and also to hear of the death of others by Consumption". William Marshall, surgeon to *HMS Alligator* in 1834, was also disturbed by the high prevalence of tuberculosis:

> Another deplorable circumstance is the great prevalence of scrofula... Facts, undeniable facts, bear me out in affirming that misery unheard of before, diseases unknown before, and deaths made fearfully more numerous than, and of a kind unthought of before, have been introduced...

In 1841, the Chief Tuhawaiki bitterly lamented the fate of his South Island tribe:

> Our parents, uncles, aunts, brothers, sisters, children, they lie thick around us. We are a poor remnant now... we had a worse enemy than even Rauparaha, and that was the visit of the Pakeha with his drink and his disease. You think us very corrupted but the very scum of Port Jackson shipped as whalers or landed as sealers on this coast. They brought us new plagues, unknown to our fathers, till our people melted away... Whole families on this spot disappeared and left no-one to represent them...

By 1855, tuberculosis was so widespread among Maori that Dr Arthur Thomson, surgeon to the 58th regiment, observed that:

> in some districts twenty per cent... bear on their bodies the mark of the king's evil... Scrofula is the predisposing and remote cause of much of the sickness among New Zealanders.

The Maori vulnerability to tuberculosis and other imported infectious diseases was seen by many European settlers as evidence of biological inferiority. In 1856 Dr William Featherstone, the superintendent of the Wellington province, declared that:

> a barbarous and coloured race must inevitably die out by mere contact with the civilised white; our business therefore, and all we can do is to smooth the pillow of the dying Maori race.

These sentiments were echoed by other leading European figures of the mid-19th century and may account for the lack of medical and social intervention during the decades that followed.

The Maori also perceived physical illness in moral terms. They attributed tuberculosis and other epidemics to the loss of "tapu" or "life-force". They believed that the old Maori gods had withdrawn their protection, angered by the supremacy of the European way of life and the abandoment of traditional Maori values. To be sick was to be possessed by evil spirits; the sufferer was sometimes driven from society, often with fatal consequences. This perception of illness as a heavenly affliction was to greatly reduce the impact of the public health initiatives of the early 20th century.

The Maori population fell from 100,000 in 1840 to a nadir of 42,000 in 1896. During the late 19th century, tuberculosis was the most common cause of Maori death and became known as "the Maori disease". Anecdotal accounts are consistent in their description of its devastating impact. Like many of his contemporaries, Bell (1890) believed that tuberculosis had a leading role in the decay of a once proud and healthy people:

> The most common disease is phthisis. Many die from this cause every year. The disease must be partially constitutional, and be aggravated by interbreeding, careless mode of living, and frequent want of proper care and nourishment... I believe that much of the lung disease could be prevented... Half-castes suffer from phthisis. I have never seen a grey-headed half-caste. Neither men nor women usually reach forty years ... It cannot be doubted but that the Maoris, as a separate race, will disappear entirely, but I believe that in future years there will be those who will be able to boast that they have Maori blood in their veins, and will be able, with pride, to trace back their descent to Maori ancestors.

For the first time, social factors had been acknowledged as important in the spread of Maori tuberculosis. In 1901, Dr Maui Pomare, a leading Maori figure and future Minister of Health, trenchantly rebutted the concept of "biological inferiority":

> Chief among the diseases I have encountered stands the dread white plague, phthisis, the exact ratio of which, to other diseases cannot be correctly estimated till death certificates are required by law. One is not surprised when we behold the abuse the poor bodies are subjected to through ignorance of hygiene and sanitary laws; the wonder is that there are not more who die of this disease. The Maori is generally looked down upon as an individual with weak lungs, but I am sure if pakehas were exposed in the same way as Maoris, they would disappear just as fast, and perhaps a little faster. Put the Maori in good healthy surroundings and he will thrive.

It is impossible to define precisely the prevalence of Polynesian tuberculosis before 1940. The notification of new cases was not, at first, widely practised. Early mortality statistics, dating from 1920 for Maori, are also incomplete. As Maori death certification was not compulsory, these figures considerably understate the true difference in mortality between the races. The Maori death-rate from tuberculosis in 1920 was recorded as 369.6 per 100,000, more than five-fold higher than in Europeans (64.8 per 100,000). In 1930 the Maori mortality rate had fallen only fractionally and in 1940 it had risen sharply to 413.2 per 100,000, now more than ten-fold higher than the European rate.

In 1935 H.B. Turbot completed the first and only investigation into the nature and prevalence of tuberculosis in the Maori population of an entire district. He chose Waiapu County in the east coast of the North Island, a rural area occupied by approximately two thousand Maori, considered representative of those elsewhere; the infant and tuberculosis mortality rates did not differ significantly from the national averages for Maori. The occupants of every Maori household were investigated; positive tuberculin-reactors and all those with clinical evidence of disease had a chest radiograph at the nearby hospital. During 1935 in Waiapu, ten Maori died from tubercuolosis, a death-rate of 494 per 100,000 and case mortality of 8.7 per cent. None was officially notified and over the three years before the survey only 14 per cent of tuberculosis deaths had been reported. The prevalence of tuberculosis was 5.7 per cent and had been similarly under-notified. These figures strongly supported the notion that Maori morbidity and mortality had been consistently understated by national statistics.

Also of interest was the documentation of social factors and their relationship to the prevalence of infection. Contact with an active case was traced or proven in 71.3 per cent of cases; in 34.4 per cent at least one other family member was also infected. Poverty, malnutrition and over-crowding were frequently identified in Waiapu County in tuberculous and non-tuberculous Maori households alike. This data appeared to vindicate further those who believed environmental factors, not racial predisposition, to be the major determinant of tuberculosis morbidity and mortality.

In fact the idea that the Maori race were genetically susceptible to tuberculosis had lost favour during the early 20th century. Disease, poverty and malnutrition had long been regarded as bed-fellows. Earlier writers had attributed the spread of infection to changes in lifestyle (from healthy open-air living to the adoption of more unhealthy European customs) and to Maori social customs including the rubbing of noses in greeting and kissing of corpses on the lips (as a farewell gesture). The importance of housing was emphasised further by Lonie (1947) who documented serious overcrowding in the homes of Maori but not European tuberculous patients.

In the socially-conscious era of the 1930s, the Waiapu data had an enormous impact. Many white New Zealanders had regarded themselves as members of a multi-racial egalitarian society and were appalled by the racial inequities detailed in the Turbot report; 60.8 per cent of Waiapu Maori with tuberculosis had received no medical aid; this was clearly contrary to the ethos of the Welfare State and stimulated the Department of Health to at last enforce provisions recommended in 1928. The birth of the welfare state in 1936 saw a concerted attack on destitution, especially Maori destitution. A major stated goal of the first Labor Government was to raise Maori living standards to European levels. In the past, the Maori people had received substantially less than their fair share of government expenditure; now they were to enjoy privileged treatment in education, employment and, above all, in the allocation of state-housing. If these initiatives did not end racial inequality, they certainly helped to eradicate the extreme poverty and malnutrition of previous decades.

All these measures contributed to a dramatic fall in Maori tuberculosis mortality between 1945 and 1955. Also of importance was the change in Maori attitudes to disease. In Waiapu County, the failure of most Maori to seek medical aid, despite adequate local facilities, was further evidence of a tragic fatalism which had hampered the control of infection from the turn of the century. Over the three years following Turbot's survey, a Maori District Nurse was intensively involved in overseeing cases, following contacts and, most importantly of all, in disseminating information throughout the district. For the first time, Waiapu Maori were systematically made aware of the mode of spread of tuberculosis and the role of preventative measures. Three years later, the Maori mortality in Waiapu had halved (from 494 per 100,000 to 247 per 100,000).

Similarly health education schemes were instituted throughout New Zealand over the next decade. In the Waikato, the revered Princess Te Puea, a leading figure in Maori education and land-development, was able to persuade Maori to attend European hospitals and doctors. In the Hawkes Bay area, R.S.R. Francis of Napier Hospital was especially energetic and is still remembered for his radio broadcasts in Maori and his addresses to parents and children throughout the region. So effective was the education campaign that in 1946 the Maori of Taranaki purchased the first mobile X-ray unit in New Zealand.

By 1954 the Maori mortality rate had fallen to 77.8 per 100,000, still seven-fold higher than the European rate. It is clear that the advent of anti-tuberculosis chemotherapy contributed to this decline. The death-rate first fell sharply in 1947, the year in which streptomycin became available in New Zealand. However a substantial proportion of this fall pre-dated the widespread use of chemotherapy and must be attributed to the improvement in Maori standards of living. Moreover the programs of the previous decade had played a crucial role in earlier diagnosis and in persuading Maori to accept European treatment.

Markers of Maori tuberculosis other than mortality convey little meaningful information before the mid 1950s. Tuberculin-positivity in Waiapu Maori aged 15 was 60.4 per cent in 1935 falling to approximately 20 per cent in 1955 (Wogan); the absence of standardised data precludes comparison with other surveys. However these and other figures seem to demonstrate a decline in tuberculous infection comparable to the fall in the death-rate. Interpretation of the notification rate is also beset with difficulty.

Throughout the 1940s and early 1950s, Maori notification cases continued to increase (521 in 1945, 634 in 1953) but not as a result of more prevalent disease. A vigorous contact-tracing program and the use of radiological screening had unearthed cases that would otherwise have escaped diagnosis. In the 1950s, BCG vaccination, radiological screening, anti-tuberculosis chemotherapy and improvements in living standards all made further inroads into tuberculosis; the epidemiological difficulties make it impossible to define the relative importance of these factors.

In 1985, the notification-rate remained more than four times higher in Maori (33 per 100,000) than in Europeans (7.4 per 100,000). It seems unlikely that genetic susceptibility contributed greatly to this difference. The epidemics of the early 19th century represented a true racial vulnerability due to lack of previous exposure. However by the late 19th century other factors had become increasingly important. During the 20th century, the decline in Maori tuberculosis followed a substantial improvement in living standards. Tuberculosis had become a medical barometer of social change.

It cannot be assumed that the present decline will continue indefinitely. Recent economic events in New Zealand have widened the gap between rich and poor. The increase in poverty and unemployment is likely to result in an upsurge in tuberculosis over the next decade. Furthermore, if overseas trends are reproduced, the advent of AIDS will be associated with an increase in tuberculosis, especially in racial groups with a high incidence of previous infection. For both these reasons, the notification-rate must be expected to rise in New Zealand, in Maori and European alike.

CHAPTER 6

Tuberculosis and Papua New Guinea: The Australian Connection

S.C. Wigley

Spurred by Australian concern about German interest in New Guinea, Great Britain declared a Protectorate over the south-east portion of the island of New Guinea on the 6 November 1884. Australia assumed administrative responsibility for the British Protectorate of Papua in 1906. This responsibility was extended in 1921 by the acceptance of a League of Nations mandate over the former German territory of New Guinea. Papua and the Mandated Territory were administered separately by Australia until 1945, when the mandate became a United Nations Trusteeship. From this time until the assumption of independence by Papua New Guinea in September 1975, the Territory of Papua and the Trust Territory were administered as a single entity, the Territory of Papua and New Guinea.

One can be sure that tuberculosis was not new to Papua New Guinea in the late 19th century, but the conditions which have prevailed over the better part of the past 100 years, and which created the circumstances which favoured spread and perpetuation of the disease, were. Extensive commercial exploitation within the country and from without, the internal and external labour trades, and the effects of World War II and its social sequels, led, amongst other things, to urban population expansion and overcrowding, to the disruption of established patterns of community living and family ties, and the isolation of individuals and communities in radically new environments. This organised social change, accentuated starkly over the years from 1945, transformed what must have been, at most, a minor endemic disease in the pre-contact era, into one which became epidemic.

The high prevalence of tuberculosis amongst Europeans and other expatriates living in Papua New Guinea at the turn of the century cannot be disregarded in the examination of this epidemiological change, nor can the contribution made by tuberculous Christian mission workers recruited for work in Papua New Guinea from other South Pacific areas where tuberculosis was well established as an epidemic disease by the mid and late 19th century.

Brief Historical Perspective

The proper antiquity of tuberculosis in Papua New Guinea is not known, but the disease must have been introduced into the country in the wake of the great migration waves from south-east Asia which are alleged to have populated Melanesia, beginning 50,000 years ago, and continuing until 2,000 years ago. It can be assumed on reasonable grounds that tuberculosis was not a problem to Melanesians at that time, and it is probable that man and tuberculosis co-existed in a way that was acceptable to both.[1]

In 1874, German trading interests settled in New Britain, New Ireland and other New Guinea outliers, and in 1878 labour was recruited from these areas to work on the German Samoan plantations. From this small beginning developed the New Guinea external labour trade which was to have a profound influence on the balance between Melanesian man and the tubercle bacillus. It was followed, in 1883, by the activities of the notorious "blackbirders" who recruited Melanesian labour from a wide area of peripheral New Guinea for work on the Queensland sugar plantations. In fifteen months 30 ships visited the area and took away some 2,600 men to work in Queensland. Sharp practice played its part, but by no means were all recruited as a result of false promises or force.[2]

Work on the plantations was hard and the hours long. Food was of poor quality and poorly prepared. Water supplies were polluted. Accommodation was overcrowded and under-ventilated. Medical care was non-existent. Approximately 25 per cent of the recruited labour died or was unaccounted for in the ten years from 1896.

Public concern led to a Board of Enquiry into conditions on the sugar fields, and the causes of such high mortality rates. Pulmonary tuberculosis was identified as a major cause. The Board recommended that all consumptive natives should be returned to their homes "at the earliest opportunity". Wide dissemination of tuberculosis in remote home villages was thus assured.[3]

The Internal Labour Trade: Labourers recruited for local employment in the old Protectorate, (German New Guinea), fared no better than those employed in Queensland. They constituted, more often than not, an involuntary labour force, and the contract labour system was indistinguishable from forced labour. Tuberculosis was common amongst them, and they lived under conditions which exposed them in large numbers to sources of tuberculous infection. German recruiting policies ensured that from the turn of the century tuberculosis was introduced into the remotest parts of the Protectorate. It is of interest to note that Robert Koch visited German New Guinea in 1910, but there is no evidence that he displayed any interest in tuberculosis there or influenced attitudes towards tuberculosis in the Protectorate in any way.

Tuberculosis in Papua

In 1871 the London Missionary Society established itself at Daru in western Papua, and by 1874 it was settled in Port Moresby. The evangelical and educational work of the mission was carried out by expatriate South Sea Island (SSI) teachers supported by a handful of British missionaries. In 1887, it was reported that 105 of the SSI teachers had died over a period of 15 years. This high mortality rate gave rise to alarmed concern. Charges of neglect of the teachers were levelled. The Reverend Dr W.G. Lawes, writing in the *Australian Medical Gazette,* May 1887, discussed the fate of the South Sea Islanders, and stated that:

> the immediate cause of death has not always been fever. There have been some cases of phthisis... and some cases difficult to diagnose.

It is known that the Pacific Islands from which the mission teachers came, Samoa, Tonga, Raratonga, Tahiti, etc., were centres of epidemic tuberculosis by 1870. And it is more than coincidental that the foci of tuberculosis along the south coast of Papua corresponded with the sites of London Missionary Society activity in the late 19th and early 20th centuries.

There are sufficient references to tuberculosis amongst Europeans and Melanesians in the *Annual Reports* to suggest that the disease was common. Between 1910 and 1923, 26 Europeans were diagnosed as tuberculous, 2–3 per cent of deaths amongst indentured labourers were due to the disease, and the death rate of tuberculous patients in hospital was over 30 per cent.

No special effort was made however, to look for tuberculosis in the native population beyond the immediate vicinity of the settlements. Isolated reports were made, but health administrators were pre-occupied with venereal disease, beri beri, yaws and hookworn, and the debate about the relationship between wearing European clothing and the inevitable development of tuberculosis.

Complacency was occasionally shaken though, and when medical patrols were asked specifically to look for tuberculosis among the native population at large, more and more cases came to light, and prevalences of up to 100 cases per 100,000 of population were found.

In the mid-1930s anxiety was expressed by some influential people in Port Moresby, including the Lieutenant-Governor, about the prevalence of tuberculosis in the Port Moresby villages, and the number of deaths from this cause. In 1936 a tuberculosis survey was carried out by Dr F.W. Clements in Hanuabada village in Port Moresby, using the tuberculin test, examination of sputum smears, and clinical examinations.[4] He found 43 cases of active tuberculosis amongst a population of 2000 people; 20 of these cases were of extrapulmonary disease. Of the pulmonary cases, 8 were smear-positive. The incidence of tuberculosis was 2.15 per cent. The limitations of Clements' methods meant that this figure was a minimal one, a view, moreover, suggested by a death-rate from tuberculosis in the village of 14 or 15 cases a year, one-third of deaths from all causes, an extrapolated estimate of tuberculosis mortality of 700 per 100,000 population

Clements' report led directly to the establishment of a hospital for tuberculous (and a few leprous) patients on Gemo Island in Port Moresby harbour. The hospital was managed by Sister Constance Paul Fairhall, a London Missionary Society nursing sister, assisted by a Samoan family, and its aim was to remove sources of infection from the villages, and provide treatment for them.

Tuberculosis in the German Protectorate in the South Seas, and the League of Nations Mandated Territory of New Guinea, 1884–1940

Annual Reports on the *Development of the German Protectorate in the South Seas* from 1900-14 drew attention to tuberculosis amongst native and expatriate populations (Europeans, Malays, Chinese and Polynesians), and to the high prevalence of positive tuberculin-reactors amongst labourers over a wide area of the Protectorate, with prevalences of up to 30 per cent being common. The foci of infection were concentrated in areas of commercial interest of the New Guinea Company. Reports noted the comparative freedon from infection of women and children in the villages, and suggested a link between infection and contact with non-indigenous inhabitants amongst whom tuberculosis was common. Innoculation with tuberculin for tuberculosis was undertaken in 1912, reflecting the remote influence in the colony of Koch's obsession with tuberculin.

Reports to the League of Nations from 1921 show that tuberculosis was rising steadily on morbidity and mortality tables. Tuberculin testing in 1923 gave positive rates of up to 34 per cent amongst adult native males. In children up to the age of 15 years the rate was 7 per cent.[5] It was believed that the chief source of infection was the Chinese. Although glandular tuberculosis was found commonly in slaughtered pigs in Rabaul, intestinal infection was thought to be of little consequence, and the pig as a source of infection was discounted.

In 1925 30 per cent of deaths in Rabaul were due to tuberculosis in an acute and rapidly fatal form "with a great tendency to dissemination".[6] It was considered that the chief cause was inadequate nutrition, and the solution to the problem lay, as far as one can see, in the

> continuance of the present policy of gradual improvement of the living conditions (of the native people)... and the development (by these natives) of an incentive towards the attainment of a higher racial status.

It was thought unlikely that the disease could be contained by the provision of sanatoria, or special hospitals. These opinions were followed by a dissertation on the psychological value of clothes to a subject race—contrasting sharply with the Papuan view, mentioned earlier, that the wearing of European clothes inevitably rendered the native vulnerable to tuberculosis.

In the 1930s tuberculosis was common in the European community in Rabaul, and amongst the native population in and around the settlements. It was reported from all districts and it was high on the mortality tables. In 1934 and 1935, limited tuberculin surveys were done in the Central Highlands of New Guinea and in the Upper Ramu Valley, both areas of recent contact. Infection rates found there ranged from zero, (in the Upper Ramu in 1934), to 1.2 per cent. This virtual freedom from infection contrasted vividly with the 23.0 per cent infection rate amongst Mount Hagen natives with some coastal contact, and the 50.0 per cent rate of the indentured native labour living in Rabaul. [7]

In 1939, the last reporting year before the outbreak of World War II in the Pacific, tuberculosis was fourth on the Territory mortality tables, and it was clear that the disease was widespread. A sad report from the Catholic mission at Vunapope, in New Britain, gives details of a micro-epidemic, at first unrecognised as such, amongst the young sisters, which led to the deaths of 23 of them over a period of ten years. The source of the infection was a young sister, the Mistress of the Novices, at the convent.

World War II in the Pacific

World War II in the Pacific involved Papua New Guinea in a degree of devastation and disruption never before experienced. What health services were in place prior to the outbreak of hostilities in the Pacific in 1941 ceased to exist, hospital patients were dispersed to the villages, and at Gemo Island, the patients, regardless of their states of infectiousness, were evacuated to villages peripheral to Port Moresby, to the east and to the west.

Tuberculosis in Papua New Guinea: the Post-war Period from 1945

The Australian Government's Provisional Administration Act of July 1945 provided for the appointment of an Administrator who assumed responsibility for both the Australian Territory of Papua and the former Mandated Territory of New Guinea. By October 1945, civil administration was resumed in Papua New Guinea and by mid-1946 it had encompassed the whole country. The Trusteeship Agreement for New Guinea was approved by the General Assembly of the United Nations in December 1946.

The health services of the Territory of Papua New Guinea were reconstructed in 1946. Tuberculosis was recognised to be an important medical and public health problem, and its management was accorded some priority in public health planning.

Port Moresby was regarded as the focal point of the infection, but the stretch of coast for a distance of 50 miles, (80 kilometres) to the east and to the west of the township appeared to be almost as bad, an assumption subsequently confirmed by epidemiological studies. Interest was expressed in knowing to what factors could be attributed the remarkable prevalence of the disease in those areas which might be regarded as the most civilised in Papua, and epitomised by Hanuabada—the "Big Village" —in Port Moresby. It was regarded as a plague spot. Early in hostilities it had been destroyed, and its inhabitants had been evacuated to peripheral villages, largely to the west of the township. Once the immediate danger had passed the villagers clamoured to return to Port Moresby. They had been allowed to do so, and the village had been rebuilt on its old site, with a total lack of supervision. The result was "the worst type of tropical slum, and a breeding place for every type of germ, from typhoid to tuberculosis". The village had reached such a state of overcrowding and filth in the early post-war years, that to burn it and establish it elsewhere was the only solution to the problem.

The rebuilding of Hanuabada village, on a different site, to the north-west of its original position, was begun in 1952. Four years later, in 1956, the village housed over 2,000 inhabitants. It was served with reticulated water and electricity, and an out-patient medical centre provided maternal and child health services, a general medical clinic, and a tuberculosis clinic presided over by a Melanesian medical assistant, John Davai, a Hanuabadan of influential standing in his own community.

Features of this era included the reopening of Gemo Island Hospital in 1946, and the reconstruction in the same year of the Lutheran and Anglican mission medical services, both of which emphasised the treatment of tuberculosis. Streptomycin was introduced into treatment programs in 1948, and during the following two years some major surgical interventions were undertaken on Gemo Island by an intrepid surgeon, and equally intrepid patients, under conditions which were far less than ideal. In 1951, a hospital development plan for New Guinea envisioned the construction of special tuberculosis hospitals. In the event three such hospitals were built.

In 1950 Dr Douglas Jamieson was appointed Specialist Medical Officer (Tuberculosis), and immediately some semblance of structure was introduced into the control program. The epidemiology of the disease began to be investigated in a systematic way, some rationality was introduced into treatment programs, using effective modern therapy, and in a co-operative venture with the Commonwealth Serum Laboratory, the earliest biological prophylactic programs were undertaken, using, initially, "wet" BCG vaccine. The formidable problems posed by its limited effective life, and its heat and light lability were overcome with great difficulty. Later the first freeze-dried vaccine produced by the laboratory in Australia was used in these programs.[8]

Between 1950 and 1955, epidemiological studies were conducted in and around Port Moresby, along the south coast of Papua, in the Gazelle Peninsula of New Britain, in New Ireland and its outliers, and in the Eastern Highlands of the mainland. A technical manual was published, and also some material on the management of tuberculosis in the individual;. mass examinations, using 35 millimetre miniature X-ray film were carried out over the latter part of this period.

The studies in the Eastern Highlands confirmed the low level of tuberculinisation first found by Heydon in 1935. They drew attention to the threat posed to the Highlanders should they become exposed to coastal Melanesians, and provided justification for insistence that Highland labourers should not be recruited for work on the coast without having been given the protection of BCG vaccination. (*Native Labour Ordinance Amendment*).

In 1954 and 1955, a series of surgical interventions was undertaken on patients at Gemo Island Hospital, without specialist anaesthesia, physiotherapy, skilled nurses, or an adequate blood transfusion service. The mortality rate from this small series was high, and the results of the operations daunting, not to say damaging to thoracic surgery in Papua.[9]

Against this background, and impressed by the number of patients who could conceivably benefit from surgery, the Director of Public Health, Dr J.T. Gunther, (later Sir John) began in 1955 to plan a program of thoracic surgery in collaboration with Australian thoracic surgeons. He was assisted materially in this plan by the Commonwealth Director of Tuberculosis, Dr H.W. Wunderly.

The program began in 1956. The visiting Australian units were self-contained in anaesthesia, physiotherapy, theatre and ward staff, and instruments. The units toured for six weeks and by the end of the year, three units had operated on 81 patients, without serious casualty. The program continued for ten years, until 1966, when it became evident that the bulk of surgery for tuberculosis had been done. In all, twenty units came to Papua New Guinea; Lae and Rabaul were drawn into the venture, and 716 operations were done on 623 patients, with a surgical mortality rate of 4.4 per cent. The thoracic surgical record was a good one—a tribute not only to the skills of the units themselves, but to the courage of their patients, and also to the vision of those who were the original planners.[10]

A physician, Dr S.C. Wigley, who came to New Guinea to select patients for the second and third surgical units, stayed on to conduct a tuberculosis survey in the Sepik District of the mainland, and was appointed Specialist Medical Officer (Tuberculosis) early in 1957, with responsibility for the management of the tuberculosis problem in Papua New Guinea.

Tuberculosis Control in the Territory of Papua and New Guinea from 1957

The philosophy of the Tuberculosis Control Program laid down in 1957 was expressed in its aim, which was to procure a reduction of the tuberculosis problem to a position of minor public health importance, in the shortest possible time.

The aim required that a comprehensive program should be mounted from the start, using biological prophylaxis on a grand scale, mass case-finding programs and intensive multi-drug therapeutic regimens, and chemical prophylaxis in appropriate circumstances. It required also that much energy should be expended on the supervision of the service, and that this should not be relaxed, no matter how favourable the immediate results of the program might appear to be.

The control program was undertaken by the Tuberculosis Control Unit of the Department of Public Health, with headquarters in Port Moresby. It was decentralised to four Regional Units in Papua, New Guinea mainland, New Guinea islands and the Highlands.

The regional units consisted of a medical officer, medical assistants, radiographers, and vaccinators. They were self sufficient, and equipped to carry out the mass examinations necessary to implement the plan. The Tuberculosis Control Unit was monolithic in its nature, and function, and elitist. It enjoyed the roles of "prime mover"; (mass epidemiological surveys, biological prophylaxis etc), "supervisor" of the essential services provided by others; for example, the general medical services, school medical services, and mission health services in the areas of diagnosis, treatment and prophylaxis; and also as "innovator", particularly in the field of treatment. This was especially true in the establishment of the out-patient treatment programs, which were set up on a grand scale, and offered fully supervised intermittent multi-drug therapy, which reached a peak patient-load in the mid 1960s. The Tuberculosis Conrol Unit was characterised by high morale.

The treatment regimen was simplified, universally applied, supplemented by appropriate and simple visual aids for use by low-level attendants, and controlled by a single authority, the Specialist Medical Officer (Tuberculosis). This eliminated the possibility of the use of unauthorised versions of the regimen.

It was recognised that fixed and elaborate units are expensive and immobilise manpower, thus nullifying the prime need of a public health service. Emphasis was placed on the mobility of the units which were expected to patrol constantly. The interest of the units was focussed on the health of the community rather than the medicine of the individual. Generally the units performed their tasks supremely well, and their members, European and Melanesian, recorded some formidable patrolling activities.

By 1963 the prevalence of tuberculosis infection was known in all areas of the country, biological prophylaxis was well established, case-finding programs were active, three tuberculosis hospitals had been built, at Finschafen in the Morobe District, at BitaPaka in New Britain, both completed in 1958, and at Embogo, in the Northern District of Papua in 1959. Substantial out-patient treatment programs were in operation, the whole programme was under intense supervision, at short and regular intervals, by the SMO (Tuberculosis), and the regional heads of units.

The Disclosed Pattern of Tuberculous Infection in Papua New Guinea

The epidemiological picture which emerged from the accumulated fragments of the work of the pre- and immediate post-war workers and the more structured efforts of the workers between 1950 and 1963, was basically a simple one. It was clear that tuberculous infection amongst Melanesians was related directly to the degree and duration of their contact with European communities, and the degree of urbanisation, or culture change which had occured in their communities. Tuberculosis was a coastal problem, and very much one of the towns, where the infection was spread diffusely through the community. In the rural areas infection was increasingly localised in the older age-groups as contact lessened in intensity, to the extent that in the remotest areas of least change it was confined to adult males. This was a reflection of the traditional movement patterns in these areas, which dictated that only the adult males would leave the rural areas to work in the heavily infected areas on the coast. This associaton reached its logical conclusion in the New Guinea Highlands (excluding an important part of the Southern Highlands), where infection rates ranged from a virtually irreducible 0.2 per cent, to a maximum of 2.0 per cent in Goroka Township, in the Eastern Highlands, in the early 1950s.

Rates in the Southern Highlands showed a curious anomaly. Above a line drawn from Lake Kutubu in the west, to Erave in the east, the rates were similar to the rates in the other highland districts, ie. they were below 1.0 per cent. Below this line the rates rose to almost 7.0 per cent, (in a sample of 3,200 people). The people living there, around Lake Kutubu, and in the Samberigi valley, are, geographically, highlanders, but culturally they have more in common with the coastal Kikori people with whom they worked and traded than with the highlanders. Many of the young men had worked in Kikori and Port Moresby, and many were employed at drilling sites in Papua by the Australian Petroleum Company. That the infection rate in this segment of the highlands community was comparatively high was thus not surprising.

Spectacular examples of the effects of contact on lightly tuberculinised groups of Melanesians included:-

1. The Goroka Highlands community, where in only two years of contact with an apparently healthy group of coastal Melanesian workers, infection rates of highland workers in the town were raised 40 times over that of highlanders in the same valley who had not had such contact (1949–1951).

2. The Bem Island community, evacuated to the Madang north coast by threat of volcanic activity on their island, where contact with the heavily tuberculinised mainland Melanesians for one year was sufficient to raise infection rates from 10 to 80 per cent.

3. A 1959 survey of Manus Island, a community subjected acutely to war, the most malignant urbanising influence, showed a dramatic rise in infection rates in the groups of this community which underwent the experience, ie. the age-groups 15 years and older. This was duplicated in the coastal Northern District of Papua, at Oro Bay.

Further studies during the decade from the early 1960s indicated that the Melanesian communities, at least in some areas, notably on the south coast of Papua, were near the end of an epidemic of tuberculosis, which may have reached its peak in the 1930s. They also indicated that although a favourable trend was apparent in the prevalence of tuberculosis in Papua New Guinea communities, there were important growing points of the disease, which would have to be restricted, if the favourable trends were to be maintained.

The growing points were: the urban areas, particularly Port Moresby, the institutes of higher education, especially the teachers training colleges, and the highlands area of New Guinea.

The Growing Points

The Urban Areas: "For too long we have proceeded on the false assumption that people would rather live in villages than anywhere, and that it is better for society if they did. The trouble is, they don't... people move into larger towns and cities..." (Adlai Stevenson, in an Address to the Economic and Social Council of the United Nations).

The phenomenon is a global one. In the towns it leads to situations which call for urban planning beyond the capabilities of authorities. The chaotic response is the shanty town, the slum, and the squatter settlement.[11]

Port Moresby, the largest by far and the prototype of the urban settlements, did not escape this universal dilemma. In the decade and a half up to the early 1970s there was a three- to four-fold increase in the population, and the city, with roughly one fiftieth of the country's population, was finding it necessary to provide facilities to manage one eighth of its tuberculous population. The prevalence of tuberculosis in the early 1970s was approximately 1.0 per cent, but in the squatter settlements it was up to four times as high.

Paradoxically, this high prevalence in the squatter settlements was set against a background of substantial reduction in the prevalence of the disease in Hanuabada village, where, thirty years after the Clements survey, not only had it been more than halved, but the nature of the disease had been substantially changed. In 1966, 2,300 villagers over the age of fourteen had been X-rayed. Twenty four were found to have lung lesions which were regarded as tuberculous, and were judged to be active and in need of treatment. With two exceptions, all had minimal to moderately advanced disease, and all were non-infectious, in that sputum smears for acid-fast bacilii were negative. The morbidity rate for tuberculosis in the village was thus a shade over 1.0 per cent. All patients completed a full course of treatment and there were no deaths from tuberculosis in the group.

Studies of the tuberculous patients in Port Moresby showed that at least 65 per cent of them were migrants from rural areas. Their importance lay in the fact that, almost invariably they belonged to large family units, their accomodation was poor, there was little or no work available for heads of households, or they were employed as casual workers in jobs with no real earning power or job security. As well, they came from areas which were poorly equipped to provide either in-patient or out-patient treatment services for the tuberculous. They resented bitterly, and actively protested against, any attempt to divide the family to implement a treatment policy designed to hospitalise only the affected member of the family. Protest took the form of default from treatment, a protest regarded seriously in the light of the obviously improving situation in the more stable areas of the city. Migrants were further handicapped by the general retreat from the old subsistence economy and the traditional social system of reciprocal giving, which was designed to lighten the burden of caring for the sick in all circumstances, and to ensure the continued inclusion of the sick and their families within the community. The urban body was less willing than formerly to accept the burden, and for valid reasons. Port Moresby epitomised to a high degree the magnitude of the social problems attending the urban drift from rural populations. The urban community was in ferment, and the by-product was a prevalence of tuberculosis some three- to four-times higher than the highest prevalence in the worst affected rural areas. This situation led to the development of innovative treatment programs the essence of which lay in making the treatment itself mobile, for the convenience of the patients and their employers.

The Institutes of Higher Education

The prevalence of tuberculosis in the centres of tertiary education in Port

Moresby in the late 1960s was up to five- to six-times higher than it was in the most severely affected rural areas. In 1968, the prevalence figures from four such institutions were as follows:-

	No. of Students	Prevalence per cent
Papuan Medical College	243	3.2
University of Papua New Guinea	250	2.4
Administration College	95	2.5
Teachers Training College	205	2.4

The difference between the Papuan Medical College and the others represents the increased opportunity for infection in the hospital situation where the students were trained.

More important than the level of prevalence among students in relation to the general prevalence of the disease, was the fact that the patients came from the late adolescent age-groups in which generally speaking outside of the institutions the prevalence of the disease was low. Since the group involved those from whom the future leaders and teachers would emerge, it presented a disturbing problem in the light of the rapid social and economic development of the country. It was particularly disturbing in relation to the school teachers, in view of the epidemiological implications of the lightly tuberculinised under fifteen age-groups in the community.

The New Guinea Highlands

In the epidemiological shape of tuberculosis, the Highlands region of Papua New Guinea is globally unique. Up to the time of World War II, 900,000 Melanesians lived in the interior of New Guinea, in what was virtually complete isolation from the coast. Whether they migrated to the area, or were driven there by more hostile elements is not known. These exuberant people were full of vitality, and protected from epidemic situations by their isolation and lifestyle. They had achieved a measure of social and political stability superior to that of the more fragmented coastal society.

What is known about the Highlands up to the late 1930s indicates that the area was essentially free from tuberculosis. Exploratory penetration of the area, begun in 1922, had been sporadic and minimal up to 1939, which year saw the last of the great New Guinea patrols from Mount Hagen in the Western Highlands to Telefomin in the Sepik District. In the report of the patrol one reads, "There does not appear to be any sign of tuberculosis amongst the natives".

Christian Mission activity had however been more intensive, and despite restrictions which had been placed on their movements in the Highlands, it was said that in the years leading up to the war, at least 1000

Melanesian missionaries were in the Highlands.

The war had little effect on the area. After 1945, modern communications broke down the isolation, the vast populations were recognised as an important source of labour, and as the pace of development quickened in the area population movements into and out of the Highlands increased.

The tuberculin testing programs in 1950 confirmed the freedom of the Highlands from tuberculosis, although there were indications in the Eastern Highlands, in the shape of minor elevations in the rates, of the influence of what little migration into the area had occurred—mainly coastal workers concerned with developmental projects, mission workers, gold miners etc. This finding had importance in the light of the fact that the immense potential labour force of the area was about to be tapped to offset a labour shortage which was threatening the economic future of Papua New Guinea.[12]

The threat to the Highlands was clear, and out of this quandary was born the Native Labour Ordinance Amendment providing for the protection of indentured labourers against tuberculosis, which threw a BCG barrier around the Highlands, through which the labourers had to pass to reach coastal employment in a highly tuberculinised environment. The twin aims of the barrier were to retard the spread of tuberculosis in the Highlands and to prevent the full expression of tuberculosis amongst this vulnerable community.

In the early 1970s the Highland communities were in a unique situation, where the potential for the emergence of epidemic tuberculosis was high. Any degree of infection, no matter how small, was serious, and if discovered the most strenuous efforts had to be made to contain it. All people formerly protected against tuberculosis, were now exposed to the disease. What had been a closed situation was now an open one. Tuberculosis was part of the price which had to be paid for the social, political and economic benefits flowing from the economic expansion of New Guinea and its reciprocal Highlands development.

Special policies were designed for the Highlands to reduce this price to a minimum.[13] It was hoped that by these means the natural evolution of the disease in a hitherto tuberculosis free community would be avoided, the natural order of events primarily being interfered with substantially by great mass-vaccination programs, leading to an expectation that new infection in the community would lead to a sufficiently high degree of anamnestic (revived) immunity response to dampen the whole process down. This would then lead to a less formidable expression of tuberculosis in the community, despite the slowly increasing incidence of the disease. The explicit corollary to these measures was that the best way to protect the Highlands was to achieve firm control of tuberculosis on the coast.

The Overview

The events following the resumption of civil administration in 1945 have been reviewed above. This overview deals with the period 1956 to 1973, with which the author is most familiar.

The seventeen years from 1956 were years of highly concentrated effort on the parts of the many who concerned themselves with the control of tuberculosis in Papua New Guinea. By no means were all graduates. The many included professional workers and lay people ranging from the lowest aid-post orderly to the graduate, expatriate and Melanesian. There was a vast input from the laity, who were encouraged by the tuberculosis control units to participate in the program by providing clerical assistance and supervising treatment programs. Generally speaking, graduates were reserved for supervisory, inspectorial and consultative roles.

Crucial to the success of the treatment programmes was the part played by the Christian mission medical services who staffed the four special hospitals at Gemo Island, at Finschafen in the Morobe District, at Embogo in the Northern District of Papua, and at BitaPaka in New Britain. They provided matchless institutional treatment programs, to which they brought endless compassion and an indispensable loving discipline.

The cardinal measure of the success of the general program, and the Missions' enthusiastic support for it, lies in the fact that all four of the special hospitals had ceased to exist as such by 1973. It was the out-patient service, regarded as an extension of the general hospital services, and enlisting as it did local comunity support, both in its initiation and conduct—without which no service was contemplated—which played the decisive role in the demise of the special hospitals, which handled their peak loads in the years 1965 and 1966.

Over the period of a decade and a half the assiduous application of the principles laid down in 1957 achieved significant reductions in infection rates in the general community and, most impressively, amongst the school children, more and more of whom were reaching adulthood without having been infected naturally. The point-prevalence of tuberculosis showed gratifying falls in those areas where control programs had been operating effectively over the period. For example, in New Ireland, mass surveys had been conducted in 1957, 1968 and 1971. The point-prevalence of the disease in 1957 was 4.1 per cent in a population of 9,300. In 1968 the prevalence was 0.2 per cent in a population sample of 54,000. The prevalence in 1971 was 0.19 per cent.

This is not to say that there were no areas of dissatisfaction in the program. The urban tuberculosis scene was threatening. Cases of tuberculosis were emerging in increasing numbers from behind the BCG barrier which had been set up in the Highlands, imposing heavy burdens on case-finding activities. The traditional beliefs of the patients and their attendants sometimes circumscribed management seriously. The difficulties with the attendants stemmed from the facts that they were in many instances at the lower levels, too close to the old culture, with little understanding of, or little belief in the validity of the aims of the control program. They did not as a rule belong to the command generation of their communities nor could they assume easily the habit of command. They found it difficult to impose unpleasant treatment regimens on the patients, or to discipline them when it became necessary. These understandable shortcomings on the part of the attendants in the early years of the program were, on the whole, a cause of great concern to many of them, but the program unfortunately meant that the attendants were least useful in many cases, where they were needed most, ie. at points of first treatment-contact. This, like most of the human problems, including those of default and absenteeism, could only be overcome, by time, patience and assiduous training.[14]

Prospect

Today's generation of Europeans is the first to be able to live comparatively safely with tuberculosis. It was a disease of European great-grandparents, grandparents and parents. Tuberculosis was not an important disease for Melanesian great-grandparents. It became one in a dramatic fashion to Melanesian grandparents, and it is still one for Melanesian parents and their children. By ensuring that what we know today is applied logically to the problem of the disease in Papua New Guinea, it is possible to ensure that Melanesian grandchildren will escape it.

The peaks of the epidemic have been passed in the coastal areas of the country. In the Highlands a peak has not yet been reached, but it should be possible to prevent a high peak ever being reached. In the coastal regions, the populations were saved from extinction, not by intervention, it must be admitted at once, but by the natural propensity of tuberculosis and communities to come to terms with one another before a situation of total uncontrollability is reached. Today's equilibrium is a precarious one, but on the whole the balance is in favour of man over the mycobacterium. The task is to preserve this balance and to augment it in a community which is moving slowly in a direction which is favourable, in the social sense, to the control of the disease.

Provided the growing points of tuberculosis are recognised, and dealt with firmly, and the pace of development is maintained in an atmosphere of stability, the outlook for the control of disease is good.

CHAPTER 7

Mycobacteriology in Australia

The earliest laboratory diagnostic work in tuberculosis in Australia appears to have been conducted by G.H.S. Blackburne in Western Australia in 1903; tuberculosis laboratories were established in the next few years at the Adelaide Hospital, the University of Melbourne, the Stock Institute in Brisbane and in 1909 in the Bureau of Microbiology in Sydney.

The first mention of atypical mycobacteria appears in papers by Reginald Webster in 1942 "who encountered strains which, on the basis of colonial morphology and animal virulence, could not be typed with confidence".[1]

Mycobacteriology in the Queensland Department of Health

David Dawson

Queensland's First Pathology Laboratory

The first laboratory tests for human diseases in Queensland were conducted around the turn of the century. On 2 December, 1893, the Stock Institute was established in Turbot Street, Brisbane, and was apparently the first facility in Australia to deal with animal diseases. The Stock Institute moved to College Road on 30 June 1899, where it became known as the Bacteriological Institute under the control of the Colonial Secretary's Department. Mr C.J. Pound was appointed the Government Bacteriologist and took charge of the new Institute. The Bacteriological Institute broadened its interests to include tests for human diseases. The plague epidemic of 1901–07 was a major concern, although Annual Reports from that time indicate that around 25 specimens were received each month for testing by microscopy for tubercle bacilli. Such tests were apparently done free-of-charge, although this was not the case for other investigations. The total examination fees paid to the Institute in 1904 was £59.

The early Annual Reports show the concern with which health officials of the day viewed phthisis or consumption. They wrote:

> The spread of consumption can be largely prevented ... The disin-
> fection of the patient's room will be undertaken by officers of the
> department within the metropolitan area.

In 1904 tuberculosis was made a notifiable disease under the Health Act. In 1908, 308 persons died from phthisis, and that year's Report drew attention to the great monetary loss being suffered as a result of the disease. It was estimated that in the period 1880-1907 the loss to the state was £5,248,760 in deaths and invalidity.

The Birth of the Laboratory of Microbiology and Pathology

In 1910 a deputation from the Queensland Branch of the British Medical Association sought the establishment of a laboratory dedicated to human diseases. The Commissioner for Public Health endorsed the proposal, and control of the Bacteriological Institute was transferred to the Department of Public Health on 16 December 1910. The Laboratory of Microbiology and Pathology (Lab M&P) was thus set up to investigate human diseases, whereas diseases in animals were to be studied at Yeerongpilly under the supervision of the Department of Agriculture and Stock. The Annual Report of 1910 reflected confidence in the success of the new arrangements.

> The scope of the laboratory has been increased very considerably, and it is anticipated that, when its re-equipment is completed, it will compare favourably with any similar institution of its size in Australia.

Dr. John Harris was appointed Director, commencing duty on 27 March, 1911, with a staff of two bacteriological assistants, a messenger and a typist. New equipment for the laboratory cost £500. The new Lab M&P apparently devoted most of its efforts to checking rats for plague (25,309 of a total of 30,514 tests carried out in 1912).

The Cilento-Derrick Era

In 1934 Dr Raphael Cilento became Director-General of Health and Medical Services. He saw the need for a medically-qualified director and Dr E.H. (Ted) Derrick was appointed in June 1935. Tests for tuberculosis continued to be carried out within the bacteriology section of Lab M&P, with an annual workload of 300–500 tests. In 1934–35, 378 specimens were tested, of which 24.6 per cent were positive. Guinea-pig inoculation was apparently introduced as a primary diagnostic test in the late 1930s. In 1941, 550 specimens were tested for tuberculosis of which 91 (16.5 per cent) were positive.

Dr. Tonge's Directorship

Dr John Tonge was appointed to the staff of Lab M&P in 1946, and was made Acting Director in August 1947 when Dr Derrick resigned to move to the newly established Queensland Institute of Medical Research (QIMR). Dr Tonge became Director in May 1948, and his appointment ushered in a new era of expanded services, and increased staff and workload. In 1949 he was granted a Rockefeller Fellowship and on 8 September left for a post-graduate study tour of the United States and the United Kingdom. It was on Dr Tonge's return in early 1951 that moves were made to begin culturing specimens for tubercle bacilli.

The Specialised Tuberculosis Laboratory

The Department's Annual Report of 1950–51 mentioned plans for a new tuberculosis laboratory to be established in the William Street building. The provision of a "walk-in" incubator, a special inoculation room, ultra-violet lights, and draught-exhaust ventilation was highlighted. Dr Tonge's report expressed concern for the safety of workers exposed to tubercle bacilli.

The new tuberculosis laboratory began functioning in September 1952 with a staff of three. With the new laboratory offering culture examinations, the workload increased: in the year 1952–53, 3,731 specimens were examined. Specimens came mainly from patients of the Brisbane Chest Clinic, with smaller numbers from country hospitals and private practitioners. All non-sputum specimens were inoculated into guinea-pigs which were examined for tuberculous disease at eight weeks. Dr Tonge wrote, "it has been found that there is little to choose between culture and guinea-pig inoculation as a means of diagnosing tuberculosis, and it is felt that as long as facilities permit, both should be used." The 1952–53 Report also made mention of the fact that sensitivity tests to streptomycin, which had previously been done only when requested, would subsequently be performed as a routine.

The Laboratory as a Reference Facility

In addition to the diagnostic services performed at Lab M&P, culture for tuberculosis was undertaken at various other institutions throughout Queensland, in particular the large Brisbane hospitals and the Commonwealth Health Laboratories in Rockhampton, Townsville and Cairns. At the instigation of Dr Tonge and Dr Ellis Abrahams (Director of Tuberculosis), isolates of *Mycobacterium tuberculosis* made in these peripheral laboratories were forwarded to the Brisbane laboratory as a reference centre. In the late 1960s the National Tuberculosis Advisory Council recommended that centralised referral systems be set up in all states.

Centralisation was completed in November 1979, and in the following year a total of 26,516 specimens were received, including diagnostic specimens from the Northern Territory and Honiara as well as cultures from Papua New Guinea.

The "Arrival" of the Atypical Mycobacteria

In the late 1950s, laboratory workers and clinicians started to take notice of the "anonymous", "unclassified" or "atypical" strains of mycobacteria. Queensland, more so than other Australian states, seemed to be encountering these strains with significant frequency.[2] Evidence accumulated that some were involved in tuberculosis-like disease, and sub-cultures were sent to Dr Ernest Runyon in the United States, to be included in his landmark studies of these "new" pathogens. It soon became apparent that the guinea-pig pathogenicity test—based on the belief that all human pathogens were also guinea-pig pathogens—was no longer valid. The realisation that certain atypical mycobacteria were the agents of serious tuberculosis-like disease in man was to have a marked influence on the functioning of the laboratory. It caused an increased interest in the taxonomy and classification of the genus Mycobacterium, and a commitment to epidemiological studies based on the serotyping of *M. avium* and related organisms.

Mycobacterial Research Unit

Towards the end of 1968 the Mycobacterial Research Unit (MRU) was set up, administered by the Division of Tuberculosis with funding from the Commonwealth Department of Health. It was established to carry out epidemiological and ecological studies related to atypical mycobacteria in Queensland. Dr Ellis Abrahams and others had already demonstrated the high prevalence of non-specific tuberculin reactivity among Queensland adolescents. Furthermore, Queensland, along with Western Australia appeared to have a comparatively high incidence of disease due to atypical mycobacteria. Mr Michael Reznikov transferred from Lab M&P to take up the position of Bacteriologist with the MRU, and Dr Robin Tuffley was appointed as Senior Research Fellow. The MRU remained functional for nine years, being concerned mostly with the serotyping of atypical mycobacteria from environmental sources. Several papers resulted, some in collaboration with workers from Lab M&P, but unfortunately the MRU did not live up to the expectations of those who had worked to have it established. However, the inspiration of Michael Reznikov was to have a lasting influence in the Lab M&P.

Serotyping

Serotyping of disease-associated isolates belonging to the *M. avium–M. intracellulare–M. scrofulaceum* (MAIS) complex was commenced in 1970, using methods introduced by Michael Reznikov following a study tour of the National Jewish Hospital, Denver, where he worked with Dr Werner Schaefer. Serotyping remains one of the specialised techniques available at Lab M&P. All antisera in use have been prepared in the laboratory, and the panel of serovars has been expanded from 31 to 45 due to the recognition of new serovars among Queensland isolates. The laboratory is one of two world reference centres for serotyping of *M. avium* and related organisms.

In collaboration with the MRU, the laboratory showed that the common serovars causing disease in humans in south-eastern Queensland were also prevalent in the environment. This was the first report of such a link between environmental and clinical isolates.

Serotyping was able to prove that isolates from consecutive patients undergoing bronchoscopy at a large Brisbane hospital were due to faulty sterilisation procedures. The technique also showed that isolates from bone marrows collected during a survey conducted at the Queensland Institute of Medical Research many years earlier, were probably contaminants and of no diagnostic significance.

All *M. avium* complex isolates from patients in Australia with acquired immune deficiency syndrome (AIDS) have been serotyped. The laboratory now has a collection of several hundred AIDS-related strains. With the co-operation of other State Tuberculosis Reference Laboratories, it is intended to serotype all disease-associated *M. avium* complexes isolated in Australia during 1988.

Sensitivity Testing

Sensitivity testing, i.e. the testing of isolates for their susceptibility to anti-microbial compounds has been an important component of the workload of the tuberculosis laboratory.

Tests were done against streptomycin in the early 1950s and over the next decade procedures were expanded to include the other so-called "first-line drugs" —PAS (p-amino salicylic acid) and INAH (iso-nicotinic acid hydrazide). Tests against other compounds, such as viomycin, cycloserine, ethionamide, ethambutol, capreomycin, and thiacetazone were carried out with resistant strains of *M. tuberculosis* and atypical mycobacteria. In 1970, rifampicin was added to the list. The Resistance Ratio Method is used, in which drugs are incorporated in Lowenstein-Jensen (LJ) medium, and the minimal inhibitory concentration for the test organism is compared with that for a known sensitive ("wild") strain.

In addition to *M. tuberculosis*, sensitivity tests have been applied routinely to pathogenic strains of atypical mycobacteria. Their value depends on the mycobacterial species involved. The conventional Resistance Ratio method has limited application. In the early 1980s, recognition of the use of drugs such as tetracyclines in treating infection with some rapidly-growing mycobacteria brought about the introduction of disc diffusion tests in Mueller-Hinton agar. Such tests, against aminoglycosides, tetracyclines, sulphonamides, cephalosporins, quinalones and beta-lactum inhibitors, are now routine for isolates of *M. marinum, M. fortuitum, M. chelonae,* etc.

The Demise of the Guinea-Pig

For around forty years the guinea-pig was used for the primary isolation of *M. tuberculosis* from specimens such as urine, gastric aspirates, tissues, etc. In its hey-day it also provided an index of pathogenicity, based on the belief that if a mycobacterium was pathogenic to the guinea-pig, it was *ipso facto* pathogenic to man. It also found use as a means of sieving *M. tuberculosis* from contaminated cultures or mixtures of atypical mycobacteria and *M. tuberculosis*. Every Monday morning, one or two people from the laboratory would venture to the animal house to carry out autopsies on the batch of animals which had been inoculated seven weeks earlier. The guinea-pigs were killed by intra-thoracic injection of a phenobarbitone compound. Towards the end of the 1970s, around 1,000 guinea-pigs were being inoculated each year. But with the low frequency of positives, questions were raised as to the cost-effectiveness of the procedure. It was decided to discontinue routine guinea-pig inoculations at the end of 1978.

Mycobacterium haemophilum

In 1978, the Kanematsu Institute, Sydney Hospital, sought assistance in identifying two unusual strains of mycobacteria which had been isolated from skin and joint lesions of immunosuppressed patients in the Sydney area. It was believed that a total of five patients had been affected. Four had received kidney transplants. The mycobacteria were fastidious and grew only on LJ medium supplemented with ferric ammonium citrate. The Brisbane laboratory had not encountered any similar organisms—they would not have been isolated on the media in routine use—but staff recalled a paper from Israel dealing with *Mycobacterium haemophilum*, a new species which required media containing blood products for growth. The organism had been isolated from superficial abscesses in a patient with Hodgkin's Disease. A culture of the new species was obtained from Israel, and comparative studies proved the Sydney isolates to be identical with *M. haemophilum*. Further isolates were received from Sydney and elsewhere in Australia, and five isolates have been made from Queensland patients. There have been very few reports of *M. haemophilum* infection from elsewhere in the world, and the collection of isolates held in the Brisbane laboratory has been distributed to workers in various countries.

Mycobacterium asiaticum

The laboratory was responsible for the initial recognition of *M. asiaticum* as a potential human pathogen.[3] This species was first isolated from the viscera of monkeys kept in a zoo in Hungary, but in 1979, isolates from a north Queensland resident were believed to be identical with *M. asiaticum*. This belief was confirmed in an international co-operative study, and by 1982, several more isolates had been encountered.

Mycobacterium neoaurum

The laboratory was associated with the first recognition of *M. neoaurum* as a potential human pathogen. The organism is a pigmented, rapidly-growing mycobacterium from soil which was first described by Dr Michio Tsukamura in Japan. The Brisbane Mater Hospital isolated a mycobacterium from blood cultures of an immunosuppressed patient with unexplained fever. The isolate was forwarded to Lab M&P, where it was tentatively identified as *M. neoaurum*, a result which was subsequently confirmed by Dr Tsukamura.

Mycobacterium ulcerans

Mycobacterium ulcerans is one of the few pathogens of man to have been first isolated by Australian workers. In the late 1940s MacCallum, Tolhurst and

Buckle from the Alfred Hospital in Melbourne were successful in isolating the causative organism from cases of severe skin ulcers on the limbs of patients from around Bairnsdale, Victoria.[4] It was later named *M.ulcerans* in a publication by Fenner, and was to be recognised as one of the more important mycobacterial pathogens in man. In parts of Africa and Papua New Guinea it constitutes a major public health problem. In the period 1957–88, the Brisbane laboratory made 30 isolates. About half have come from patients living around Cairns, North Queensland. Interesting cases include two which arose after a prick from a pineapple leaf, and another which developed following a bite from a spider. The laboratory has served as a source of cultures and clinical summaries for researchers in various countries.

Mycobacterium bovis

The Department's Annual Reports show that *M. bovis* was encountered as a human pathogen in Queensland in the 1930s. Identification would have been based on animal pathogenicity tests. In the post-1950 era, occasional strains were grown on culture, but it must be realised that the LJ formulation used in those early days was not optimal for *M. bovis* because it was not supplemented with sodium pyruvate and contained glycerol. In 1977 pyruvate-containing medium was introduced as a routine, and this brought about an increase in the frequency with which *M. bovis* was isolated. Eight cases were identified in 1979-1980. At the time of writing, only one or two cases are being seen each year.

The laboratory participated in the *M. bovis* isolation trials conducted by the Australian Society of Microbiologist's Special Interest Group in Mycobacteria in 1986–87. The studies were designed to identify the most sensitive culture methods for *M. bovis* from animal tissues. The laboratory performed poorly in the first trial, due to the fact that the culture media employed contained glycerol, to which most *M. bovis* strains from animals are sensitive, even in the presence of sodium pyruvate.When glycerol was removed from the medium for the second trial, the Brisbane laboratory returned optimal results.

In December 1993 the laboratory will celebrate its centenary marking its evolution from the Stock Institute to a WHO Reference Laboratory in Mycobacteriology.

Tuberculin as a Diagnostic, Epidemiological and Case–Finding Agent

K.J.M. Carruthers

In 1890 Koch announced his discovery of tuberculin and at the same time made a preliminary statement about the therapeutic effect of tuberculin in infected and diseased guinea-pigs. In his own account of his incomplete work on tuberculin, he observed that the healthy (ie. uninfected or infected but not diseased) individual reacts either:

> not at all or scarcely at all... but the case is very different when the disease is tuberculosis; the same dose of 0.01 cc injected subcutaneously into the tuberculous patient caused a general reaction as well as a local one.[5]

The local reaction was an area of induration and erythema of the skin at the site of injection, the general reaction being characterised by fever, arthralgia, nausea, vomiting and weakness. Koch immediately recognised the value of this reaction to tuberculin and said "I think I am justified in saying that the remedy will therefore form an indispensible aid to diagnosis". However he considered that the potential curative properties of tuberculin far outweighed its promise as a diagnostic agent. In the event, tuberculin gained more lasting recognition as a diagnostic and epidemiological tool. In 1965 Myers went so far as to claim that the tuberculin test was "man's greatest victory over tuberculosis", a claim which few would now support. In practice the test has proved to be of more limited value, and the interpretation of results not always as straight-forward as had been anticipated.

The greatest value of the tuberculin test is as an epidemiological measure of infection within a community. In 1920 Robertson[6] conducted a survey of the prevalence of tuberculosis among miners and ex-miners and their families in Bendigo. In all, 451 adults and children were examined using the Mantoux test. Positive reactors were given sputum tests for tubercle bacilli. The result was that proven tuberculosis was found in 55 (12 per cent), 36 being sputum smear positive, and 5 positive on guinea-pig innoculation. The remaining 14 had extrapulmonary disease. There were also 31 (7 per cent) with suspected tuberculosis. This survey clearly demonstrated the value of the tuberculin test as a screening procedure leading to subsequent diagnosis by clinical, radiological and bacteriological means.

In 1949 another tuberculin survey in Bendigo was reported by Kerr. At that time the mortality rate from tuberculosis was 59 per 100,000 compared with 41 in Melbourne and 35 in Geelong. Positive reactor rates (per cent of those tested) were as follows:

	Male	Female
Primary school children	3.5	3
High School children	5.5	5.5
Workers aged 15-35 years	33	18
Workers aged 36-60 years	65	55

In 1950, Pinner reported a voluntary survey in Canberra (population 15,100) and Queanbeyan (6000).[7] Over 80 per cent of the population responded. The results (again expressed as a percentage of tuberculin positive of those tested) were:

Age (years)	Male	Female
0-14	4	2.7
15-19	11	10
20-34	45	46
35-59	71	47

These surveys, in two quite different communities, showed that positive tuberculin reactor-rates increased dramatically with age, probably due partly to the presence of infection in the workplace and partly to higher rates among children in earlier years, those children having reached adult age by the time of the survey.

During the period 1951–1953 R.M. Mills of the Institute of Child Health, University of Sydney, carried out three studies on the source and rate of tuberculous infection in infants and children in Sydney and demonstrated the value of tuberculin testing as an adjunct to case finding.[8] In a study of children admitted to the Royal Alexandra Hospital for Children, 246 children who were Mantoux-positive and who had not been vaccinated with BCG, were followed up. A probable source of infection was established for 109 of the 123 children born in Australia, and for two of 33 migrant children. Among the Australian-born, a probable source of infection was established for two-thirds of those who were Mantoux-positive but who had no clinical manifestations of tuberculosis, and also for two-thirds of those with clinical disease other than tuberculous cervical adenitis. A probable source of infection was established for only one of these. Thirteen adults associated with the children studied were found to be suffering from previously unsuspected active pulmonary tuberculosis.

The second survey reported was made possible by the courtesy and co-operation of A.E. Machin, former Director of the School Medical Service.[9] In this survey, Mills studied the presence of tuberculous infection and its source in primary schoolchildren. Mantoux tests were carried out on some 6,000 primary school children and those who reacted to the test, together with the members of their families, were invited to undergo examination for evidence of tuberculous infection. In an inner industrial

area, 7 per cent of the children reacted and a probable source of infection
was established for just over one-third. Nine adults with radiographic
abnormalities suggestive of tuberculosis were referred for further investigation. In an outer suburban residential area only 4 per cent reacted and
again a probable source of infection was found in just over one-third, five
adults being referred for further investigation. It was also noted that
tubercle bacilli had been recovered from milk from dairies in the area in
1952.

In the third survey[10] Mills studied a group of 141 infants and young
children who reacted to a Mantoux test before reaching the age of two
years with particular reference to prognosis. Seventy-four of the 141 were
patients in the Royal Alexandra Hospital for Children at the time of the
Mantoux testing, and 67 were examined at an anti-tuberculosis clinic
following contact with an adult suffering from tuberculosis ("clinical contacts"). The outstanding factor affecting prognosis was the presence of
miliary tuberculosis or of tuberculous meningitis. Of 48 "hospital patients" not suffering from miliary or meningeal tuberculosis at the time of
the survey four either died or developed tuberculous meningitis subsequently. Of 67 "clinical contacts" not suffering either of these conditions
one subsequently died of tuberculous meningitis. A human source of
infection was recorded for 49 of the 74 patients.

Epidemiological tuberculin surveys are still carried out in all Australian States, although with the cessation of BCG vaccination in school
children in the mid 1980s these surveys may well cease. In Western Australia a series of epidemiological tuberculin surveys was carried out on
schoolchildren (10–19 years old) between 1960 and 1983 (*Reports of the
Commissioner of Public Health*). The percentage of positive reactors for these
two age groups fell from 10.8 and 24.8 to 1.9 and 1.6 respectively during
the 24-year period, this reduction being achieved despite the migrant and
refugee children who comprised a significant proportion of the population. In 1978 the reactor rates for the same two age-groups were 1.9 per
cent and 2.6 per cent respectively for all schoolchildren tested, but 25.2 per
cent and 42.0 per cent respectively for Vietnamese refugees. These figures
show that, apart from refugees from south-east Asia, tuberculous infection
in Western Australian children and youth is now very low indeed,and in
fact in 1985 only 0.3% of 5,366 school children tested in Perth were found
to be tuberculin positive. A similar situation can be expected throughout
Australia.

An increasing awareness of the complexities of tuberculin testing, and
the desirability of standardisation of technique and interpretation
throughout Australia led the National Tuberculosis Advisory Council to
establish a sub-committee on tuberculin testing. The sub-committee was
charged with the task of producing a booklet on tuberculin testing. In 1970

the Commonwealth Department of Health published *The Tuberculin Test,* an illustrated booklet described as a "review and recommendations by the National Tuberculosis Advisory Council". The sub-committee favoured a 10 I.U Mantoux test. Suggested degrees of reaction were negative, less than 5 mms; weak positive, 5 to 9 mms; intermediate positive, 10 to 14 mms; and strongly positive, 15 mms or more. Although the latter two suggest infection with tubercle bacilli this possibility is not excluded by finding only a weak positive reaction and comparative Mantoux tests may be indicated. As Sir William Refshauge said in his foreward "not the least advantage of this publication is its recommendation of a standard Australian epidemiological tuberculin test".

Original Mycobacterial Sin

*E.W. Abrahams**

Fazekas de St Groth and R.G. Webster used the startling phrase "original antigenic sin" to describe an immunological phenomenon which they had discovered while investigating the antigenic effect of influenza vaccines. When immunity due to a specific vaccine is boosted, not by the homologous but by a cross-reacting vaccine, the newly formed antibodies react better with the primary antigen than with the antigen actually eliciting the response. It would seem, in fact, that in considering immune responses to closely related infections in the viral field, due consideration must be given to the order in which infections occur as well as to their nature; it follows therefore that the interpretation of tests which depend upon such immune responses may be less simple than has been thought. It is suggested that a similar state of affairs may exist in the mycobacterial field.

It is now accepted that in warm and tropical areas many persons who react to tuberculin tests do so not because of infection by tubercle bacilli but by allied organisms, most probably other mycobacteria. Schoolchildren in Queensland have, in general, greater reactions to avian than to human tuberculin. After vaccination with BCG they still show a predominance of avian reactions. A group of children who had been vaccinated (with BCG) shortly after birth were tested with avian and human tuberculin up to 16 years after vaccination. There was a significant excess of children with greater human reactions. It is suggested that the first mycobacterial infection may set the antigenic pattern. Secondary infection by an antigenically similar mycobacterium would then not alter the pattern of response.

---

* *Tubercle* 1970. 51, 316. (Abridged version edited by A.J. Proust)

The Diagnostic Use of Tuberculin: a 1931 Perspective

In the *Medical Journal of Australia* (17 October, 14 November 1931) F. Guy Griffiths, senior physician at Royal North Shore Hospital and W. Cotter Harvey, junior physician at Royal Prince Alfred Hospital, Sydney, published their views on the then controversial use of tuberculin as a diagnostic agent in tuberculosis.*

Griffiths recommended its use in cases of suspected chronic pulmonary tuberculosis in which tubercle bacilli could not be found in the sputum. He advised against its use in febrile and toxic patients or in suspected cases of tuberculous meningitis. Griffiths used 0.01 cc of old tuberculin, the dilution varied from one in ten to one in a hundred. In all cases the patient's temperature must be recorded for 24 hours before and subsequently for 48 hours. If the reaction was severe the patient should rest in bed.

Griffiths described two types of reaction; a local erythema measuring 2 to 6 cm was positive ("local reaction"). A more severe local reaction (induration and blistering) together with a brief fever was strongly positive ("general reaction"). In some cases there may be a local reaction at the site of the disease, for example pleural pain and cough in cases of pulmonary tuberculosis or pain and swelling at the site of non-pulmonary disease. Griffiths summarised his views on the value of the test:

> A local reaction shows that infection has occurred, a general reaction shows the infection is still active and may show its location.

Cotter Harvey in a typically forceful article set out his views in the 14 November 1931 issue. He described his method of doing the Mantoux test using 0.1 cc of diluted old tuberculin, and he was more specific about what constituted a positive reaction, he was more dogmatic about the significance of the tuberculin test.

> A positive reaction would have a wheal 0.25 cm in diameter and a strongly positive reaction would have a wheal 1 cm in diameter surrounded by erythema... The cutaneous tuberculin tests tell us whether infection with the tubercle bacillus has occurred and not whether the patient is suffering from tuberculosis... it indicates a focus of infection somewhere in the body but this focus may be active, latent or healed.

Bovine Tuberculosis in Relation to Public Health in Australia

A.J. Proust

Bovine tuberculosis was doubtless introduced in the early years of the settlement at Sydney Cove. Due largely to year-round grazing in the open air and a much lower density of cattle per acre than in Europe, bovine tuberculosis was probably uncommon in the first hundred years of European settlement in Australia. The discovery of the tubercle bacillus and the public disputation about the pathogenicity of the bovine tubercle, stimulated, particularly in Victoria, sporadic surveys of dairy cattle, using the tuberculin test, and of beef cattle, based on carcase inspection at public abattoirs. The reported prevalence of bovine tuberculosis varied widely as between districts and states. Measures to control bovine tuberculosis were aimed principally at preventing human infection. Carcases were inspected at public abattoirs and the diseased were condemned or if feasible, the diseased lymph nodes were excised and the carcase passed for human consumption. Dairy farms and holding paddocks for beef cattle were inspected at intervals and beasts with clinical evidence of tuberculosis were either destroyed or witheld from sale. Even these simple measures were not uniformly enforced and pasteurisation of milk was done only on a limited scale. Trivett in his study of tuberculosis mortality in New South Wales 1876–1903 maintained that when these measures were strictly enforced there was a dramatic decline in tuberculosis mortality in the age-group 0–4 years between 1886 (when the Dairies Supervision Act was proclaimed) and 1895.[11]

> All dairymen and milk vendors must be registered under the Act and the sale of milk by unregistered persons is strictly forbidden. Their premises must be kept in a sanitary state and cases of infectious disease must be notified immediately. Naturally the sale or supply of unwholesome milk is not allowed... to this Act may be attributed the wholesome reduction in infantile (tubercular) mortality which has been so noticeable in the present discussion. The infantile tuberculosis mortality was lowered by 51 per cent in Sydney during the decade 1886–95 and by 35 per cent in rural areas where the Act was less enforceable.

In the *Australian Medical Gazette* of 20 January 1911, J.B. Cleland reported that 1,219 of a total of 17,171 cattle (7.1 per cent) slaughtered in Perth and Kalgoorlie abattoirs in 1906–07 showed evidence of tuberculosis. In the following year only 1,085 of 25,563 (4 per cent) slaughtered at the same abattoirs were diseased. While these figures were much lower than in European reports, Cleland expressed concern that even 4 to 7 per cent of free-ranging cattle in Western Australia were tuberculous. Cleland tabulated the sites and extent of tuberculosis in 43,734 cattle slaughtered for meat for human consumption in Western Australia 1906–08:

Total with tubercular lesions	2,302	(5.2%)
The sites of tuberculosis		
Lungs	1,790	
Head glands	1,206	
Abdominal organs	139	
Generalised	53	
Udders	2	

Cleland's presentation provoked an interesting response from Dr Guy Griffiths of Sydney. He was interested in:

> Dr Cleland's remarks on the prevalence of tuberculosis among cattle that had enjoyed all their lives such an abundance of fresh air and sunlight. This seemed of immense importance in relation to the treatment of tuberculosis in human beings. Again Dr Cleland's ideas of the way in which milk may be infected with tubercle bacilli by the dung of tuberculous cows had only to be heard to be accepted as probably correct although it has usually been considered that tubercle bacilli were absent from the milk of tuberculous cows except in the small number of cases where the udder was affected.

(This was soon shown to be false; tubercle bacilli were found in the milk of up to 40 per cent of tuberculous cows with apparently healthy udders). Dr Griffiths continued:

> However on the absence of spume in cattle with pulmonary tuberculosis I must altogether disagree. In my experience a cow coughed out far more spray than did the most careless human being.

Dr Griffiths heartily agreed with the suggestion that all tuberculous cattle should be destroyed. While he regarded them as a comparatively minor source of danger to human beings, they were very dangerous to other cattle and constituted an enormous loss to the grazier and dairy farmer. These comments by Dr Griffiths, who was a leading tuberculosis physician, illustrated the developing interest in the public health and veterinary problems posed by bovine tuberculosis in Australia.

In 1930 the Commonwealth Department of Health issued a comprehensive report on *Bovine Tuberculosis in Man and Animals in Australia*. The Report concluded that the bovine strain was rarely if ever found in adult human pulmonary tuberculosis. It estimated that 25,000 children would develop infections of the bovine strain; the mortality from bovine tuberculosis in humans was relatively low but it could cause prolonged disability especially if the skeletal system was involved. Most cases however did not proceed beyond a localised lymphadenitis. The prevalence of bovine tuberculosis was highest in Victoria and lowest in Queensland. The prevalence of the disease in Australia was significantly lower than in most comparable developed countries. The mortality from bovine tuberculosis in infants had fallen in New South Wales since Public Health Acts had been passed, improving the hygiene of dairies and the health of dairy herds. The Report considered evidence based on tuberculin testing of dairy herds, carcase inspection at abattoirs, bacteriological examination of milk and physical examination of cattle; the final estimate was that 5 per cent of beef cattle and 8 per cent of dairy cattle in Australia were tuberculous. The annual economic cost to the farmers of Queensland, New South Wales and Victoria was an estimated £750,000.

The consensus was that bovine tuberculosis should be controlled but not necessarily eradicated; contamination of milk with tubercle bacilli could be reduced to "a safe level" because children could resist small doses of bovine tubercle bacilli, even if repeated. The Report recommended tuberculin testing especially of stud herds, compensation for animals destroyed because of tuberculosis, pasteurisation of milk sold by commercial dairies and the establishment of laboratories to monitor the quality of milk and especially the presence of tubercle bacilli.

Progress was slow and it was not until 1948 that compulsory tuberculin testing of commercial dairy herds became universal in Australia. During the 1950s, compensation for animals slaughtered because of tuberculosis also became accepted and these measures, together with pasteurisation, virtually eliminated bovine tuberculosis from dairy herds. Bovine tuberculosis in humans by the 1960s was a negligible public health problem.

National Bovine Tuberculosis Eradication Program

*R. Layland ***

In 1968 the Commonwealth and States Veterinary Committee was established and a subcommittee was appointed to plan and supervise the eradication of tuberculosis and brucellosis in the national herd. The principle motivation was concern that Australian beef might be refused access to overseas markets. Beef exports were then valued at about $1000 million annually. Public health authorities within Australia were also concerned about the incidence of brucellosis in abattoir workers.

By July 1970 a co-ordinated Australia-wide campaign was launched, involving tuberculin tests and blood samples for brucella agglutinins. The campaign was a joint venture between the cattle industry and State and Commonwealth governments.

Each State was subdivided into well-defined areas which were classified into one of five categories according to the prevalence of bovine tuberculosis; as the herds in an area were tested and retested, then that area might be reclassified according to the test results.

* edited by I.S. Cameron Stephen

The basic approach was to test every beast and slaughter the positive reactors with generous compensation to the owners. Herds which were negative were declared provisionally free and confirmatory testing carried out at a later date. Herds with reactors were retested after positive reactor cattle had been slaughtered. Movement and sale of cattle from infected or potentially infected herds were strictly controlled.

By mid-1986, only 290 of Australia's 177,000 cattle properties were classified as infected; free or provisionally free (less than 1 reactor per 1000 head) areas contained 22.7 million cattle or 93 per cent of the national herd. Tasmania was "tuberculosis and brucellosis free" while New South Wales, Victoria, South Australia and large portions of Queensland and Western Australia were "provisionally free". The aim is to achieve provisional freedom from bovine tuberculosis by 1992; this goal, short of complete eradication, means that there would be no infected herds nor restrictions placed on cattle movements. A major problem in the larger states is the presence of feral animals which are often extensively infected with tuberculosis. Control measures continue to safeguard a tuberculosis-free milk supply.

Dr Reginald Webster

A.J. Proust

Reginald Webster was born in Melbourne in 1889 and educated at Wesley College, a contemporary of Harry Wunderly and Robert Menzies. He graduated from Melbourne University second only to Charles Kellaway who became an internationally recognised immunologist and first Director of the Walter and Eliza Hall Institute. Webster gravitated to pathology at the Royal Melbourne Hospital and was appointed clinical pathologist at the Children's Hospital in 1914 and served that hospital for 57 years.

During the Great War tuberculin was in short supply so Webster supplied it until production at the Commonwealth Serum Laboratories was established. One of his major interests was tuberculosis. His techniques for isolating the tubercle bacillus from sputum, gastric washings, biopsy material, cerebrospinal fluid, urine, pleural fluid and pus were painstakingly thorough and highly successful.[13] He isolated the tubercle bacillus from the cerebrospinal fluid of all 65 children who died from tuberculous meningitis at the Children's Hospital during the period 1938–41. He isolated the tubercle bacillus from the urine of 116 patients with various forms of tuberculosis other than clinically recognisable renal tuberculosis; he taught that tuberculosis was a multi-system disease, not just pulmonary or skeletal or meningitic. His skill at isolating the tubercle bacillus was such that physicians were reluctant to pronounce a case "inactive" until Webster had failed to obtain a positive culture. Among his many achievements was his bacteriological examination of Australian service personnel during World War II who were shown to have a pulmonary lesion, possibly tuberculous, on mass miniature radiography (MMR). [14]

In 1932, Webster published a study of the relative incidence of human and bovine tuberculosis based on patients seen at the Children's Hospital, Melbourne[15]. He had earlier furnished Dr W.J. Penfold with 60 cultures recovered from tuberculous children at the same Hospital and classified by Penfold with respect to human or bovine type.[40.] Webster's paper added a further 86 cultures obtained from 81 children (5 cultures were of cervical glands and tonsils in the same child; he added five cultures from bone and joint tuberculosis in adults which were excluded from the survey).

Webster's technique was initially in the majority of cases to inoculate a guinea-pig with the material from the tuberculous lesion and recover material from a lesion in the guinea-pig for culture on Dorset egg media.[16] In this way he avoided contaminants proliferating on the culture media. Only when he thought the patient's lesion was likely to produce uncontaminated material did he inoculate the media directly from the patient. "The striking contrast between the profuse verricose pigmented growth of the 'eugonic' human strain, its characteristics developed to a maximum on the glycerine medium, and the flat pigmented 'dygonic' bovine strain, its growth retarded and perhaps inhibited by the presence of glycerine, enabled a provisional identification with respect to type to be made without difficulty in the vast majority of cases. In the few in which cultured characteristics appeard to be equivocal, the virulence test in the rabbit determined the issue". However, all cultures were subjected to the virulence test; an emulsion was made from the culture and injected by intracardiac injection in the anaesthetised rabbit. Bovine strains induced fatal disseminated tuberculosis in 11 to 14 days. The rabbit was autopsied to confirm that death was due to bovine tuberculosis. Rabbits inoculated with strains identified as human by its cultural characteristics lived for an indefinite number of weeks but were usually sacrificed at six weeks and autopsied. A localised lesion in the pericardium was present and as a rule there was limited dissemination in the lungs and kidneys, much less marked than in the bovine rabbits.

Bone and Joint

In Webster's series, all 22 children with bone and joint tuberculosis (and the five adults with similar disease) were shown to be suffering from the human strain of tuberculosis. Similarly all 4 cases in Penfold's series were caused by the human strain.

Webster concluded that bovine tuberculosis played at most only a minor role in bone and joint tuberculosis in children in Australia. This was in contrast to the report submitted to the Royal Commission on Bovine

Tuberculosis (1911) in the United Kingdom when 20.5 per cent of 598 cultures recovered from bone and joint tuberculosis were identified as bovine.

Cervical Glands and Tonsils

Of 24 cultures recovered from cervical glands, 17 were bovine and seven human strains. Of seven cultures from tonsils, four were bovine and three human.

Bronchial Glands and Lungs

Of Webster's 27 cultures, all were of the human strain. Penfold on the other hand identified 25 cultures, four as bovine and 21 as human.

Webster commented that:

it was anticipated that human strains would predominate in this group, respiratory tuberculosis of bovine origin being very uncommon.

He quoted W.T. Munro in Scotland who remarked that:

recovery of the bovine tubercle bacillus from the sputum was sufficiently rare to command attention.

The numbers of specimens from mesenteric glands (four bovine, nil human) and from cerebrospinal fluid (nil bovine, two human) were too small for analysis. However coupled with Penfold's similarly small numbers, 71 per cent of mesenteric gland cultures were of the bovine strain and 86 per cent of the cerebrospinal cultures were of the human strain.

The only significant divergence between Webster's series and that of Penfold was in respiratory tuberculosis. Webster's 27 cultures were all of the human strain as were all 71 sputum cultures from adults from Health Laboratories of the Department of Health in several states (*Report on Bovine Tuberculosis in Man and Animals in Australia*, 1930, Commonwealth Department of Health). Of Penfold's cultures from bronchial glands, lung tissue and sputum, four were of bovine origin.

Radiography and Pulmonary Tuberculosis

A.J. Proust

X-rays were probably produced without being recognised as such, by a small group of scientists who transmitted electrical charges through rarified gases in glass tubes in the 1870s. William Crookes "damaged" photographic plates doing such experiments in 1879.

In 1895 Wilhelm Roentgen was investigating the luminescence that cathode rays produced in certain substances and on blocking the cathode rays with cardboard, he was surprised that the luminescence persisted. He assumed that another more penetrating ray was being emitted by the cathode tube; he named this the X-ray and after further experiments announced his discovery before a meeting of the Physical Medical Society of

Wurzburg in Germany of 23 January 1896. The new X-rays easily pene-
trated the soft tissues of the body and their medical application was
quickly recognized.

Roentgen's experiments were repeated within months in Australia and
New Zealand. On 4 March 1896, T.R. Lyle, Professor of Physics at the
University of Melbourne produced X-ray photos of a human hand. These
early X-rays were produced by a generator, an induction coil and a
Crookes' tube. The induction coil converted low voltage direct diffuse
current into high voltage alternating unidirectional current which was
then passed through the Crookes' tube (a glass bulb from which virtually
all air had been evacuated).

Less than a year after Roentgen's original paper Oudin and Barthelemy
at Nancy in France had reported their observations of the heart beats and
movements of the diaphragm and Bouchard in the same year (1896) described his observations of X-rays of a case of pulmonary tuberculosis. In
1906 Hugh Walsham and G. Harrison Orton of the Electrical Department
of St. Bartholomew's Hospital published *The Roentgen Rays in the Diagnosis
of the Chest* (H.K. Lewis, London). Walsham and Orton described the
essential equipment necessary for X-rays of the thorax—a Crookes' tube,
an induction coil, some form of high voltage transformer, a fluorescent
screen, and for radiography, a photographic plate. They described the five
positions employed for a complete radiographic examination of the chest:
the anterior and posterior examinations, the right anterior oblique and left
posterior oblique examinations and the left lateral. Walsham and Orton
noted several important abnormalities in pulmonary tuberculosis: the
movement of the diaphragm was restricted on the affected side, opacities
were observed in the apices, and the cardiac shadow is "smaller than
normal and placed more vertically in the chest". Alterations in the shape
of the chest wall and "a peculiar slope of the ribs giving a roof-tile appearance is often seen associated with chronic lung disease". Cavities in the
lung were easily seen, usually surrounded by consolidation. Areas of
fibrosis and calcification and hilar lymphadenopathy were described.

Primitive X-ray departments were established in Sydney Hospital
(1900) and St Vincent's Hospital, Darlinghurst (1905). In Australia, by 1910
X-rays were being taken principally of limb fractures. In Sydney X-ray
examinations of the chest were rarely made until after the World War I; in
1915 of 813 X-rays taken in St Vincents Hospital, 424 (52 per cent) were of
injured or fractured limbs, and only 84 (10.3 per cent) of the chest.

Dr H.M. Hewlett gave the first annual lecture of the Australian and New
Zealand Association of Radiology on 7 April 1938.17 His personal association
with radiology began at the Children's Hospital, Melbourne in 1896.

> I was always keenly interested in photography and electricity and the late
> Dr William Snowball suggested that I take up the new photography.

He set up his apparatus in a corner of the mortuary. He first used a Coolidge tube which allowed for the insertion of an ammeter and voltmeter in 1914, thus taking the guesswork out of timing exposure. According to Hewlett:

> even in those early days (1903, in Europe), extensive use of X-rays in pulmonary tuberculosis had led to the following conclusions: (1) in no single case in which physical signs were present did the X-rays fail to detect mischief; (2) in some cases in which no physical signs were detected the rays showed deposits and subsequently physical signs appeared; (3) the rays frequently demonstrated that the disease was more extensive than the physical signs indicated.

World War I gave a great impetus to radiology and chest X-rays became commonplace. The Potter-Bucky grid greatly enhanced the quality of chest X-rays by reducing the radiation scatter. In 1935 the tomograph was introduced from Germany but little use was made of sectional radiography up to 1938 in Australia.

Mass Miniature Radiography (MMR)

In August 1938 Dr H.W. Wunderly, in Adelaide, began a survey of young women with a view to detecting early cases of pulmonary tuberculosis. Positive tuberculin reactors were radiographed on full-size film. Early in 1939 Pagel, in England, noted a report of mass chest X-ray surveys of German police and Nazi SS troops, 100,000 in all, using 35 mm photofluorography. He referred to this in his regular correspondence with Wunderly. Stevens described the sequel:[18]

> By April 1939, Wunderly had constructed, in his private rooms in Adelaide a primitive miniature radiographic unit, using an existing fluorescent screen, a fabricated tunnel and a Leica camera attached to it by adhesive tape. It is understood that the camera tunnel rested on a kitchen table, and was, of course, not adjustable to suit the varying heights of his patients. It is probable that he may have, at that early stage, used a simple form of a technique, to be routinely employed later, of adjusting the height of the patient on a platform relative to a fixed height of X-ray tube and camera tunnel. Perhaps he used a series of his medical textbooks to achieve the appropriate height for each patient! Wunderly, acting as his own technician, obtained a series of miniature chest radiographs of the young women he had under study. He established that, on the 35 mm film, he could demonstrate evidence of chest lesions which he confirmed by direct chest radiography.[19]

It is recorded by Walker in *Australia in the War of 1939-45* that:

> realising that this method might be of value in the examination of recruits on enlistment or in surveys of the general public, he (Wunderly) brought it to the notice of Colonel S.R. Burston, later Major-General and DGMS, who was the DDMS of the 4th Military District and on May 4, 1939, also wrote to Dr J.H.L. Cumpston the

Director-General of Health. The actions of Dr Wunderly, who was later to serve Australia with distinction as the Commonwealth Director of Tuberculosis in the formative years of the Commonwealth and States Tuberculosis Arrangements, must be regarded as the starting point for the development of miniature radiography for tuberculosis case-finding programs in Australia.

In 1938 Dr C.E. Eddy (of the Commonwealth X-ray and Radium Laboratory) was asked to meet Wunderly together with Dr J. O'Sullivan and Dr Eric Cooper. It was decided to ask Eddy to build a prototype machine, and miniature radiographs from this machine were considered to be of superior quality to those seen overseas. As a direct result of this the first machine was delivered to the army on 23 December 1939 and in less than two months all 22,000 members of the 6th Division AIF were X-rayed and 109 cases of active tuberculosis were detected. The results were so impressive that all servicemen and later government munition workers were subjected to mass chest radiography. Australia was the first allied country to use mass radiography for tuberculosis case-finding.

Cotter Harvey made two comments on this early exhibition of the value of mass radiography:[20]

> The most important advance in preventive medicine ... will be the surveys of whole groups or even whole communities by mass X-ray photography... A mass survey does not pretend to offer final diagnosis. Its object is to select for more careful study a relatively small number of persons from a large population of presumably healthy individuals.

Stevens concluded that:

> Sir Harry Wunderly, Colonel Cooper and Dr Eddy were the major contributors to the development of miniature radiography in Australia.

Compulsory mass miniature chest radiography was the principal case finding method used in the Australian Tuberculosis Campaign. Initially the surveys applied to all members of the population aged over fourteen years.

It is difficult to prove just how effective mass radiography was in the tuberculosis campaign. However it is undeniable that the decline in notification rates during the campaign (1950–73) was over four times that of the decline in the previous 23 years, 1927–50. More specifically, this accelerated decline was delayed until 1959 in Queensland and 1963 in Victoria when compulsory surveys were introduced in these two states. Various studies in Victoria and South Australia showed that voluntary surveys covered at most 50 to 60 per cent of the population. Moreover Abrahams in Queensland showed conclusively that the yield of active cases was significantly higher in that section of the population which did not respond promptly even to a compulsory survey. Prompt attenders at surveys yielded relatively few cases; those who attended only on receiving notices that their non-attendance might lead to prosecution yielded more cases while the highest yield was in those who attended only under the immediate threat of prosecution. In 1969 the rate among those who co-operated promptly was 0.30 per 1,000 films compared with 2.92 per 1,000 among the non-cooperators. In the seven years from 1963 when compulsory surveys were in operation Australia-wide, they discovered 5,805 active cases, representing 33 per cent of the 17,717 pulmonary cases notified. In addition many thousands of persons with abnormal chest X-rays due to inactive or healed tuberculosis were brought under the surveillance of chest clinics. Furthermore there was evidence that the pulmonary tuberculosis discovered on mass surveys was less advanced than that presenting as symptomatic tuberculosis between surveys or discovered by other case-finding methods. Early diagnosis limited the spread of infection and improved the chances of a complete cure with less interference with the patient's employment. The aim was to survey the whole Australian population every three years and this was generally achieved up until 1968; the decline in yield or discovery rate per 1000 films by 1968 was about 75 per cent compared with 1950.

By 1970 the yield of active cases was less than 0.3 per 1,000 films and cost-benefit analysis suggested the winding down of mass surveys was overdue. The benefits of mass surveys were undeniable during the first 15 years of the campaign. The drawbacks were now becoming apparent; the community began to show hostility to compulsory exposure to irradiation which was double or treble that of large modern static units.

The total attendances at mass surveys to 1970 were recorded at 29 million. The surveys were then concentrated in high risk groups and finally discontinued in 1975.

MMR in Victoria

R.S.A. Marshman

The X-ray apparatus used initially in the Victorian surveys consisted of 35 mm lens camera units which were installed in the South Melbourne Town Hall, another in the Sacre Coeur Private Hospital in Coburg and the third in Geelong. There was also a similar unit in the Central Chest Clinic in Little Lonsdale Street which was used for contacts of active cases, other special groups (such as pre-employment) and the general public. Later transportable units were used together with one unit installed in a bus.

Later, 70 mm Odelca mirror camera units were installed in specially built caravans which were towed all over Victoria. The Odelca mirror camera units were combined with Nanophos X-ray units and were much more satisfactory than the 35 mm units; the films were of better quality and the patient received less radiation. Occasionally loans were made of up to four units by the Anti-Tuberculosis Association of New South Wales and the NSW Department of Health. This was arranged by Dr Allan King who was the Commonwealth Director of Tuberculosis 1960–63. There was a great deal of publicity prior to a survey, costing up to £12,000; nobody could claim they were unaware the survey was taking place. For example, in the Essendon-Coburg mass X-ray campaign the electoral rolls, which coincided with the survey areas, were used and as people attended the units, their names were ticked off. In addition, in Essendon the whole school population was tuberculin-tested.

The Last Roundup in the Nation's Capital

A.J. Proust

I joined the staff of the Canberra Community Hospital in 1954 and observed the compulsory miniature mass radiographic surveys (MMR) conducted in 1956, 1959, 1962 and 1965. The 1965 survey yielded so little previously unrecognised tuberculosis that seven years elapsed before another survey was mooted. The National Tuberculosis Advisory Council at its 1972 meeting discussed MMR and recommended a final round of compulsory surveys throughout Australia. Specifically in regard to the Australian Capital Territory and Canberra, the council noted that the population had increased from 96,000 to 169,000 over the seven years since the last survey, that Canberra had a higher percentage of migrants than the national average and that a more complete register of high risk groups (people with abnormal chest X-rays and a positive Mantoux) could only be maintained by another survey. The recommendation to carry out a compulsory survey was submitted to the Minister of Health, Sir Kenneth Anderson, and approved by him on 15 March 1972.

Due to changes in the community attitude towards compulsion (probably the result of conscription for Vietnam) and especially compulsory exposure to radiation, there was public disquiet about this survey. The argument in favour of maintaining "compulsion" in MMR was supported by Queensland research which had shown that the prevalence of tuberculosis in the 80 per cent of the adult community who responded immediately to a survey was low; in the remaining 20 per cent who responded only at the second or third request, the prevalence was eight times higher. Hence a MMR must be compulsory otherwise half of the cases of tuberculosis and probably other abnormalities would be missed. In addition there was community concern about fall-out from the French nuclear tests at Mururoa. This was not going to be an easy survey to sell. Plans were made to grant exemptions more readily than in the past, to pregnant women or to women who thought they were pregnant, to housebound invalids, to those whose work exposed them to radiation (for example those working with isotopes in the Commonwealth Scientific and Industrial Research Organisation, Australian National University and other laboratories) and to those who could produce evidence of a chest X-ray during the previous 12 months; this latter exemption was widened to include anyone claiming to have had a chest X-ray within the previous two years. Finally alternate arrangements were made (but not publicised) for those people who had an unreasonable but apparently genuine fear of radiation; these people could have a Mantoux test and only if the result was significantly positive (10 mm or more) were they required to have a chest X-ray. As many as possible of those seeking exemption were screened briefly by a clinic nurse for symptoms of productive cough, weight loss or a family history of or exposure to tuberculosis. (Some seeking exemptions were to change their minds and request a chest X-ray as the survey progressed).

A list of adults was drawn up from the Electoral Rolls and the Aliens Register; this was then computerised for easy reference. However, thousands of workers and shoppers from Queanbeyan visited Canberra every day as well as large visitor and "floating" populations not represented in the Electoral Roll. Finally there were an estimated 3,000 diplomats, family members and staff who did not appear on any roll. An estimate was made of the target population of about 80,000.

In December 1972 a Labor government was elected and despite its anti-nuclear stance, the new Minister of Health, Dr Everingham, promptly approved the recommendation for a compulsory MMR survey and the necessary notice was signed by him and appeared in the Commonwealth Gazette of 10 February 1973. The survey was to begin on April 9 and end on June 6.

Within the next month the *Canberra Times* reported that the American College of Radiology, the American College of Chest Physicians and the Food and Drug Administration had jointly called for an end to mass surveys using mobile miniature X-ray units. The reasons given included radiation exposure was unacceptably high, the expected yield of tuberculosis was too low and alternative methods of case-finding were available, notably tuberculin tests, so that only significantly positive-reactors were required to have chest X-rays. On 19 March 1973 the Society for Social Responsibility in Science wrote to the *Canberra Times* supporting the American policy and calling upon the government to cancel the proposed survey. On 27 March Mr McKellar, a Liberal MP, defended the decision to proceed with the survey; he quoted figures for cosmic and natural background radiation in Canberra, estimated at 100 millerads per annum and contrasted this with the additional 60 millerads sustained by a single MMR film. To add to the turmoil, the French were poised to explode another nuclear device and well known anti-nuclear activist and Nobel Laureate, Dr Linus Pauling arrived in Australia; his statement that "each added amount of radiation causes damage to the health of human beings" was repeated in the media for several days. The pressure on the Labor government to abandon the survey mounted as the anti-survey activists accused it of hypocrisy for pursuing the French to the International Court of Justice in the Hague, seeking an injunction to force a halt to the explosion of nuclear devices at Mururoa and on the other hand, the same government was compelling all adults in the nation's capital to be unnecessarily irradiated. The chest clinic and the Tuberculosis Division of the Health Department received hundreds of calls over the months of March and April, some of them abusive. At 1 am about three days before the survey was scheduled to begin, a man purporting to be a senior journalist of a metropolitan paper rang me at home asking me to respond on the Minister's behalf to a statement by Dr Pauling. I responded by saying I was not authorised to respond on the Minister's behalf whereupon he assured me the Minister had given him my telephone number. I terminated the conversation.

Despite all this agitation and turmoil the MMR units from the Anti-Tuberculosis Association of New South Wales arrived and the survey began. The MMR staff did an excellent job and after 14 working days had taken 32,700 70 mm films and were well-ahead of schedule. Total exemptions granted to that date were 1,440, 63 per cent because of evidence of having had a satisfactory chest X-ray within the past two years, 19 per cent because they were absent from Canberra for the duration of the survey, 10 per cent because of pregnancy and the remaining 8 per cent because of recent heavy radiation exposure due to their occupation or diagnostic radiography. Total refusals were 210, about one quarter of whom were eligible for exemption, another quarter accepted tuberculin tests and a chest X-ray if positive and 96 were hard core refusals (about 0.3 per cent of the 32,900 who had up to that point received a chest X-ray request notice).

The survey continued and gradually the refusal rate, exemption requests and criticism eased, due mainly to the imperturbability of the staff of the MMR units and the unflagging courtesy of the chest clinic staff to the public. The attitude of the Department of Health spokespersons and of the chest clinic staff was that every precaution was taken to avoid unnecessary or harmful radiation, and in view of the potential benefits of early diagnosis of a curable condition, compulsion was essential for the success of the survey as a case-finding tool.

The survey was completed on schedule on 6 June. The quality of the 70 mm films was uniformly excellent and there were fortunately only minor technical hitches. The films were processed and read in Sydney by the Anti-Tuberculosis Association and returned to the chest clinic who then

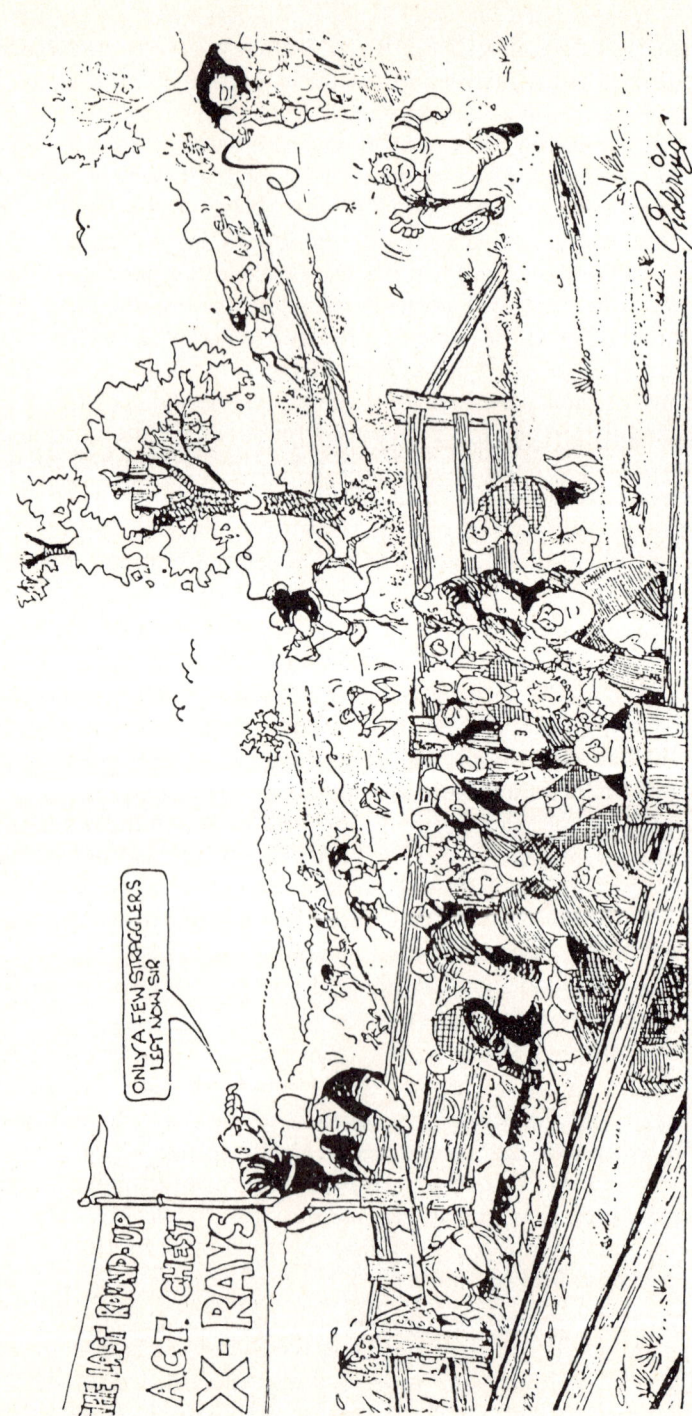

recalled those people whose films were abnormal.

The final results of the survey were:

Total number of request cards sent	82,534
Total persons x-rayed	61,546
Additional persons attend at own request	7,023
Total x-rayed	68,569
Total exemptions	8,253
Total refusals	210

8,877 persons on the Electoral Roll were absent from Canberra long-term or had left permanently and 143 had died. Thus 3,279 or 4 per cent remained unaccounted for.

Of those X-rayed, 619 or 0.9 per cent were recalled to the Chest Clinic for further investigation. The final diagnoses were:

		Abnormalities per 1,000 X-rays
Active or suspected active pulmonary tuberculosis	13	(0.19)
Previously unknown significant inactive pulmonary tuberculosis	220	(3.20)
Intrathoracic neoplasms	21	(0.30)
Chronic obstructive lung disease	127	(1.85)
Cardiac abnormalities not previously suspected	50	(0.73)
Intrathoracic cysts, goitres	24	(0.35)
Sarcoidosis	7	(0.10)
Miscellaneous (pneumonitis, pneumoconiosis, fibrotic scars of undetermined origin)	8	(0.10)

In summary the total significant abnormalities recorded were 470 or 6.82 per1,000 of those X-rayed. The vast majority of the community responded and the yield of previously undiagnosed and mostly asymptomatic disease was considered to have justified the survey.

There were some flashes of humour during the survey. The *Canberra Times* published a cartoon depicting cowboys attempting to round up some fractious cattle to join their mates in the cattle yards—entitled *The Last Great Roundup*!

CHAPTER 8

Evolution of Treatment

A.J. Proust

Sanatoria

The concept of the "open air cure" was promoted by Aesculapius who was the Greek god of medicine.[1] Sick people flocked to his temples which were on mountain tops or in secluded valleys in the middle of pine groves. Bathing, resting, breathing exercises and "taking the waters" of nearby sacred springs comprised "the cure". Over two thousand years were to elapse before the concept was revived by an obscure English physician who practised in a village near Birmingham. In 1840 Dr George Boddington published his essay entitled *The Treatment and Cure of Pulmonary Consumption on Principles Natural, Rational and Successful*. For the first time, a well qualified physician—he held degrees and diplomas from St Bartholomew's Hospital, London, Edinburgh and Erlangen in Bavaria—addressed his mind solely to the cure of tuberculosis. Up to this time, no one had thought in terms of a cure for tuberculosis; the diagnosis was a sentence of death which was confirmed in 20 per cent of patients within six months and delayed for up to five years in a further 50 per cent. George Boddington dismissed the current "treatments" such as purges and bleeding as worse than useless. His theory revolved around the virtues of open air and a fresh country environment, far from the industrial smogs. He also proposed a thoroughly good diet including a glass of wine daily to stimulate the appetite; he advocated graded exercise from a gentle walk to vigorous horse riding, then early to bed in a room with wide-open windows or on the verandah of the purpose-built sanatorium. Finally he provided live-in nursing supervision and regular medical attention. All this was quite revolutionary especially when proposed by a physician from the provinces; the venture failed financially despite some modest success with patients who "took the cure".

A German physician, Dr Hermann Brehmer, established a sanatorium in the mountains of Upper Silesia in 1854. He also preached about the virtues of pure mountain air and the benefits of graduated exercise. His sanatorium was a success due partly to the health insurance scheme introduced by Bismarck, the first Chancellor of Germany; this enabled ordinary working people to "take the cure" as well as middle class and wealthy people who paid higher tariffs for more luxurious accommodation. However all patients followed the same regimen of open-air relaxation, nutritious diet and graduated exercise under medical supervision. Other sanatoria sprang up in Germany, Switzerland, North America and eventually in Australia and New Zealand.

The Early History of Sanatoria in New South Wales *

Tuberculosis mortality in the Australian colonies (apart from Western Australia) peaked in the last two decades of the 19th century.

> It was the one complaint against which medical men seemed to have no armoury and for which they could recommend only two palliatives—the one, Koch's tuberculin and the other the open-air treatment in sanatoria distant from (urban) settlement.[2]

This may have influenced the apathy of politicians and the indifference of most physicians to what was an enormous public health and social problem. During the period 1890-96 in New South Wales there were 7254 deaths from phthisis (pulmonary tuberculosis) and probably 10,000 from all forms of tuberculosis; the total tuberculosis mortality in all the Australian colonies was probably about 40,500 during this period 1890–96, allowing for the much higher mortality in Victoria. As a proportion of the present-day population, the equivalent mortality would be 223,000. The highest death rates were in the age group 20–35 years, prompting Dr George Lane Mullins, assistant physician at St Vincent's Hospital, Darlinghurst, to write:[3]

> Tuberculosis strikes down those in the prime of life, runs a chronic course and causes permanent incapacity for occupation. Surely the restriction of this terrible disease is one of the most pressing questions in preventive medicine.

St Vincent's Hospital opened in 1857 in Tarmons, the Pott's Point home of Sir Charles Nicholson, a distinguished Chancellor of the University of Sydney.[2] In the years at Tarmons, 136 patients with tuberculosis were treated and during the first twelve years after the hospital moved to Darlinghurst the Hospital admitted 214 consumptive patients, of whom 72 died. The Sisters of Charity saw that there was a great need to open a hospital for consumptives and in 1886 they established St Joseph's Consumptive Hospital at Parramatta. The role of St Joseph's Hospital was the treatment of tuberculosis and Dr W. Brown and Dr H.G. Phillips were engaged to attend the patients. When St Joseph's proved too small, in 1889 the Sisters built a new 50-bed hospital next door, installing modern equipment. They also opened a hospice in Darlinghurst in 1889

---

* Catherine O'Carrigan is a member of the Sisters of Charity religious order, a teacher and medical historian; she has published *Some Facets of Public Health in Nineteenth Century New South Wales* (Department of Child Health, Royal Children's Hospital, Brisbane, University of Queensland Press 1983). Sister O'Carrigan made available relevant sections of her MA thesis and her paper on phthisis.

where tuberculosis patients were admitted. In 1892 St Joseph's was moved to much smaller premises at Auburn because Cardinal Moran wanted the Parramatta premises for a school.

St Vincent's Hospital at Darlinghurst continued to treat consumptives; between 1882–95 416 tubercular patients were admitted of whom 90 (21 per cent) died. In the thirteen years 1895-1907, there were 532 patients admitted with tuberculosis of whom only 52 (9 per cent) died. This latter group, at least, must have consisted mainly of patients with early disease which were amenable to the sanatorium regimen with tuberculin therapy in selected cases. What was unusual was that a centrally situated city hospital was devoting so many bed-days (estimated at 5000 each year) to the treatment of tuberculosis. In Edinburgh, Dr George Philip was doing precisely the same; the famous "Edinburgh Plan" for the prevention, treatment and control of tuberculosis stressed the need for consumptive patients to be treated as close to their homes as possible, thus maintaining family bonds.

The only other institution for tuberculosis patients in Australia was founded in 1877 by Colonel Goodlet, a remarkable medical philanthropist; initially his sanatorium was located at Picton and later transferred to nearby Thirlmere, where it assumed the name, Home for Consumptives. The Home treated some 960 patients (during the period 1886-93), the great majority of whom were very ill and 226 of the in-patients died. By the mid 1890s the Thirlmere Home for Consumptives was experiencing financial difficulties in spite of a public committee having taken over its financial management in 1893[2]. Catherine O'Carrigan distinguishes the role of St Joseph's as a hospital for the treatment of salvageable tuberculosis patients from that of the Thirlmere Home as a hospice for incurable advanced cases.

In 1897 there was, throughout the British Empire, the remarkable celebration of Queen Victoria's Jubilee. A great ground-swell of public philanthropy developed to commemorate her life and a significant proportion of this enthusiasm was directed at the treatment of tuberculosis. A special fund was established to help tuberculosis sufferers and specifically to establish a consumptive hospital in New South Wales. The fund was called the Queen Victoria Homes for Consumptives Fund (QHFC Fund). Pearn[4] described the public meetings with committees of prominent citizens and leading doctors which sought donations; a charity stamp was issued to raise funds, ultimately benefiting the fund by nearly £3000 . The fund was able to take over the Home for Consumptives at Thirlmere in 1898 and in 1903 the Queen Victoria Home for Consumptives was opened at Wentworth Falls in the Blue Mountains west of Sydney. Many prominent Sydney physicians were associated with the QVHC fund and the sanatorium at Wentworth Falls and Pearn mentions Dr Sydney Jones,

Dr Scott Skirving, Dr Cecil Purser and Dr Camac Wilkinson who were active in the establishment of the Fund and Dr Sydney Jamieson, Dr George Rennie and Dr McIntyre Sinclair who provided honorary clinical services to patients at Wentworth Falls.

South Australia

The James Brown Memorial Trust was established in Adelaide in 1892. James Brown was a wealthy grazier who died in 1890; his widow established a trust to honour him. The Trustees decided to build a sanatorium at Kalyra after the Supreme Court ruled in 1893 that "a home for consumptives, a home for the aged blind and a home for crippled children are fit and proper objects for the Trust".[5]

The Kalyra Sanatorium was fortunate in attracting well qualified physicians as medical superintendent such as Dr C. Reissman during the early 1900's and then Dr J. Walter Browne (1914-44).

The results of the sanatorium regimen are well-summarised in the Annual Reports of Kalyra Sanatorium. During the year 1913–14,190 patients were treated in the 40 bed sanatorium, the average duration of stay being 105 days. Thus Kalyra avoided being a repository for advanced cases as at the Tasmania sanatorium at Hobart and Wallaroo outside Perth. There were 100 male and 90 female patients treated at Kalyra in that period. On discharge the status of the patients was classified as arrested (18%) improved (51 per cent), unimproved (27 per cent) and "other" (4 per cent). This latter group included cases finally diagnosed as non-tuberculous as well as tuberculous patients admitted briefly for education in personal hygiene so they could be treated with safety at home. The term "arrested" meant the absence of any evidence of active tuberculosis together with negative sputum bacteriology. The ten year follow-up showed that 24 per cent were classified as "arrested", 48 per cent improved and only 28 peer cent not improved. These results appear most impressive except that the classification of the tuberculosis on admission was not included and the failure to include deaths meant that the "good" results applied only to long-term survivors, most of whom were probably at stage one (early asymptomatic pulmonary tuberculosis) when admitted originally to the sanatorium. Like Dr Brehmer in Silesia, Dr J. Walter Browne, medical superintendent at Kalyra, obtained better results (54 per cent arrested) in stage one patients than in symptomatic stage two patients (6 per cent arrested) or advanced stage three patients (only 2 per cent arrested).

Tuberculin therapy had been used in the early 1900s by Dr C. Reissmann. He reported significantly better results in patients with stage one disease treated with tuberculin (79 per cent arrested) than in a control group (62 per cent arrested). Dr Browne was unable to reproduce these results; he achieved arrested status in only 57 per cent of tuberculin-treated stage one patients. Dr Browne expressed considerable doubt about the efficacy of tuberculin therapy but no doubt about its capacity to harm patients.

Victoria

In Victoria the first large sanatorium was the Heatherton Sanatorium; Gresswell Sanatorium was opened much later, in 1933. An excellent history of Gresswell Sanatorium was compiled by Dr Keith Cowen who was on the medical staff for many years.

Gresswell Sanatorium was built in the middle of a Crown reserve of 500 acres about 12 miles from Melbourne. Dr Cowen was a patient in Gresswell in 1939 and like many of his medical colleagues with tuberculosis, rehabilitated himself gradually by working there as a medical officer and later, in 1945, joining the Tuberculosis Branch of the Victorian Department of Health; he was appointed Medical Superintendent of Gresswell in 1956 and Deputy Director (Sanatoria) in 1961. Gresswell was built on the "open air" principle with pavillion-type wards and verandahs.

Dr Cowen described the medical management:

> the basic idea was rest, both mental and physical, followed by a long period of graduated exercise and work... always with the idea that the purpose of treatment was to return to the community individuals able and prepared to take an active part in family life, recreation and work and so educated that they would not be a source of infection to others.

Discipline was strict and the whole atmosphere was paternalistic and authoritarian; rules were made to be kept, and recalcitrant patients would be made to feel the disapproval of both staff and patients. However life was not without its lighter and happier moments. An active social club provided occupational and recreational activities including cinema shows, a library and musical programs.

A modest amount of surgery was done, about 60 thoracoplasties during the period 1933–40, the patients being temporarily transferred to the Austin Hospital. About 10 per cent of patients were treated by artifical pneumothorax. Hence the vast majority of Gresswell's patients took the simple "rest cure" until chemotherapy was introduced about 1950. Patient morale rose dramatically when the combination of effective chemotherapy and more active surgical treatment, fully operative by 1950, resulted in the recovery of the majority of patients. The death-rate which had been almost 20 per cent of all patients admitted in 1936 fell to only 1 per cent in 1953. The very success of the treatment of tuberculosis at Gresswell finally forced its closure in 1970. This closure came only 16 years after tuberculosis beds in Victoria reached a peak of 1,216 in 1954.

Another reason for the closure of Gresswell and similar sanatoria all over Australia and other Western countries was that medical care suddenly became much more sophisticated and expensive. It was no longer cost-effective to up-date expensive radiology departments, operating rooms, microbiology and biochemical laboratories, physiotherapy and occupational therapy departments in these sanatoria which despite the efforts of their medical staff remained outside the mainstream of medicine.

A Personal Experience

John Storey of Canberra describes the lengthy battle he had with pulmonary tuberculosis from the age of seventeen (1944).

> After suffering from the childhood illnesses so common in the 1930s, measles, mumps, tonsillitis followed by scarlet fever, then the more serious diphtheria, I entered the workforce at the age of 14 years and the following year was transferred from Ballarat to the Victorian Railways Stores Depot in Spotswood, Melbourne. I boarded in the western suburbs and played football and cricket. At the age of 16 years I joined the RAAF Air Training Corps and led an active social life, dancing several nights a week. In June 1944 I was boarding in Williamstown, sharing a room with another youngster of my own age. My bed was near the window which opened onto a verandah sleepout where a relative of the boarding house proprietor slept. We rarely saw this man who had special meals on his own. He used to cough a lot at night and I used to keep the window open between our beds. I later found out this man had chronic TB of the lungs. I didn't stay there more than about 3 months and moved to another boarding house. I then developed a chronic cough, had night sweats and frequency of urination at night. I lost one and a half stone from 11.7 to 10.0. My new landlady insisted that I see her doctor in Williamstown and he sent me for a miniature X-ray. While awaiting the result I went home to Ballarat and on seeing my condition my mother took me to our family doctor who promptly admitted me to the Ballarat Base Hospital. Chest X-rays and sputum tests proved positive for tuberculosis and I was transferred to the tuberculosis chalet in a rear corner of the Hospital grounds. The treatment at this time (1944) was mainly bed rest and good food; the food was good especially in view of wartime rationing which was in full swing. We had two compulsory rest periods each day, morning and afternoon, and these were strictly enforced, no talking or even reading or radio was allowed. Sputum was tested weekly. If the disease was mild, then the treatment was bed rest and good food. If the disease was in only one lung, then artificial pneumothorax (AP) and phrenic crush was the treatment. If it was more advanced then surgery was recommended. If the disease was advanced in both lungs, there was little hope of recovery and you eventually ended up in a single room. Otherwise we were in two bed wards and by necessity became a closely bonded community.
>
> We all had a disease which the public could not or did not want to understand. A year or more in the Chalet was par for the course

so we made our own amusements; we had our own sense of humour which some nurses found hard to understand but accepted when they realised our sense of isolation. No attempt was made to stop us smoking; I once offered to give it up if it would hasten my recovery but the doctor told me to please myself so I kept on smoking. Dr G.T. James was the specialist and was always available. Sister E. Cooper was the Matron and she ruled the roost but in a nice way. We were wheeled out in our beds on to the verandah every day unless it was raining and windy. During summer we often slept on the verandah overnight.

After several months Dr James decided I was to have an artificial pneumothorax (AP) as the tuberculosis was confined to the apex of my right lung. An AP is a form of treatment by which the affected part of the lung is collapsed by air introduced through a needle into the pleural cavity, the space between the lung and the inside of the chest wall. This air is gradually absorbed so "refills" are made at regular intervals to replenish it and maintain the collapse of the lung. The theory was that the collapse of the lung hastened healing. I used to lie on my good side, the needle would be inserted between the ribs until it was in the pleural space and then the air introduced under slight pressure. I used to feel a little breathless after the "refill" but otherwise there were no ill effects.

After 13 months in hospital I was discharged and attended regularly for chest X-rays and "refills". I was given a special pension, the Tuberculosis Allowance, by the Victorian Government and it was more generous than the invalid pension, thus my parents could afford to keep me at home with good food. My parents built a special sleepout out the back for me.

All went well for 6 months until I developed a pleural effusion on the side of my AP. I was readmitted to hospital and the AP was combined with regular aspirations of the fluid, in other words the fluid would be siphoned off and then replaced by air. This caused me a lot of distress and eventually the AP refills were abandoned; I continued to have the fluid aspirated. After a few months the pleura over the affected lung thickened up and the fluid dried up and Dr James decided that the affected lung was being effectively collapsed by the thickened pleura. That was in 1946 and the position is unchanged in 1988—the pleura is quite thick over the whole of the right lung, thus compressing and partly collapsing the underlying lung.

My second spell in the chalet lasted 17 months and on my second discharge I had been "taking the cure" for a total of 3 years since the diagnosis was made. I was nearly 21 and I attended a Red Cross rehabilitation program involving toy making, weaving and leather work. I lived on the Tuberculosis Allowance for 5 years and took a series of part-time jobs, mainly in the Hospital, until I was able to qualify for the PMG Department. I then studied at night and passed the Leaving Certificate and finally qualified as an accountant. I finished my career as an accountant in the Public Service in Canberra. I led an active sporting life, training football teams and playing lawn bowls.

I attend the Chest Clinic at regular intervals and my chest X-ray and lung function remain satisfactory. I have been told that my unaffected left lung has compensated for my partially and permanently collapsed right lung.

Tuberculin and Some Other Therapies Used in the Treatment of Tuberculosis

A.J. Proust

In 1890 Koch announced he had produced "a material" called tuberculin which when injected into animals previously uninfected with the tubercle bacilli, produced a degree of immunity; more importantly, he claimed it could bring advanced tuberculosis in guinea-pigs to a complete halt. Such confident statements, coming from Koch caused a sensation but doubts were raised when Koch refused to give any details about "the material" or how it was produced. Further experiments by Koch were said to show tuberculin was of some value in human tuberculosis, and the clamour finally obliged Koch to release some information.

The confused and controversial history of tuberculin therapy began with Koch's initial reluctance to release details of his method of preparing tuberculin; it worsened with the early exaggerated claims of its efficacy by colleagues of Koch, based on inadequate animal experiments and human therapeutic trials. It was compounded over the next 20 years by conflicting reports based on tuberculins of varying potency and purity administered to patients whose tuberculosis was not classified according to generally accepted criteria. Koch prepared highly purified tuberculins which were said to be 30– to 50–times more potent than the raw English tuberculins. Koch complained:

> it was discreditable to bacteriologists that they have not long since prepared the same tuberculins as mine after the information published by me. Instead they waited to get my formula and joined with others in complaining I had not told them what to do.

Dr J.W. Springthorpe of Melbourne visited Koch's laboratories in Berlin in March 1891 and secured supplies of Koch's tuberculin. He published his experiences with tuberculin therapy in 99 patients in 1891–92.[6] He classified his patients in the same five stages of disease as the physicians in Berlin. Stages one and two were early asymptomatic and more advanced with symptoms, respectively; he claimed 19 of the 52 in these stages were cured. Stages three to five were far advanced and Springthorpe claimed three of the 47 patients in these groups improved and were able to return to work. Using the criteria of bacteriological conversion, Springthorpe's results were poor; only one of 38 bacteriologically proven cases of pulmonary tuberculosis showed sustained negative bacteriology after the usual course of three months of twice weekly tuberculin injections. Clinically, the results were much better; 13 of 38 patients with proven disease gained weight of between 7 and 22 pounds and the same proportion lost their fever. In conclusion, Dr Springthorpe wrote "there seemed good grounds for the belief that in tuberculin, we have met with a real and important advance in the treatment of tubercular disease". He urged continued investigation and careful recording of results. He noted that one could expect reasonably good results in patients with incipient disease while one would fail in the great majority of patients with far advanced disease. He stressed that the individual's resistance was an important factor and counselled against over-confidence on the one hand and outright condemnation on the other. "For myself, so interesting is the work, so pleasurable the feeling that now at last we can exercise an influence directly on the tubercular process, already curing some, relieving others in a manner and to a degree which was formerly impossible for me, that I am satisfied to go on helping to gather the facts from which surer deductions of the future will come —reporting failures as well as successes and confident we are upon the right track even though we shall not reach the goal for some time to come".

Another great proponent of tuberculin therapy in Australia in the first two decades of the 20th century was Dr W. Camac Wilkinson, lecturer in medicine at the University of Sydney and honorary physician at Royal Prince Alfred Hospital. In 1908 Dr Wilkinson published the *Treatment of Consumption* which was a treatise on the natural history of tuberculosis as well as a detailed exposition of tuberculin as a therapeutic and, less importantly, a diagnostic agent in tuberculosis.[7] Dr Wilkinson claimed to have been a pupil of Koch in 1884 and supported Koch's views that "man was the essential source of infection (in tuberculosis) ... and that there was no well-attested instance (where) the bovine tubercle has ever been found in cases of ordinary consumption in man". Like all physicians of his era, Wilkinson laid great stress on the diagnostic value of the physical signs in the lungs.

> He who never misses an early stage of tuberculosis ... should be the life-long friend of many grateful patients. It is far more important not to misread the signs of early disease than it is to make the most accurate guesses as to the size and content of cavities... because in the latter case the patient dies rapidly while the physician looks on helplessly.

Sputum examination for acid-fast bacilli was a helpful but not specific diagnostic aid: "Is it right merely because tubercle bacilli are found in the sputum to make the diagnosis of tuberculosis?" Wilkinson recognised the value of tuberculin as a helpful diagnostic aid both through its local reaction of erythema and induration at the site of injection and its general systemic reactions such as fever and myalgia.

Tuberculin and tuberculin therapy were the main themes of his book. "Tuberculin is the name given to a class of toxic products of the tubercle bacillus grown upon an artificial medium". He listed eight different types of tuberculin according to source (human or bovine) and to method of manufacture (filtered, evaporated or pulverised). Each had its special value in diagnosis or treatment: bovine tuberculin evaporated to one-tenth of its volume was a particularly powerful therapeutic tuberculin.

The aim of tuberculin therapy was a progressive process of active immunisation via a naturally produced antitoxin, that is, tuberculin stimulated the body's active production of antitoxin; to produce the antitoxin, the body cells must be in a relatively healthy state. The early failures of tuberculin therapy by Koch and others were due to a lack of understanding the mode of action of tuberculin; its efficacy was limited by the body's ability to produce antitoxin—an active natural endogenous antitoxin compared with diphtheria antitoxin which was passive, exogenous and produced independently of the body's cell activity. Koch failed to recognise this and applied tuberculin in toxic patients where its efficacy was at best very limited and at worst highly detrimental.

Wilkinson stressed the importance of discriminating between "pure" and "mixed" tuberculous infections. He noticed that during influenza and other viral epidemics tuberculous patients often died rapidly from the viral infection. If tuberculin therapy was applied to patients with mixed infections (bacterial as well as viral) they suffered marked general reactions which were ascribed to tuberculin but were actually caused by the non- tuberculous coexisting infection. Koch erred by using tuberculin in such patients. Wilkinson chose his patients for tuberculin therapy carefully excluding those with "mixed" infections.

Wilkinson explained how he exploited hypersensitivity to tuberculin (the ability to produce marked local and general constitutional reactions) in diagnosis; he used only minute doses of tuberculin, increasing it in gradations until he was satisfied he had excluded the presence of tuberculous infection. In tuberculin therapy, on the other hand, he used high doses in patients with "pure" tuberculous infections, overcoming hypersensitivity with a resultant heightened immune response. He claimed he achieved double the proportion of "arrested" or "improved" results of standard sanatorium care. His results were better because he used various forms of tuberculin specific to the type of disease, at higher dosages and at more frequent intervals.

Wilkinson summed up his results:

> I have herein presented 115 cases in the first stage of tuberculosis ... of the 110 cases treated fully since 1902, I know of the deaths of only three (one of acute malaria, one of splenic anaemia and one after laparotomy for acute intestinal obstruction or acute pancreatitis). I have not heard of a single case dying of pulmonary tuberculosis. At the worst I can claim success for tuberculin treatment in 80 per cent of (early) cases since 1902.

Throughout this and other chapters on tuberculin therapy, Wilkinson made some extraordinary claims:

> Pulmonary tuberculosis can be cured with certainty by means of tuberculin... Is it mere chance that while in other hands scores of cases passed from the first to the third stage within three years, not a single case can be recorded against me in which under tuberculin treatment, the disease has passed from the first into the second stage.

However, occasionally he adopted a more cautious position, stating that "In the treatment of this disease, even with tuberculin, we dare not be overconfident".

Wilkinson dominated the Australian medical literature on tuberculin therapy for over 20 years; his last contribution was in the *Medical Journal of Australia* in 1924. Nobody was able to achieve his level of success with tuberculin; perhaps he used his knowledge of the natural history of tuberculosis to select cases which were most likely to remit.

There are few other such well-documented clinical trials of tuberculin therapy in the Australian medical literature. One concludes that there was rapid disillusionment with tuberculin therapy in Australia as in England, punctuated by occasional bursts of enthusiasm by individual physicians.

BCG in Victoria

R.S.A. Marshman

BCG vaccination commenced in Victoria in October 1947. A "wet" Canadian vaccine was used and in the 1948–49 *Report of the Tuberculosis Services* it was stated that 2,000 vaccinations had been administered, chiefly to the nursing staff of sanatoria and public hospitals and to young family contacts of infectious cases. The Central Tuberculosis Bureau established a contact-clinic on 1 August 1949 to examine all contacts of infectious cases and where indicated to administer the Frapier BCG vaccine flown out from Montreal. The vaccine had to be used promptly as usually there were only three days between its arrival and expiry date. Initially local ulceration and axillary lymphadenitis were not uncommon until expertise in administering intradermal vaccine was acquired.

The Australian vaccine manufactured by the Commonwealth Serum Laboratories (CSL) was available from 24 December 1948; it was also a "wet" vaccine prepared by Dr Edgar North. In 1954 the freeze-dried vaccine was prepared by CSL and excellent conversion rates of 87 to 95 per cent were reported by Dr James in Melbourne and Dr Kerr in Bendigo.

Assessment of Calmette's Vaccine (BCG) in Australia: 1926—1927

The Australian Archives contain a file of official correspondence on Calmette's BCG.

Dr T G Morgan of the CSL received BCG cultures from the Pasteur

Institute on 28 January 1926. The cultures were passed through 3 to 8 subcultures and then administered to guinea pigs; the guinea pigs remained well and at autopsy no evidence of tubercles was found. Dr Morgan askedDr Cumpston whether he should proceed with further animal experiments eg. on monkeys or calves. Dr Cumpston wrote the single word "Delay" in the margin.

Dr W.J. Penfold, Victorian Government Pathologist, visited Europe in 1926 and in his report dated 23/2/27 expressed caution about the use of BCG. In Germany very large doses of BCG vaccine had proved lethal to guinea pigs. Fagin in Warsaw similarly reported some deaths in guinea pigs inoculated with large doses of BCG and although at autopsy she could find no tubercles in tissues, she was able to culture acid-fast bacilli from tissue biopsies.

Penfold reported that these results did not conflict with Calmette's own experiments but the Medical Research Council in the United Kingdom was very concerned.

The wide-scale use of BCG in neonates in France had been completely safe over four years. Deaths due to tuberculosis did occur in vaccinated infants but "it could be shown in many cases that the infants had been exposed to tuberculosis prior to vaccination".

Dr C.L Park, Chief Medical Officer, Australia House in London sent a memo to Dr Cumpston dated 29/3/27. When in Geneva Dr Park had consulted Dr Biraud, medical officer-in-charge of the League of Nation's Health Office and discussed with him the results of recent clinical trials of BCG vaccination in 45,000 new-born infants in France. These infants had been subdivided into two groups:

1. Those with known domestic or maternal contact with tuberculosis; BCG vaccine was administered. Mortality from all causes in the first year of life was 76 and 65.5 per 1,000 respectively.
2. Those with known domestic contact with tuberculosis; no BCG vaccine was administered. Mortality from all causes in the first year of life was 240 per1,000.

BCG Vaccine: Its Use in South Australia
Philip Woodruff

From 1905 Calmette and Guerin at the Pasteur Institute in Paris had examined strains of tubercle bacilli–in many cases altered in the laboratory by various methods aimed at attenuating their virulence or pathogenic-ity—with a view to producing a protective vaccine. Their aim was a vaccine which would protect recipients against the consequences of infec-tion with tubercle bacilli. Calmette and Guerin observed that tubercle bacilli which had passed through the alimentary canal showed some evi-dence of diminution of pathogenicity. They therefore cultivated their strain of bovine tubercle bacilli by serial passage on a solid medium consisting of potato impregnated with bile. The organism certainly became less virulent for experimental animals. After some 230 serial subcultures had been made on this medium, they decided to find out whether the organism had become sufficiently attenuated to have completely lost its capacity to produce tuberculous lesions in test animals, but had retained sufficient of its original characteristics to produce a positive tuberculin reaction. This proved to be the case. The next step was to find out whether animals converted from tuberculin negative to positive by this organism had at the same time acquired significant ability to resist subsequent challenge by virulent tubercle bacilli.

By the year 1920 Calmette and Guerin were entirely satisfied that their treated organism did satisfy the three essential requirements for a protective vaccine against tuberculosis, that is:

- it brought about tuberculin conversion,
- it failed to cause tuberculosis,
- it regularly provided a protective effect against tuberculosis in test animals.

Thus was BCG produced, and aptly named after its two originators.

In France, the new vaccine, coming from the Pasteur Institute and bearing Calmette's name, was received with enthusiasm as an important contribution to the prevention of tuberculosis. The Anglophone world remained sceptical. There were those who saw that widespread vaccination of humans with BCG would certainly invalidate the tuberculin test as a tool in the diagnosis of tuberculosis. To make this loss worthwhile would require convincing demonstration of very significant protective value from the vaccine. And might not this artificially attenuated organism revert at any time, or gradually over time, to its original virulence? Extensive research programmes were set up in many countries to provide answers to these questions.

One of the first tasks of Dr M.J. Holmes, the first Commonwealth Director of Tuberculosis, was to investigate the safety and efficacy of BCG vaccine. His report in 1928 described the work of Calmette and Guerin, and the results of a meeting of world experts at the Pasteur Institute in October 1928, called by the President of the Health Committee of the League of Nations. The conference concluded that BCG vaccine was harmless, and that it produces in both vaccinated children and cattle "a certain degree of immunity against tuberculosis". However further research was necessary to enable the commission to pass final judgement on the value of anti-tuberculosis vaccination with BCG. Holmes concluded that:

> until full investigation has been made into this matter it would not seem advisable to take any steps for the use of BCG vaccine as a public health measure in Australia.

These investigations continued for another decade and then World War II intervened.

In 1943, at the height of the war in the Pacific, great concern was expressed in Adelaide at the hazard faced by staff members in hospitals caring for tuberculous patients. Dr D.R.W. Cowan, in reporting on the work of the chest clinic at the Adelaide Hospital in that year, noted that 95 student nurses had undergone conversion from tuberculin negative to tuberculin positive. He did not doubt that this conversion had taken place as a result of exposure to tuberculous patients, recognised or un-recognised, in the course of these nurses' hospital duties. The report states:

> The scheme (already applying to staff at the Adelaide Hospital) was extended to all employees of Morris Hospital and Bedford Park Sanatorium whereby they are given regular Mantoux tests, and leave on half pay is granted for recuperative purposes in cases of a Mantoux positive following a Mantoux negative.

In the years following, the numbers of tuberculin-conversions, espe-cially among student nurses, caused Cowan increasing concern, especially as numbers of these young women (student nurses at this time were all young women) developed primary tuberculosis in succeeding months, and a small proportion of these went on to develop progressive pulmo-nary tuberculosis, and in some cases fatal generalised miliary or menin-geal disease. In 1943, 647 student nurses had Mantoux tests at the chest clinic; 95 of these underwent conversion from Mantoux negative to posi-tive during that year; in 1944 among 807 tested, 41 converted; in 1945–46 (eighteen months) 40 of 500 converted; in 1946–47, 70 of 1366 converted; and in 1947–48 the figure was 125 out of 1416.

This last year, 1947–48, was different from its predecessors. A special note stated that of the 125 conversions 69 were due to natural infections, and 56 were brought about by vaccination with BCG. Cowan was now satisfied both by reports in the literature and by his own observations while visiting Britain and Europe, of the safety and the protective value of BCG vaccine. He had expressed the view to Nancy Atkinson in the De-partment of Bacteriology in the Institute of Medical and Veterinary Science at the University of Adelaide, that it would be a great advance to have available in Adelaide a supply of BCG vaccine for use in protecting nurses, medical students and selected family contacts. Atkinson assured him that she could obtain a culture of the BCG organism from England, and that there was no reason why the vaccine should not be prepared in her laboratory. Cowan's report to the Director General of Medical Services describes this new venture:

> An interesting feature of this year's work has been the increasing   .
> use of BCG vaccination as a protection against tuberculosis.
> Something like 500 vaccinations have been done with satisfactory

immediate results. The vaccine is being prepared by research workers Miss Erica Page and Miss Dawn Allen in the laboratories of the Institute of Medical and Veterinary Science, under the supervision of Dr Nancy Atkinson. That there is nothing wrong with the vaccine prepared in Adelaide or in the method of its use is evidenced by the fact that none of the persons vaccinated has come to any harm, that the vaccination "takes" have been good, and that there has been a regular conversion of the Mantoux reaction from negative to positive.

Dr Nancy Atkinson wrote of this venture in the *Adelaide Medical Students' Society Review* in 1949. She has been good enough to allow me to quote it in full:

Human inoculation with BCG vaccine prepared in this department was introduced to Australia for the first time about two years ago (1947). The project was carried out under the auspices of the Faculty of Medicine, which set up a special reference committee for the work. We had the collaboration of Dr. D.R.W. Cowan on the clinical side.

A strain of the BCG organism (Bacille Calmette Guerin) was obtained from England and preserved here by drying. The culture was tested for pathogenicity in guinea pigs and found satisfactory. Therefore vaccine was prepared and tested for ability to change the Mantoux reaction of guinea pigs from negative to positive and to confer on them increased resistance to experimental tuberculous infection. In these tests the vaccine proved effective enough to go on to human inoculation. The first human vaccination was performed by Dr Cowan by multiple puncture on Miss G.E. Page, who had prepared the vaccine, the concentration of which was 5 mg wet weight per ml. Miss Page became Mantoux positive within four weeks and has remained positive. Vaccine for general human use was prepared in a separate building in which no other bacteriological or pathological work was done; all equipment was devoted only to BCG work. The first group of human volunteers (30) was then vaccinated by the multiple puncture method, using a specially designed gun giving forty simultaneous pricks. This vaccine also contained 5 mg. wet weight per ml. The local reactions to vaccination were very mild and all volunteers were Mantoux positive six weeks after vaccination. Later tests showed that the majority were still Mantoux positive at six months, but several were negative at 12 months. Another group of volunteers was vaccinated with stronger vaccine containing 20 mg. wet weight per ml. Local reactions were much stronger than in the previous group and all who returned for the Mantoux test in six weeks were positive. Later tests showed that all who returned for testing were Mantoux positive at six and twelve months. All vaccinations have subsequently been made by the multiple puncture method.

A more accurate method of standardising vaccine by dry weight was evolved and all subsequent batches of vaccine were standardised by this method. The concentration of vaccine finally selected and found suitable was 5 mg. dry weight per ml. Seventeen batches of this vaccine were made and used to inoculate more than nine hundred persons. With vaccine less than ten days old, 780 persons were inoculated, of whom sixty three failed to return, ten gave a doubtful positive Mantoux reaction, and 707 gave a positive reaction at six weeks and six months. About 150 vaccinations were done with vaccine kept at 4 degrees Celsius for about four weeks. Of these persons 20 failed to return, one gave a weak Mantoux reaction, and the others gave positive Mantoux tests in six weeks.

As an extension of this work we have tried to preserve BCG vaccine by freeze-drying. If vaccine could be preserved so that it remained potent for long periods, greater uniformity of vaccine would result, supplies would be more likely always to be available, and complete tests in guinea pigs to prove the safety of the vaccine could be carried out before use. After nine months a marked decrease in viability had occurred in the wet vaccine and in the vaccine dried from distilled water. No obvious change was detected in vaccines dried from serum or peptone water. Frozen vaccine and vaccine dried from 5 per cent lactose showed little decrease in six weeks. Of the dried products the 5 per cent lactose preparation seemed the most satisfactory.

We are indebted to the NH and MRC for grants partly supporting the work on antibiotics, salmonellas, and BCG vaccine and to the Phoebe Ferris bequest to the University of Adelaide for funds to commence the work on BCG.

BCG played an important role during the National Campaign against Tuberculosis in protecting adolescents, young adults, and those especially exposed at home or at work to the danger of tuberculous infection. It served to remove the threat of progressive primary tuberculosis in these groups, and thereby to give substantial protection against miliary and meningeal tuberculosis. It also seems certain to have increased substantially the resistance of many young adults to post-primary infection with the tubercle bacillus. The impact was widespread: by 1972 the Commonwealth Serum Laboratories had issued more than nine million doses of BCG. Some of this vaccine had been exported to New Zealand, Papua New Guinea and Pacific Islands, but by far the greater part of it had been used in protecting young Australians.

Some other Forms of Treatment

A.J. Proust

In 1904 Dr Duncan Turner consulting physician to the Victorian sanatorium at Mount Macedon published his book, *A New Treatment of Consumption and other chronic chest disease* (G. Robertson & Co., Melbourne, 1904). The "new treatment" was lengthy and energetic twice-daily whole body massage using liberal quantities of warm cod-liver oil. The recommended duration of each massage was 15 to 20 minutes. Dr Turner quoted Sir James Simpson of Edinburgh, the pioneer in the use of anaesthesia in childbirth who, on a visit to the woollen mills at Galashiels in Scotland, was told by Dr Macdougall, the factory medical officer, that the operatives were strikingly free of consumption and this was attributed to their absorption of lanoline through their skin while handling the wool during the processing of fabrics. Dr Simpson later wrote:

> if oil applied incidentally was capable of preventing or arresting phthisis, the same effects should be obtained with greater certainty if it were applied methodically with the same regularity of a medicinal agent.

He used the cod-liver oil massages in conjunction with the standard sanatorium regimen of nutritious diet, bed rest and then graduated exercise. The treatment combined the beneficial effects of the oil with the stimulant effects of the massage. First of all the patient was sponged with a warm bicarbonate of soda solution followed by "a sponge with a little spirit, whisky or brandy. When night sweats are heavy or the temperature high, I add Quinine to the oil". He also used guaicol or creosote mixed with the oil and if the patient objected to the odour, he added oil of citronella.

Dr E.H. Smalpage's Cure*

On 31 March 1925 Dr Smalpage wrote to the Minister of Health, Sir Neville Howse, stating that after six years of experiments and research into tuberculosis, he had succeeded in producing a serum and antitoxin which he had used with great success in treating patients with tuberculosis. He was prepared to place all the evidence before the Minister and he had already given all the details of the production methods to Dr W.J. Penfold of the Commonwealth Serum Laboratories (CSL). However CSL advised the Minister that the procedure for making the extract was "so vague as to amount only to a suggestion as to the course to be followed". Dr Smalpage refused to give more specific directions for making his serum and he promptly applied for patent rights. On 24 October 1925 Dr Smalpage wrote to the Minister requesting "a bond of £100,000 due when his claims were amply proven". The Federal government sensibly requested Dr Smalpage to provide full details of the manufacturing process to CSL which would then determine its identity, stability and safety. Dr Smalpage was also requested to provide details of his treatment of patients with tuberculosis.

Dr Smalpage replied by claiming that the whole of his research results was in the hands of a research committee established by the University of Sydney and the Medical Research Council in London. The University of

---

* From Commonwealth Archives.

Sydney denied any such research committee existed. Dr Smalpage was then invited to work at the CSL with the object of furthering his research which he claimed basically involved lysis of the tubercle bacillus using a splenic extract and then injecting this into horses and later obtaining an equine anti-serum. However the relationship between Dr Smalpage and CSL was stormy. He repeatedly offered to hand over his production methods and then reneged. He offered to make a generous gift of his vaccine to the nation and then withdrew his offer the following week, demanding £5,000 compensation unconditionally irrespective of the success or failure of his vaccine. All attempts by CSL to "fragment" the tubercle bacillus using a splenic extract failed.

Dr Smalpage's claims were given wide publicity in Australia and overseas and the Commonwealth government felt obliged to establish a clinical trial of the anti-serum, supervised by committees of leaders in tuberculosis in each state. The committees unanimously reported that no patient derived any benefit from the course of treatment.

Dr Spahlinger's Serum*

A. J. Proust

Dr Spahlinger was a European of uncertain origin and details of his medical qualifications are unknown. He established a clinic in Geneva shortly before World War I where he administered a serum or vaccine to tuberculosis patients and claimed he had achieved a cure. His claims attracted world-wide attention. In 1924 he described his serum as "incomplete" in that the horse was bled and the serum separated before the horse had achieved the optimal anti-toxin level. He explained that he had been financially embarrassed by the war because his source of wealthy patients from England and America had dried up. The inference was that when he obtained a "complete" serum his results would be even more spectacular.

In August 1924 Dr H.W. Wunderly of Adelaide was appointed an honorary commissioner by the South Australian Government to investigate Dr Spahlinger's treatment. He met Dr Spahlinger in Geneva and was given access to his records (case histories, chest X-rays, bacteriological results and temperature charts). Dr Wunderly made careful notes about 50 patients during his two visits to Spahlinger's clinic in 1924 and 1925.

Dr Wunderly was satisfied that all the patients had bacteriologically proven tuberculosis. Of the 30 patients whose records he had examined in December 1924, four had died before his return in April 1925. Despite this Wunderly was "of the opinion that the clinical results of his (Spahlinger's)

---

* From Commonwealth Archives.

treatment of tuberculosis were remarkably good". He noted that one advantage of Spahlinger's treatment over tuberculin therapy was the former could be safely administered to advanced cases when tuberculin was contra-indicated.

Spahlinger was not prepared to divulge details of the methods of manufacture of either his serum or vaccine to the health authorities in the United Kingdom who were prepared to conduct a controlled trial. His claims caused a lot of excitement in Australia where pressure was brought to bear on the government to import the serum and vaccine to treat some of the ex-servicemen with active tuberculosis. But his refusal to co-operate with the health authorities in England convinced the Repatriation Department in Australia that his claims were bogus.

Artificial Pneumothorax

A.J. Proust

In 1882 Dr Forlanini, an Italian physician, wrote concerning the sound physiological and mechanical reasons why the introduction of gas into the pleural space, producing an artificial pneumothorax and collapse of the underlying lung, should be beneficial in cavitary pulmonary tuberculosis. He proceeded cautiously over the next ten years, introducing nitrogen into the pleural space through a large-bore needle; the procedure was repeated at frequent intervals as the gas was absorbed. By 1910, the procedure was well established in Europe but the problem of pleural adhesions, preventing effective collapse, limited its use. In 1913 Jacobaeus in Stockholm solved this problem by dividing the adhesions under direct vision, using a thorascope. The Great War intervened and it was only in the 1920s that artificial pneumothorax (APX) was used extensively in Britain and even later in Australia and New Zealand.[1]

The objective of collapse therapy of pulmonary tuberculosis was to compress and immobilise the lung, wholly or partially, to close cavities in the underlying lung and enable the diseased lung to heal. The decision to induce APX was made only after the patient was given a trial of conservative sanatorium regimen; if progress after three months or so was unsatisfactory and the cavitary disease was limited to one lung, preferably in the apex, then APX was increasingly considered. In some cases, especially where repeated haemoptyses occurred, it was considered at an earlier stage. When the disease was advanced and obviously spreading to the opposite lung, particularly in the mid and lower zones, APX was absolutely contraindicated; it was rarely used in children or elderly people.

Artificial pneumothorax was a safe procedure and, although initially painful despite local anaesthesia, a skilled physician could induce an effective APX gradually over several weeks and most patients adapted to the regular refills necessary to maintain collapse without complaint. The

APX was usually maintained if effective and uncomplicated for about three years and, in the majority of cases, tubercle bacilli disappeared from the sputum, the cough virtually disappeared and the patient put on weight as appetite and well-being improved. When indicated, the APX was gradually diminished by smaller and smaller refills.

Certain Considerations of Artificial Pneumothorax in the Treatment of Pulmonary Tuberculosis *

Dr Sargeant, of Waterfall Sanatorium, Sydney, pointed out that assessment of the value of any treatment method in pulmonary tuberculosis was difficult as spontaneous improvement under sanatorium conditions was common and because the placebo effect was powerful in such a dreaded disease.

Patients must be carefully selected for artificial pneumothorax (APX); preferably the patient should be less than 50 years of age and of a placid disposition and the tuberculosis confined to one lung. Cavitation is the principal indication. Acute exudative disease, even if confined to one lung, presents a problem to the doctor—should the patient be given absolute bed rest in the hope of achieving some clearing before inducing APX, despite the risk of the disease spreading to the contra-lateral lung? However APX of a lung which is acutely diseased carries its own risks and if it is delayed too long, there may be extensive pleural adhesions present when it is finally attempted. In the more chronic cases, APX may be difficult to induce satisfactorily because of pleural adhesions.

The routine use of chest X-rays and fluoroscopy is absolutely essential in the management of the patient with APX. Radiological evidence of chronic fibrotic lesions associated with pleural thickening, mediastinal displacement and thick-walled cavities suggest that even if APX can be induced it will almost certainly be incomplete and achieve an unsatisfactory result. In such cases, an APX may be attempted as one may be surprised at the success in an unlikely case; if it fails, then thoracoplasty may be considered.

There are several points about the technique of inducing APX. A blunt Reviere needle should be introduced into the pleural cavity through the anterior axilla or in the subclavicular region. An initial introduction of 300 ml. of air is followed next day with 350 mls and with subsequent increases to 700 or 800 mls. The usual interval between refills is about ten days. A negative intrapleural pressure should be maintained at least during the early stages. The use of positive intrapleural pressure increases the risk of

---

* A summary of a paper by Dr B.A. Sargeant. Waterfall Sanatorium. *Med. J. Aust.* 1938. 1,912. Edited by A.J. Proust. Copyright © the *Medical Journal of Australia*. Reprinted with permission.

air embolism, pleural effusion and displacement of the mediastinum and it will also cause the patient discomfort in the chest. A satisfactory collapse having been obtained, it is usual to continue the APX for at least three years.

Complications include vaso-vagal reactions ("particularly in female patients"), pleural shock ("varies in severity from faintness to actual death"), air embolism and surgical emphysema. Pleural effusion is a common and important complication. It will be heralded by a sudden diminution in the amount of air that can be introduced at a refill and by a slight febrile reaction. Aspiration may have to be combined with air replacement.

Thoracoplasty

The first tentative steps towards surgical collapse by rib resection (thoracoplasty) were taken about 1885 by German and French surgeons. In 1907 Brauer and Friedrich began removing ribs 2 to 9, initially in one stage, later in two stages as mortality rates in one stage operations were unacceptably high. However, Sauerbruch in Germany was the acknowledged master of the para-vertebral thoracoplasty, removing ribs 1 to 11 in one or two steps; the mortality-rate was 25 per cent and the cure-rate 35 per cent. Alexander in the United States modified the operation limiting rib resection to a partial 7 rib operation, with great success.[1]

It was James Officer Brown who established the first Australian thoracic surgical unit at the Alfred Hospital, Melbourne in 1941. The team of Officer Brown, surgeon, and Orton, anaesthetist, also worked at the Austin Hospital where there had been an increase in interest in the surgical treatment of pulmonary tuberculosis by thorocoplasty largely due to the appointment of Dr Hilary Roche as medical superintendent of that hospital. Dr Roche had been in charge of a tuberculosis sanatorium in Switzerland and had returned to Australia at the outbreak of World War II in Europe. He and Officer Brown soon joined forces in the management of the many tuberculosis patients in the Austin Hospital.

> Servicemen who developed pulmonary tuberculosis in Victoria during World War Two were treated in a sanatorium at Bonegilla under the charge of Dr (later Sir Harry) Wunderly who sent an increasing number of these patients to Heidelberg for surgical management... This team of Roche, Orton and Officer Brown made rapid strides in the surgical treatment of pulmonary tuberculosis in Australia... (After 1945), a system of consultation between staff of the Tuberculosis Division of the Victorian Department of Health, consultant physicians and Officer Brown (was instituted). Officer Brown was appointed consultant surgeon to the Tuberculosis Division and he held this appointment for thirty three years and was a foundation member of the National Tuberculosis Advisory council which was established in

1949. The regular consultations held in the various Sanatoria and at the Austin Hospital were of great educational value for the many who came to listen and learn. The first form of anti-tuberculosis chemotherapy, streptomycin, was introduced about this time and increased the number of patients in whom surgery could be of benefit. It was not long before there was a six month waiting list for surgery at the Austin Hospital despite the efforts of four teams ... we must acknowledge today that even had his (Officer Brown's) life's work ceased at this point (the surgery of pulmonary tuberculosis), he would still have been a great man to whom the community owed an enormous debt.[8]

In May 1945 at the annual meeting of the Royal Australasian College of Surgeons, Officer Brown presented a paper on "The Place of Surgery in the Treatment of Pulmonary Tuberculosis".[9] The paper was followed by a discussion in which M.P. Susman (Sydney) H.W. Wunderly (Adelaide) and Hilary Roche (Melbourne) took part.

Officer Brown emphasised the importance of sputum-conversion which greatly improved the patient's prognosis and reduced the risk of infection; without it return to work was unlikely. Artificial pneumothorax (APX) and thoracoplasty had important roles to play in cavity closure and hence sputum-conversion in carefully selected cases. Effective artificial pneumothorax was simple and safe. Of every 100 patients, air could be introduced into the pleural space in only 80 and in only 40 of these would an effective pneumothorax without adhesions be achieved. The complications of pneumolysis (section of adhesions) were empyema, haemorrhage and atelectasis. Of his 148 patients undergoing pneumolysis, 11 developed empyemata and three died. Officer Brown proposed that a two-stage limited thoracoplasty in carefully selected patients was the best means of achieving cavity closure where APX was inapplicable or had failed. The most important complication was spread of tuberculosis to the opposite lung which could be prevented by pre- and post-operative physiotherapy. Officer Brown summed up his experience thus:

> Modern thoracoplasty results in sputum conversion in about 75 per cent of well-selected patients with an operative mortality of less than 5 per cent.

The discussion which followed was led by M.P. Susman who said APX was not "simple and safe". A complicating empyema could be horrendous. Dr H.W. Wunderly reviewed his first 200 patients at Bonegilla Military Hospital; 124 (62 per cent) required some form of collapse therapy. In 104 APX was induced, only in 14 was the pleural space completely free of adhesions. In 13, induction was impossible due to adhesions and of the 90 complicated by adhesions, almost 80 were referred for pneumolysis (surgical section). The final speaker was Dr Hilary Roche who described at length closed suction drainage (Monaldi) which overcame the mechanical factors which tended to keep cavities distended and in addition it removed the caseous lining of the cavity. Roche proceeded to describe the technique of this procedure in which he was obviously experienced. Collapse therapy in various forms was the first specific therapy for tuberculosis which held out any hope to the patient of "a cure" which enabled him or her to return to work. The results were initially poor by our present-day standards; only about one-third of patients recovered sufficiently to return to work. As surgical expertise improved, the results improved and 60 or 70 per cent returned to work. However with the advent of effective chemotherapy in the early 1950s, all forms of collapse therapy fell from favour.

Personal Experience

H. Sloan, (Tuross, South Coast, NSW)

I was diagnosed as having active tuberculosis of the lungs in Melbourne in 1942. The main symptoms were weight loss and drenching night sweats. My general practitioner sent me to a clinic where, in addition to chest X-rays, I was examined in front of a fluorescent screen. No sputum tests were done.

As there was no financial assistance to TB sufferers in those days, my wife and I decided to go to Brisbane and live with my wife's widowed mother. I was then a temporary Commonwealth public servant and I was given extended sick leave. In Brisbane I was advised by a local general practitioner to take three months complete bed rest and I was then allowed up, gradually taking exercise. After 12 months I was well enough to resume work in the Department's Brisbane office. However, within two months my condition worsened and I was sent to Dr Alex Murphy (later Sir Alex) who advised me to have the left lung collapsed by thoracoplasty (1944).

The operation was done at the Brisbane General Hospital in two stages. The first stage was done by Dr Neville Sutton and my only memory of that was considerable post-operative pain. I can remember imploring the nurse to give me more morphine. Later I developed an empyema which required regular drainage through a needle and syringe. This delayed the second stage operation, performed by Dr Lee, which was eventually carried out while the infection was still present in the chest. I don't recall that I had as much pain with the second operation but I do remember waking up and thinking I might not be much longer for this world. I was given blood transfusions and was on the critical list. However, I gradually recovered and after five or six months I was discharged with a drainage tube still in my chest as the empyema was still present.

I resumed work again in 1945 about two and a half years after the initial diagnosis. I must have made a good recovery because in 1946 I was appointed permanently to the Public Service.

In 1959 I attended the Brisbane Chest Clinic for a routine check up. I was admitted to Chermside for a bronchoscopy and active TB was found in the bronchial tube of the collapsed lung. I was then given a course of three drugs, streptomycin, PAS and isoniazid, all the time completely at rest in bed for three months, then allowed up a few weeks prior to discharge. I was encouraged to eat and I put on two stone in weight. I was cleared by the CMO to go back to work after two months at home. About December, 1960 I was promoted to Canberra and have attended the Canberra Chest Clinic each year since, even though I now live down the South Coast.

Looking back over the years I believe I have been fortunate. My only regret is that the drugs which I was given in 1959 were not available when I was first diagnosed in 1942. My bronchial tube and upper spine became displaced and curved and this resulted in repeated chest infections. Since retiring in 1973 I have been able to live in reasonable comfort.

CHAPTER 9

The Rise and Fall of Surgery in Pulmonary Tuberculosis in Australia and New Zealand

Rowan Nicks

The discovery of the tubercle bacillus by Robert Koch in 1882 and the demonstration of the tuberculous lung lesions in the living patient by Konrad Roentgen in 1896, established the essential foundation for the understanding of the disease. Carlo Forlanini introduced artificial pneumothorax to collapse the diseased lung and this method of treatment was being cautiously adopted in Europe by 1910. In Australia it was not in general use until the late 1920s. In Germany Paul Frederick and Ferdinand Sauerbruch introduced thoracoplasty, a surgical method of collapsing the diseased lung, in the first decade of the twentieth century; its introduction here was delayed until the 1930s.

Thomas Fiaschi of Sydney and his colleagues, just prior to World War I, had the vision to introduce Samuel Meltzer's important advances in anaesthesia, using intratracheal insufflation-ventilation of anaesthetic gases; in this way the lungs were kept distended and were prevented from collapsing when the chest wall was opened. This promised to remove the main obstacle to the development of chest surgery in Sydney but his plan was frustrated by his retirement from the staff of Sydney Hospital and the declaration of war in 1914.

Experience of chest wounds in World War I led to the development of chest surgery in Europe and America. Ferdinand Sauerbruch created a chest clinic in Berlin, American surgeons founded the American Association of Thoracic Surgery in 1917 and the British established a centre for thoracic surgery in London where some Australian and New Zealand surgeons trained in the 1930s and brought back an interest in chest surgery. Development of special centres in Australia and New Zealand were hampered by the smallness of the populations, the individualism of leading doctors and the difficulty of organising professional teams on an honorary basis. Problems of chest surgery interested many of the best surgeons in both countries, but the majority inherited a fear of acute respiratory distress and asphyxia which might follow the opening of the chest and they avoided it as a dangerous area.

Maurice Susman, who established chest surgery in the Sydney Hospital, Royal North Shore and Prince of Wales Hospitals, was the pioneer in Sydney. C.J. Officer Brown, of the Alfred and Austin Hospitals, and Hugh Trumble in Melbourne, Konrad Hirschfeld in Queensland, Fred Clark in

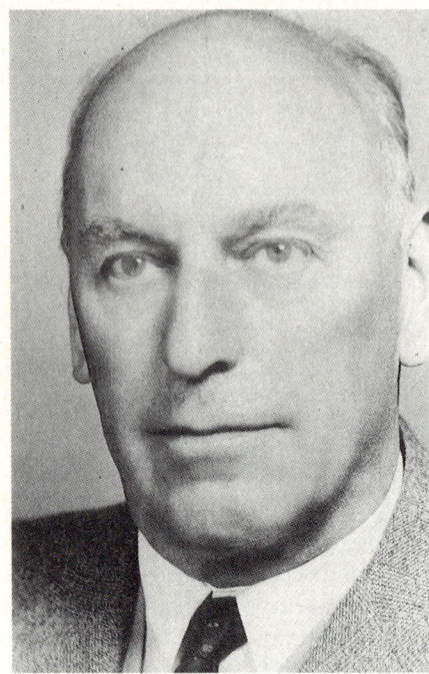

Sir James Officer Brown.
(Photo courtesy of History of Medicine
Library, Royal Australasian College of
Physicians).

Western Australia, Henry Newland and his colleagues in South Australia, and Peter Braithwaite in Tasmania are but some of the pioneer Australian thoracic surgeons. In New Zealand, Sir Douglas Robb in Auckland, Sir Gordon Bell in Dunedin, Eric Luke in Wellington and David Mitchell in Palmerston North were the pioneers.

During the war, civilian thoracic surgery remained dormant for the most part except for C.J. Officer Brown and his colleagues in Melbourne and Douglas Robb in Auckland who both established units and carried out general and tuberculosis thoracic surgery in their clinics. The armed forces in Australia had organised chest units staffed by well trained physicians and surgeons, nursing sisters, scientific personnel and anaesthetic staff. They worked in compact teams at Concord and Heidelberg Hospitals as well as in each combat zone and the New Zealand armed forces were organised likewise. These organisations for military chest patients would be the models for the creation of civilian chest services in Australia and New Zealand after the war.

The flowering of thoracic surgery in the post-war era was due to the summation of several factors, firstly the adoption of the organised unit so successful in the war, led by highly motivated and skilled surgeons and anaesthetists working closely with physicians for a specific goal. The second factor was the mushrooming growth of medical science and technology, advances in surgical and anaesthetic equipment and finally the emergence of specific anti-tuberculosis chemotherapy. The rapid dissemination of advances and experience between surgeons through journals, visiting one another's units and at meetings of the thoracic surgical section of the Royal Australasian College of Surgeons was also important. In this way they persuaded their more conservative colleagues to recognise the new horizons of thoracic surgery.

Establishment of Main Units in Australia and New Zealand

The modern Australian story began with C.J. Officer-Brown, a general surgeon who developed an interest in lung surgery in the 1930s and established the first Australian thoracic surgical unit at the Alfred Hospital in Melbourne. In 1940 he brought Robert Orton to the Austin Hospital as his assistant. In 1941 Officer Brown occupied himself entirely with thoracic surgery at the Alfred, the Austin and the hospital at Heidelberg. He made two important friendships, Paul Gebauer, a young chest surgeon from Cleveland, stationed at the Fourth American Hospital in Melbourne in 1942 and Hilary Roche, a chest physician who was superbly competent to manage pulmonary tuberculosis, having gained a wide experience in Britain, Switzerland and Canada. The unit at the Alfred Hospital was complemented by another established by John Hayward and Ian McConchie at the Royal Melbourne Hospital shortly after the war. This was was built on the work of Edgar King and took on an important teaching and clinical research role.

In 1939 the New South Wales Government established a chest block at the Royal North Shore Hospital with its own operating theatre for surgery of tuberculosis and other chest diseases, and in 1955 the thoracic surgical unit was formally established there with M.P. Susman as surgeon and Ian Monk as assistant surgeon. Maurice Susman had to struggle for recognition for his specialty. He wrote in his retirement that his main difficulty was lack of support mainly from physician colleagues. Ian Monk (1915–78) who took up a post-war appointment as assistant surgeon at the Royal North Shore Hospital in 1948, with subsidiary appointments at Prince Henry Hospital and the Red Cross Hospital, Bodington, contributed greatly to tuberculosis surgery in New South Wales.

St Vincent's Hospital established a 42-bed unit in 1950 with Harry Windsor as surgeon and Geoff McManis as physician working together as a team. Harry was a well trained, ambitious and enthusiastic surgeon with a flair for communication, who had been awarded a Nuffield Scholarship to train in Britain after the war. When he came back to St Vincent's Hospital he was appointed honorary assistant surgeon and surgeon to the Repatriation Hospital, Concord, and to the Anti-Tuberculosis Association of New South Wales. Together with McManis he developed surgery for tuberculosis and other chest diseases and then expanded into the whole field of cardiothoracic surgery.

Russell Godby (1912–69) of the Bodington Red Cross Hospital in the Blue Mountains provided the drive and the physical requirements for developing a vigorous surgical service for tuberculosis where Monk and his colleagues carried out 700 pulmonary resections between 1952 and 1956 with two deaths—an extraordinary achievement.

In Royal Prince Alfred Hospital, in the era of dominant physicians and autocratic general surgeons, surgical specialism was slow to be accepted. John McMahon, a general surgeon interested in chest surgery and an excellent technician, carried out the chest surgical work referred to him by physicians as a part of his large surgical practice. The Chest Clinic was directed by Cotter Harvey whose dominant interest was tuberculosis, and by Maynard Rennie. On return from World War II where he had been a prisoner-of-war, Cotter Harvey led a crusade for the eradication of tuberculosis in Australia. The success attending this great objective was largely due to Cotter Harvey, Earle Page, Harry Wunderly, Darcy Cowan and others. Rowan Nicks from the Green Lane Hospital, Auckland, was appointed surgeon to the newly formed unit in the Page Chest Pavilion in 1957 but by this time the Pavilion, which had been originally built for tuberculosis was being modified to accommodate the cardiothoracic surgical unit and the Hallstrom Institute for Cardiology. Tuberculosis was declining in importance, thoracoplasty was rarely performed and resection for tuberculosis was being phased out. Operations were now confined to specific complications of tuberculosis and cancer of the lung.

The chest unit at the Prince of Wales Hospital, Randwick, which had been a major Repatriation chest centre since World War I, was established as a fully equipped thoracic surgical unit with M.P. Susman in charge. F.W. Ross, who succeeded Susman as surgeon, reported in 1970 that of 173 resections carried out between 1959–63, there had been no deaths and only one patient still had a positive sputum.

In South Australia there had been an interest in thoracic surgery since the time of John Davis Thomas and his work on hydatid disease. Henry Newland (1873–1969) who provided a link with Listerian times developed an interest in chest surgery during World War I. With colleagues he had operated on sporadic chest cases referred to him after the war while Gilbert Brown (1883–1960) developed the anaesthetic service. D'Arcy Sutherland, an ambitious surgeon of singular drive and ability returning from service in the Royal Australian Navy during World War II, established the thoracic surgical unit. He was persuaded by Darcy Cowan (1885–1958), Director of Tuberculosis, to train as a chest surgeon and was awarded a Nuffield Travelling Scholarship. He went to England at the time of the introduction of effective anti-tuberculosis therapy and treatment by resection of the disease under the umbrella of streptomycin and PAS rather than thoracoplasty. With Mary Burnell as his anaesthetist, he developed a full service for tuberculosis chest diseases and then expanded his interest into cardiac surgery as tuberculosis surgery declined.

In Western Australia, Fred Clark (1898–1970), a robust, adventurous, larger-than-life figure, originally from Melbourne, was appointed to the Royal Perth Hospital in 1925. Seeing the need for chest surgery in Western Australia in 1929 he visited Tudor Edwards and Ivan Magill at the Brompton Hospital with his anaesthetist, Gilbert Troop. They started operating on tuberculosis patients in Wooroloo Sanatorium in 1937. In 1945, when a chest unit was formed, he and Archie Simpson, an ex-naval surgeon from Newcastle-upon-Tyne carried out regular sessions in the Royal Perth Hospital on patients who were temporarily transferred from the sanatorium.

In Tasmania, Peter Braithwaite was the pioneer and founder of the unit in the Royal Hobart Hospital. Apart from T.B.C. Muir (1899–1975) the medical superintendent who carried out chest surgery for tuberculosis and other chest diseases during the war years, surgery for tuberculosis was in a parlous state immediately after the war. Returning to Hobart from active service where he had developed an interest in chest surgery and feeling that this was being practised with indifferent success, Braithwaite formed a liaison with his war-time comrades John Hayward and Ian McConchie at the Royal Melbourne Hospital. He was sent to train with them, then appointed to the new Royal Hobart Hospital in 1950.

In Brisbane and Rockhampton, Morgan Windsor did a considerable amount of chest surgery in the 1950s. In the two years 1952–54, 162 surgical procedures were performed on 102 patients; 43 thoracoplasties, 30 lucite plombage, 27 resections mainly lobar and segmental and six Monaldi drainages. In the 27 resections there was no mortality.

In many ways the New Zealand story was similar to that of Australia. Experienced general surgeons with an interest in chest surgery were carrying on chest operations referred to them by chest physicians in the traditional way. The foundations of New Zealand cardiothoracic surgery in Green Lane Hospital and in the Auckland Hospital were roughly contemporaneous and paralleled one another. In Auckland, Chisholm McDowell, a Brompton-trained physician at the Green Lane Infirmary, persuaded Douglas Robb (1897–1974) to carry out chest operations and he was appointed surgeon to the newly formed chest unit in 1942. He was joined by Rowan Nicks in 1947 on his return from service in the Royal Navy and post-war training at the Brompton Hospital. Eric Anson (1893–1969) provided excellent anaesthetic service with Alexander Warnock and Jack Watt as his assistant.

In Dunedin, Sir Gordon Bell carried out sporadic chest operations until after the war when Alan Sutherland established a trained specialist service. John Borrie, who was appointed surgeon when the unit was established in 1950, was the real pioneer of thoracic surgery in the south. In Wellington, Eric Luke and physicians Gilbert McLean and Eardley Button established the service. They were succeeded by James Baird and Timothy Savage. Thoracic surgery in Christchurch was carried out by L.A. Bennett and H.E.H. Denham in the General Hospital and Cashmere Sanatorium until Heath Thompson was appointed to a special unit at the Princess Margaret Hospital.

David Mitchell established a chest unit in Palmerston North in 1930 and was responsible for training a generation of young surgeons including Barratt-Boyes, Jim Baird and Tim Savage.

Personal Recollections

At the time of my appointment to Green Lane Hospital in 1947, patients were apprehensive about thoracopolasty—that "ribbing operation" as one patient put it. In the early 1950s, as confidence grew in chemotherapy, especially when isoniazid was added to streptomycin and PAS as triple therapy, the whole picture changed to one of confidence and hope. There was no longer fear that wounds would not heal after resection or of the disease spreading with surgery. With advanced anaesthesia and the introduction of the drug curare, permitting controlled respiration, resection was safely carried out under an antibiotic umbrella. The wounds healed normally, leaving residual disease in the lungs to be resolved by prolonged chemotherapy. Partial thoracoplasty was reserved now for patients in whom there was scarring in the residual lung and was carried out with the objective of tailoring the pleural cavity to fit the lung and allow normal respiration.

This was a happy era in which surgical teams flourished, surgeons, physicians, resident staff, nurses and all ancillary staff worked together inspired by a common goal and patients were grateful for their skill and kindness. One cannot help reflecting that this related to the warm personalities involved and the spirit of co-operation built up in the armed forces. When it became clear that the drugs killed the bacteria and actually cured tuberculosis and that this could be done in the vast majority of patients without operation, surgery was phased out except to deal with specific complications, including life-threatening haemoptyses or infection and the complication of cancer. Surgeons now directed their energy, skill and team spirit acquired during these years working among patients with apparently hopeless tuberculosis, to developing a service for general chest, oesophageal and modern cardiovascular surgery.

Recollections of the Surgery of Tuberculosis

Peter Braithwaite

I had been Regimental Medical Officer of the 2/12 Battalion AIF from 1939-42, then Surgeon 104 Australian CCS for the rest of the war. In 1945, I became surgical registrar of the Royal Hobart Hospital, then surgeon superintendent until 1948. During this time I had six months study leave in Melbourne. My interest was aroused by a series of pathology slides shown by Edgar King, when I realised that these pathological lungs were operation specimens.

In 1948 the Royal Hobart Hospital advertised for a trainee in thoracic surgery who would later take up full-time or part- time employment at the hospital. I applied, was appointed and spent 1949 with John Hayward and Ian McConchie at the Royal Melbourne, Heidelberg and the Austin Hospitals, as well as weekly meetings with Jim (later Sir James) Officer Brown who had under his wing two other trainees, Morgan Windsor and Ken Morris.

My training was financed through the Department of Tuberculosis. The instigator was Harry Wunderly, the Commonwealth Director of Tuberculosis, who was determined to get the surgery of tuberculosis off the ground in Australia. I returned to Hobart at the end of 1949 and took up my appointment. At that time (1950) the state of play was:

- Brisbane: Konrad Hirschfeld and Morgan Windsor
- Sydney: Mick Susman and Ian Monk at North Shore, Harry Windsor at St Vincent's and Repatriation;
- Melbourne: John Hayward and Ian McConchie at Royal Melbourne, Austin and Repatriation, Jim Officer Brown and Ken Morris at the Alfred and the Austin where we all met weekly;
- Adelaide: D'arcy Sutherland
- Perth: Fred Clark;
- Hobart: Peter Braithwaite

I was the only one who had not been to the Brompton. We were a small group, most of us had started surgery during the war or just after. We were all learning, all teaching one another, "writing the book". Overseas experience gained by one would be shared with the others.

In Sydney Hospital in 1951, during a meeting of the College of Surgeons a Thoracic Section of the College was formed and the following year in Melbourne, fourteen of us, together with Bob Shaw from Texas, met behind locked doors round the council table in the college headquarters and had the first and perhaps the most famous of our "confession sessions". In turn round the table each member had to confess the biggest mess he had made of anything since our last meeting. How we vied with one another; what friendship, what honesty!

Selection of cases for surgery was very similar in all states. There would be regular conferences, mostly weekly, between physicians, surgeons and radiologists, where cases were presented, discussed and the type of surgery decided. Initially, the type of interference suggested was designed to assist a tuberculous abscess cavity in the lung to heal by allowing it to relax, by pneumothorax or thorocoplasty. This had been the traditional surgical approach. Cases at these conferences were put up for thoracoplasty. Some of us felt that resection of the affected part would be more certain of sputum-conversion and would conserve good healthy functioning lung. Antibiotics and modern anaesthesia allowed us to undertake resection.

At first, cases considered suitable had disease confined to a single lobe or a whole lung, then gradually more and more complex multiple segmental resections were undertaken.

In Tasmania, the Director of Tuberculosis, Dr Tommy Goddard, had introduced compulsory mass X-ray which found the cases, picked up early operable cancer and helped deal with hydatid disease. This made the work load heavy and regular. When a case of tuberculosis was tentatively selected for future surgery, the name was put in a slot as far as six months ahead. Sometimes the patient had improved enough to avoid surgery when his time came.

If a case was bilateral, the worst side was operated on first. The other side always improved, sometimes enough to avoid operation. Morale of patients and relatives underwent a remarkable change from initial apprehension to grateful acceptance. Typical were the reactions of Frances and Ivy.

Frances had been in bed until a few days after her operation when I told her she could get up now. She was pretty startled. She'd been in bed four years and thought she was there for life. Poor Ivy had had a bad time for years. I asked her if she would like an operation. "Oh, could I doctor? I thought I was just waiting to die".

In Tasmania, the population numbered half a million, were easily accessible and we had mass chest X-ray. One surgeon to half-a-million was a better proportion than the other states had. It was not surprising then that when I left for a College of Surgeons meeting in New Zealand in 1956, there were only two patients awaiting operation for tuberculosis in the state.

Of course, there were more to come but the back had been broken.

The Training of a Thoracic Surgeon in Australia 1953-56

Lindsay Grigg

In 1947, as a third-year medical student, I was fired by a challenge in a speech by that great British surgeon, Sir Gordon Gordon-Taylor, that thoracic surgery was the frontier of exploration for advancement in surgery.

The following year, at the Royal Melbourne Hospital, I saw John Hayward repair a diaphragmatic hernia caused by a motor vehicle accident and, so help me, my career was determined. I saw cardiothoracic surgery as demanding the most consistent combination of applied anatomy and physiology of any branch of surgery, an assessment I have never had cause to retract. No-one could have predicted the path along which this challenge would lead me and I had no true appreciation at the time of the momentous advances which even then were just beginning to stir. Endotracheal anaesthesia, blood transfusion, dissection lobectomy and pneumonectomy together with the World War II experience of chest trauma (including cardiac injury) were now combined with antibiotics and, perhaps of paramount importance, relaxant anaesthesia to make thoracic surgery remarkably safe. As I graduated, streptomycin became available. During my second post-graduate year, Russell Howard successfully repaired his first tracheo- oesophageal fistula whilst I was a resident medical officer at the old Children's Hospital in Melbourne. In 1953 I was plunged into the thick of things as medical officer to John Hayward and Ian McConchie in the thoracic surgery unit at the Repatriation General Hospital, Heidelberg.

The work was predominantly tuberculosis, bronchiectasis and lung cancer; it was demanding, tiring and often bloody. But these years were a watershed. In 1953–54 I learned bronchoscopy—the real thing, rigid bronchoscope and local anaesthesia—the management of artificial pneumothorax and empyema and long-term chest drainage, but above all the day-to-day ward work and the interpretation of chest X-rays. I could scarcely have had better mentors—my surgical chiefs, ably backed by Nairn Elder, Doug Gauld, Tammy Steele and Alastair Campbell. So often, situations were only truly appreciated in retrospect. The Friday chest meeting discussed management of individual patients, particularly assessment for and later the results of surgery. Debate was keen, occasionally acrimonious, but these were men forging whole new systems of management as streptomycin, PAS, isoniazid and the new antibiotics dramatically changed the character of lung disease. Artificial pneumothorax rapidly gave way to thoracoplasty. In the wards there was the continued dedicated pragmatism and skill of nurses like the indomitable Gina Hayes and physiotherapists like Peg Gooden. But the watch-word was team-work under chiefs who were demanding taskmasters but nevertheless exercised a constant concern for their staff. Neither John Hayward nor Ian McConchie permitted us to start a long operating session without leaving the main hospital building and having a decent meal in the mess, the walk in the open air being part of the protective therapy. Both were superb teachers, Ian, laconic, dry and brilliant; John, dogmatic, master of the Socratic method and equally brilliant. One could not but learn. All his nicknames were variants of Jack, but he appeared to love "Coronary Jack". For all his foibles, including calculated tantrums, he loved to point out that his systolic pressure had never been recorded above 120.

I left the unit for 18 months while I completed my FRACS, yet that was long enough (1955–56) for the face of the surgical treatment of pulmonary tuberculosis to change almost beyond recognition. Artificial pneumothorax was virtually of historic interest, even surgical collapse therapy was becoming rare—who could possibly regret the passing of having to haul on the scapula during a first-stage thoracoplasty?—and segmental resection and the removal of isolated tuberculomas had become the order of the day. Bronchography was of increasing importance in both tuberculosis and bronchiectasis, in order to define the precise bronchial anatomy and permit accurate dissection. The lobe or lung, hilum encased in a fibrous cuirasse like reinforced concrete, was becoming a thing of the past as drugs halted the infection process more effectively.

I will close with a final reference to pulmonary tuberculosis. Rampant acute pulmonary tuberculosis, sometimes complicated by haemoptysis, still occurs in our community, chiefly amongst migrants. It is not sufficient to hope to be able to cope with these problems de novo. No chest surgeon or physician can now hope to obtain the tuberculosis experience of our pioneers. We need to ensure that they have at least read what these remarkable doctors achieved and to learn the principles they derived from their experience. There is an urgent need once more to stress the basic pathology and the natural history of the disease if the work of our pioneers is not to have been in vain.

Sir Douglas Robb: a Brief Biography
Athol Wells

During the decades after the First World War, surgery for tuberculosis in New Zealand came into its own, as it had elsewhere in the Western world. In the 1920s, artificial pneumothoraces began to be induced in hospitals throughout the nation. In the latter part of the decade, phrenic nerve interruption was increasingly performed and by 1932 extrapleural thoracoplasty was a well-recognised part of the surgical armamentarium. In the 1930s, the indications for these procedures were refined but there were no further important developments until resection surgery was attempted at Green Lane Hospital by Douglas Robb.

Every great venture has small beginnings: the present site of Green Lane Hospital was occupied from 1890 by "The Costley Home for the Aged Poor". In 1914, open-air shelters for tuberculosis patients were added and the complex was renamed "The Auckland Infirmary". Further shelters were built regularly and care of these patients became an important function of the institution. In 1933, Dr Chisolm McDowell was appointed as visiting medical tuberculosis officer and modernised the approach to treatment. In particular, the induction of pneumothoraces became commonplace.

In 1938, six new wards were built at the infirmary to relieve overcrowding at Auckland Hospital and shortly afterwards it was decided to integrate these into a general hospital. In 1943, Green Lane Hospital was formally opened by Peter Fraser, the New Zealand Prime Minister. The advances in tuberculosis surgery had not been lost on the medical establishment. McDowell had urged the hospital board to appoint G.D. Robb as the first senior surgeon to the newly formed Thoracic Surgical Unit in 1942. Even before the new hospital was opened, the infirmary lounge had been converted to a makeshift theatre.

Douglas Robb (1899–1974) was later regarded by many as New Zealand's first medical statesman and was to play a leading role in the evolution of Green Lane Hospital as a centre of surgical excellence. He was born in Auckland shortly after his Scottish parents had emigrated, and was educated at the Auckland Grammar School where he attained second place in the New Zealand Junior University Scholarship Examination. His experiences in childhood imbued him with a stern self-discipline and a strong sense that matters of principle were of greater importance than financial or social success, a perspective that he never abandoned during a long and sometimes stormy career. After graduating from the Otago Medical School in 1922, he became an anatomy demonstrator and then a house-surgeon at Auckland Hospital. In his final year as a medical student, he contracted a tuberculous pleuritis and this recurred during his post-graduate training in England (1923–1928) and again after this return to Auckland. He was in poor health for much of the time but this did not prevent his passing the FRCS examination in 1926 and working as senior resident at the East Suffolk and Ipswich Hospital until his departure for New Zealand.

In 1928, he started in private practice in Auckland, and, from 1929 to 1935, he served two terms as an assistant surgeon at Auckland Public Hospital. At the end of this period he was dropped from the hospital staff and was not reappointed when positions were reviewed. During the previous six years, he had antagonised the hospital board and some of his surgical colleagues by an uncompromising pursuit of excellence. He had audited techniques used in cancer surgery at Auckland Hospital and had graded and openly criticised his seniors. This was bitterly resented and did nothing to rally support for his reappointment in 1935. His position was weakened further when he admitted authorship of a series of exceedingly scathing articles attacking the Auckland Hospital Board, published anonymously in *The New Zealand Herald*. In his defence, he was later to say that:

at almost every stage I was naive enough to think, for much longer than anyone else did, that I had been rather a helpful fellow, who had at least come up with some ideas.

He regarded the era as:

one of rather naked personal power politics, in which considerations of medical progress were by no means uppermost...

Throughout this period Robb remained unwell. In 1935, immediately after his marriage, he developed cavitation of his right lung; this persuaded him to undertake a sea-voyage to England. While in London he worked for several months at the Brompton Hospital; this, his first experience of thoracic surgery, was to enable him to perform a small series of thoracoplasties for tuberculosis over the next few years. However his time at the Brompton was cut short by the recurrence of his symptoms; these were not controlled by phrenic nerve interruption. The following year, after his return to New Zealand, arrangements were made for him to undergo a thoracoplasty in Sydney but in the interval his symptoms settled, never to return.

These various setbacks had prevented Robb from establishing himself in the forefront of his profession. Ironically, however, they led indirectly to the great triumphs of his later years. The refusal of the Auckland Hospital Board to employ him left him free to take up the position of senior surgeon to the newly formed Thoracic Surgical Unit in 1942, a year before Green Lane Hospital was opened. This was to be the turning point of his professional life.

However Robb had one further obstacle to overcome before embarking confidently upon thoracic surgery. His practical experience in this field amounted to a few thoracoplasties performed in the 1930s and the observation of various procedures at the Brompton Hospital. This had not prepared him for the technical difficulties of his new specialty. Fortunately he had a very capable colleague. As well as training as a physician, Chisolm McDowell had assisted the great English surgeon, Tudor Edwards, in thoracic procedures performed at the Brompton in the late 1920s and early 1930s. His guidance while assisting in theatre, during the early years of the Thoracic Surgical Unit, allowed Robb to attempt procedures that lay outside his repertoire. On at least one occasion, during a severe pulmonary artery haemorrhage in theatre, McDowell's immediate practical assistance averted disaster.

As Robb himself was to recall, "those were days of great endeavour, of anxiety, and of advance into what was to us pretty new territory. I had not been abroad to see work of this sort since 1936 and much of it was new; a great deal therefore had to be surmised, gleaned from journals, and worked out by ourselves on the spot".

The earliest resectional surgery at Green Lane Hospital was entirely in keeping with this vital and innovative approach. Over the previous decade, resectional procedures for tuberculosis had been reported only sporadically in the medical literature. Until the celebrated Massachusetts series of 1943 (Churchill & Klopstock) the result had been uniformly discouraging. Robb, however, was not deterred.

The first resectional surgery for tuberculosis in New Zealand was performed in December 1944. A 19 year-old woman had had major lung haemorrhages during the previous year, associated with loss of volume and cavitation of the right lower lobe. The procedure, a right lower lobectomy, was uncomplicated and the patient remained well during the next six months. However a bilateral apical infiltrate then appeared and the disease progressed rapidly until death, almost a year after the surgery.

The second case had a happier outcome. A 27 year-old man was found to have a tight tuberculous stenosis of the left main bronchus, resulting in copious sputum production. The disease was confined radiologically to the left lung, which was extensively involved. A left pneumonectomy was performed. Twelve months later, no relapse had occurred; no details survive of longer-term progress.

Three further resections were undertaken early in 1945. A woman aged 26 underwent a left pneumonectomy for a tuberculous left main stem bronchial stenosis with extensive involvement of the lung; she survived for only four months. A left pneumonectomy was carried out on a 32 year-old woman with upper lobe atelectasis and involvement of the left main stem bronchus. The patient died of staphylococcal infection 22 days after the procedure. A fifth patient underwent a left lower lobectomy and lingulectomy for tuberculous bronchiectasis; active tuberculosis was confirmed in the resected material. The post-operative period was uneventful; details of further progress are not recorded.

As with early resection surgery elsewhere, these results gave rise to considerable misgivings. Three of the five patients had perished within 12 months of surgery. While it might be argued that these patients had advanced disease and were unlikely to survive with conservative treatment, the outcome was extremely disappointing. Perhaps as a result, no further resectional surgery was attempted until 1947, by which time favourable results had been reported in several large series. Candidates for surgery were accepted only after consideration by a "Combined Chest Committee", which included Robb, McDowell, Dr John Hinds (chest physician) and Mr Rowan Nicks (appointed as thoracic surgeon in 1947). Resection was confined to those complicated cases unsuited to simple collapse measures; the committee believed that resection was unjustifiable in cases suitable for thoracoplasty.

As reported by Nicks[4],between 1947 and 1951, 33 lobectomies were performed for tuberculosis. Eleven of these followed unsuccessful thoracoplasties, nine were for lower lobe cavities. Other indications comprised bronchiectasis (5), contralateral fibrosis and thoracoplasty (3), tension cavity (2), tuberculoma (2) and tuberculous cyst with asthma (1). Four patients died 2–5 years after the procedure, three of them as a result of tuberculous empyema from bronchopleural fistulae. Sputum-positivity had persisted in one instance. However 28 of 33 patients (84 per cent) were free of disease, 2–6 years later.

Over the same period, 31 pneumonectomies were completed for bronchostenosis (14), failed thoracoplasty (6), bronchiectasis (5), empyema (2), residual disease and empyema following lobectomy (2) and destroyed lung (2). Five patients (16 per cent) died two to six years following surgery. Two remained sputum positive after surgery, but in 24 (77 per cent) the disease remained quiescent. In four cases, segmental resection was performed, with or without a concurrent lobectomy. One was complicated by a bronchopleural fistula requiring lobectomy, but there were no deaths and all became sputum negative. Segmentectomy was not routinely performed at Green Lane Hospital, except when the disease was very well encapsulated. The higher risk of a bronchopleural fistula was regarded by the committee as unacceptably hazardous. Overall, a bronchopleural fistula (resulting in empyema and, often, in spread to the other lung) was responsible for over half of the post-operative deaths. From 1947 to 1949, the hemi-thorax was not collapsed at pneumonectomy; thereafter, a limited thoracoplasty (with removal of segments of three to seven ribs) was completed at resection. Nicks attributes the absence of late post-operative empyema in 1950 and 1951 to this precaution.

Plainly the routine use of streptomycin (available in New Zealand from 1948 onwards) and, later, PAS and isonicotinic acid, also reduced the risk of post-operative recurrence; 82 percent (56 of 68) of patients were clinically and radiologically free of disease, 2–6 years after a resection procedure. A mortality, over this period, of 13 per cent (9 of 68) represented a considerable advance over the 25 per cent mortality recorded in resection series before 1947.

After 1951, Robb took little further part in resection surgery for tuberculosis. As was the case elsewhere in the Western world, these procedures were performed at Green Lane Hospital throughout the 1950s, but less frequently, as anti-tuberculosis chemotherapy became more effective. Sadly, no detailed account of this period survives. For Robb, the spotlight had shifted to cardiac surgery, the field in which his greatest contributions were made.

Robb played little part in the surgical advances of the early 1960s (carried through by Brian Barratt-Boyes and David Cole) and in 1964 retired from Green Land Hospital; the final years of his career were marked with public distinction. In 1960 he was made a Knight Batchelor for services to surgery, university education, the Medical Council of New Zealand and the New Zealand Medical Research Council. Later that year, he was elected to the Presidency of the British Medical Association for a two year term. Among his other offices in the 1960s, he served as Chancellor of Auckland University, Chairman of the Medical Council of New Zealand, and the Sir Arthur Sims Commonwealth travelling professor. He also played a leading role in persuading the government that the second medical school in New Zealand should be sited in Auckland.

Robb remained fully active until his sudden death in 1974, aged 75. Well before the end of his career, he had achieved widespread recognition as a driving force behind medical reform. In his many writings, and throughout his life, he remained a champion of the underdog and a trenchant critic of the second-rate. This did not always endear him to the medical establishment, especially during his early career. Diplomacy was not among his gifts and he was ever impatient of the misuse of influence and status. In the end, however, his achievements in surgery, in medical education and in public life spoke for themselves. Perhaps no medical man of his era did more to change the shape of New Zealand medicine.

CHAPTER 10

The Chemotherapy Revolution of the 1950s

A.J. Proust

Many chemical agents came into vogue in the treatment of tuberculosis and were then discarded in the first half of the 20th century—iodide salts, creosote, copper and mercurial compounds. Creosote preparations for tuberculosis were still on the shelves of the hospital pharmacy of Royal Prince Alfred in Sydney in 1948. The most serious contender for efficacy was sanocrysin, a double thiocyanate of gold and sodium. It was administered in variable doses by the intravenous route; side effects were common, often serious and occasionally fatal. After being in use for ten years, Amberson in the United States mounted a controlled clinical trial which showed no evidence of efficacy and much evidence of serious side effects. Even so sanocrysin faded into disuse only slowly.

Rich reported that sulphonilamide exerted a weak inhibitory effect on the tubercle bacillus in the laboratory in 1938. This heralded the exciting era of effective chemotherapy.

Selman Waksman,[1] originally a biochemist and later professor of soil microbiology at Rutgers University in New Jersey isolated actinomycinin 1940 and streptothricin in 1942. In 1944 he isolated streptomycin from two strains of actinomyces. Waksman enlisted the help of Professor W.H. Feldman a pathologist and Dr. H.C. Henshaw a physician at the Mayo Clinic to do the essential animal laboratory work and late in 1944—the same year as its discovery—Feldman and Henshaw reported that streptomycin was well-tolerated by guinea-pigs and exerted a "strikingly suppressive effect on the pathogenic proclivities of the human variety of *M. tuberculosis*". By September 1945 a limited clinical trial in 34 patients, using low doses of streptomycin, showed a suppressive but not rapidly bactericidal effect. A large co-operative trial by Waksman, the Mayo Clinic, the Veterans Administration and the American Trudeau Society concluded in 1947 that streptomycin was able to eradicate tuberculosis under some conditions in guinea-pigs, its efficacy in human tuberculosis was promising, that drug resistant strains emerged quickly thus limiting its long-term use, and both vestibular and auditory functions of the 8th cranial nerve suffered toxic effects. This progress in just over three years from discovery was remarkable. Undoubtedly a major advance had been made in the treatment of tuberculosis in humans.

In the United Kingdom the Medical Research Council sought supplies of streptomycin even before the multi-centre trial results were reported in the United States. The Medical Research Council trial was meticulously planned and set the standard world-wide for chemotherapy trials of anti-tuberculosis drugs. The first MRC trial was reported in October 1948 and demonstrated marked clinical improvement within the first three months, however relapse and drug resistant organisms commonly occurred at six and nine months. Streptomycin was shown to be life-saving in tuberculous meningitis and miliary tuberculosis.

The companion drug sought by both American and British investigators was actually known, para-amino salicylic acid (PAS); it had been shown in 1944 to be weakly bacteriostatic against the tubercle bacillus but had been overlooked during the excitement engendered by streptomycin. In 1949 the MRC began the first of its classical controlled trials, comparing a streptomycin-treated group against a PAS-treated group and a streptomycin and PAS group. This trial showed conclusively that the combination of streptomycin and PAS when the latter was used in high dosage prevented the emergence of resistant organisms and allowed longer and more effective regimens to be used. By almost eliminating endobronchial tuberculosis, the two-drug regimen lowered dramatically the complication of broncho-pleural fistula following resection for tuberculosis.

In 1949 J. Bell Ferguson, V.G. Bristow and P.R. Bull summarised the results of tests in Victoria in an article, "Streptomycin in Tuberculosis".[2] In August 1947 the Victorian government made available a sum of £5,000 for the purchase of streptomycin. The first supplies were used at the Austin Hospital but later limited quantities were made available to Gresswell, Greenvale and Heatherton sanatoria. A total of 43 patients, carefully selected by a group of consultants, were treated at the Austin and a further 70 patients at sanatoria and chalets throughout the state.

> The results were striking; 81 (72 per cent) improved radiologically and 90 (80 per cent) improved clinically. Of the 43 patients treated at the Austin Hospital, 34 (79 per cent) maintained improvement and the remaining 9 relapsed (3 died). Streptomycin was used successfully in 19 patients in preparation for surgery.

The authors concluded that:

> streptoymcin does not and should not be expected to replace the well-tried methods of bed rest and the various well-tried procedures of collapse therapy. Rest is still the keystone of successful treatment of tuberculosis.

Dr R. Munro Ford[3] reported from Adelaide six cases of pulmonary tuberculosis treated with streptomycin 0.5g to 1.0g daily for 8–12 weeks There was some clinical improvement but bacteriological conversion did not occur.

In 1952 a simple chemical agent burst dramatically on the already fast moving tuberculosis scene. Isonicotinic acid hydrazide (isoniazid) was developed in the laboratories of Hoffman–La Roche in Basel, Switzerland. In 1950 and in January 1952 its anti-tuberculosis activity in man was reported from Sea View Tuberculosis Hospital in New York by Robitzek, Selikoff and Ornstein. In October 1952 Proust and Beacham reported in the *Bulletin of the School of Medicine,* University of Maryland,[4] its use in 20 patients with pulmonary tuberculosis at Baltimore City Hospitals in the United States. Only one of the patients failed to respond to streptomycin and PAS, and the others improved clinically, with reduced cough, sputum production and fever. Ten of the 20 were smear-negative after 3 months; however only 5 showed radiological improvement. Emergence of isoniazid resistant bacilli occurred in about 50 per cent of those who were still sputum-positive at 3 to 4 months.

The first report of isoniazid in the *Medical Journal of Australia* was in the correspondence columns (February 1953). Proust[5] described his observations of four cases of tuberculous meningitis and miliary tuberculosis in Johns Hopkins Hospital, Baltimore. All were critically ill despite streptomycin intramuscularly and intrathecally and PAS orally. Within a few days of oral isoniazid, all four patients became afebrile and showed marked clinical improvement.

Early in 1953, Proust, Beacham and Allen reported further on their experience with isoniazid, PAS and streptomycin.[6] Then, in Spetember 1953, Dr R. Munro Ford[7] reported on 25 patients treated at the Morris Hospital, Adelaide; 22 received isoniazid and PAS and 3 isoniazid and streptomycin; their progress was reviewed at 3 and 6 months. He reported that:

> improvement occurred during the first few weeks and this was maintained for the next two months but after three months 14 of the 22 patients on isoniazid and PAS and 2 of the 3 patients on streptomycin and isoniazid relapsed to their original state.

Of the 25 patients, 21 were smear-positive initially and at six months 16 of the 21 were still sputum positive, all the cultures showing resistance to isoniazid. In his summary Dr. Munro Ford wrote in part

> it appears that PAS at least is incapable of preventing the emergence of strains of isoniazid resistant tubercle bacilli especially in the presence of chronic cavitary pulmonary disease in patients who have received previous chemotherapy.

Heyworth and Nobbs[8] reviewed 800 cases of tuberculosis notified in Queensland and treated in 1958 and followed up five years later. As a general rule these patients had been admitted to hospital for three months of triple chemotherapy and then continued with dual chemotherapy for a total duration of two years. About 9 per cent required some additional surgical treatment; 40 of the 70 patients had surgical resection of some type, nearly always segmental resection or lobectomy. The remaining 30 had collapse therapy, usually artificial pneumothorax or pneumoperitoneum; only four required thoracoplasty. (All forms of collapse therapy had been abandoned by 1967 in Queensland and resections had also become rare). The results of the 1958 treatment regimens were excellent; 67 per cent were free of active disease at five years, only 3 per cent had relapsed, 21 per cent were dead (only one quarter due to their tuberculosis) and 9 per cent lost to follow-up. The majority of relapses were due to lack of compliance on the part of the patient; in most cases the regimen prescribed was adequate but was taken irregularly by the patient; in some cases irregular drug-taking was associated with alcoholism.

From this review one may assume that by 1958, in Queensland, triple chemotherapy (streptomycin, PAS and isoniazid) was prescribed for all newly-diagnosed cases for at least the first three months and two-drug chemotherapy was then prescribed for a total duration of two years. The drugs were given in single daily doses.

In 1967 Bayliss[9] summed up how he viewed the role of surgery in pulmonary tuberculosis:

> For patients in whom the organisms are sensitive (to first line drugs), surgery should not be necessary—the question of surgery could arise in the few patients in whom the organisms are resistant to all three first line drugs—there is also the occasional patient on whom surgery is performed for reasons not strictly medical.

By 1965 triple chemotherapy was achieving 90 per cent "cure-rates" two years after treatment had ceased. However of these three drugs, one was definitely the poor relation—PAS. Streptomycin was, after all, administered only for three or four months; PAS along with isoniazid was usually self-administered for the second stage of 21 months. Isoniazid was no problem either to patients or doctors. PAS on the other hand was never popular with either. The dose was large and unpleasant to swallow; indigestion and hypersensitivity reactions were common and it required great patience, perserverence and time on the part of physicians, nurses and above all patients to complete a course of PAS without serious interruption. In many cases, perhaps as many as 40 per cent, chemotherapy was less than ideal because of failure on the part of the patient to co-operate and of the physician to secure that co-operation in self-medication with PAS in the second stage of chemotherapy.

In July 1968 the first edition of the *Treatment of Tuberculosis with particular reference to Chemotherapy* was published by the Commonwealth Department of Health incorporating the recommendations of the National Tuberculosis Advisory Council. The introduction read as follows:

> These recommendations on treatment are intended for Australian conditions and assume the free availability of drugs and other treatment facilities. Under these conditions a 100 per cent conversion to negative bacteriology should be the target. The recommendations... are intended as a guide and are not to limit the treatment of the individual case.

The principles of treatment in 1968 as recommended by the advisory council included admission to hospital in all cases for assessment and the first phase of chemotherapy; the drugs recommended as "first line" were streptomycin, isoniazid and PAS, all of which were administered for the first 3 months or longer until conversion occurred; isoniazid and PAS were then continued during the second phase for the remainder of the two-year period. Treatment should be based on sensitivity testing and advice was tendered on handling "slow responders", "chronic positives" and those with drug-resistant disease. Close supervision of drug taking was stressed; reference was made to fully supervised intermittent chemotherapy for unreliable patients, such as alcoholics.

The treatment document as it was called was only about 1,500 words in length; when read more than 20 years later it is still highly relevant. It was so successful that it was reprinted and was soon followed by much more detailed booklets.

Soon after the first treatment document appeared, ethambutol began to displace PAS as the companion drug to streptomycin and isoniazid. Ethambutol is primarily bacteriostatic or at most only weakly bactericidal; however it is well tolerated and preferred by patients to PAS. It is also a useful drug in drug resistant tuberculosis.

In 1957 a new strain of streptomyces (*S. mediterranei*) was isolated from a soil sample by Sensi in Italy. The culture showed high bactericidal activity against Gram-positive and some Gram-negative bacteria and also against *M. tuberculosis*. The crude active product was called rifamycin and six years elapsed before a derivative of rifamycin SV was shown to be highly active against mycobacteria and capable of sustained serum levels in man after oral administration, hence suitable for clinical trials in human tuberculosis. It was given the name of rifampicin (rifampin in the United States).

Limited clinical trials of regimens containing rifampicin began in Europe in 1966, however there had been a poverty of long term clinical trial reports and in addition there had been conflicting reports about the possible hepatotoxicity of rifampicin. After the 20th meeting in Canberra of the National Tuberculosis Advisory Council in June 1969, a closely co-ordinated multicentre Australian trial was undertaken. The protocol was prepared in July 1969 and the first patient entered the trial on 5 August and the final patient was admitted on 20 February 1970. The first paper which concentrated on assessing the hepatotoxicity of rifampicin was published by Proust in July 1971[10]. Among the 54 patients in the trial and an additional 226 patients treated with a rifampicin regimen by the same physicians, about 3 per cent of the patients developed evidence of toxic hepatitis and an additional 11 per cent evidence of abnormal liver function which did not interfere with treatment. The author concluded:

It is considered in retrospect that the incidence of such side effects could have been materially reduced by more careful patient selection, by reducing the dosage of rifampicin and by paying close attention to any complaint by the patient of anorexia or nausea.

It appeared that in the context of the patient selection criteria for the Australian trial, the incidence of hepatic toxic effects was acceptable. The inference was that when the patient complained of even mild dyspepsia, a temporary lowering of the dose of rifampicin would often obviate more serious side effects.

A second report which evaluated the clinical, bacteriological and radiological response, was published in October 1972 by Proust and Evans[11]. This evaluated the therapeutic efficacy of the rifampicin containing regimen. The regimen achieved a 100 per cent conversion rate in disease due to *M. tuberculosis* sensitive to all three drugs; where the *M. tuberculosis* was resistant to at least two of the standard first line drugs, rifampicin combined with at least one other effective drug achieved bacteriological conversion in 93 per cent of 29 patients; a conversion rate of over 40 per cent was achieved in 22 patients with disease due to atypical mycobacteria.

The results of the Australian rifampicin trial were well-received; the planning, the protocol and co-ordination of physicians and chest clinics right across Australia was of high quality and the results were well presented and promptly reported.

In 1973, O'Connell, Campbell, Cowen and Verins published another important paper on the treatment of tuberculosis with rifampicin[12] . The previous clinical trials of rifampicin concentrated on cases of drug resistant disease or treatment failures from other regimens; most new antibiotics and chemotherapeutic agents are used on such cases. Such trials do not necessarily require controls; if the new drug is effective where older drugs have failed then the new drug proves its efficacy. However a trial comparing a new drug-containing regimen with an established regimen in the treatment of newly diagnosed disease is of great value. Regimen one consisted of rifampicin, isoniazid and ethambutol and regimen two contained the well-established and proven streptomycin-isoniazid-PAS. After three months regimen one was reduced to rifampicin-isoniazid and regimen two to PAS-isoniazid. Twenty five patients entered regimen one and 23 regimen two. There were no significant differences between the groups in regard to age, sex or severity of disease. Regression analysis showed a significantly more rapid conversion of sputum cultures in regimen one. Significantly more toxic effects were noted in regimen two from which eight patients were withdrawn as against only one in regimen one.

This trial was significant because it indicated that regimens containing rifampicin had converted in a significantly shorter period than the standard regimen. But even more importantly the regimen one was accompanied by a much lower incidence of side effects than regimen two. This trial did much to hasten the phasing out of PAS in Australia as a first- or even second-line drug.

The rifampicin trials sharpened the clinical acumen of participating Australian thoracic physicians especially with regard to observing and reporting the side effects of anti- tuberculosis drugs. In retrospect one rare but potentially fatal hypersensitivity reaction to rifampicin was overlooked in the trial. One patient among the seven who died during the trial was reported as dying from "acute gastroenteritis and renal failure". The patient was well enough to be travelling on holiday when the sudden completely unexpected collapse occurred followed by death. Autopsy could not be arranged; the death was almost certainly due to the then unreported hypersensitivity renal syndrome.

While no instance of thrombocytopenia was reported during the two-year trial, the mechanism of reporting side effects remained in place for several years and by 1975, six cases of rifampicin-induced thrombocytopenia with one death were reported among the estimated 3,000 Australian patients treated with rifampicin up to July 1975. In July 1970 a case of rifampicin-induced thrombocytopenia was reported in England and in December 1971 the first report of thrombocytopenia in Australia was received at the Tuberculosis Division of the Department of Health. During the period 1971–75 another four cases of thrombocytopenia were reported and one case of purpura without thrombocytopenia. The cases were predominantly female (five female and one male), the usual companion drugs were isoniazid and ethambutol and in all cases there were premonitory symptoms of drug intolerance or hypersensitivity reactions, especially nausea and fever.

In an effort to reduce the incidence of the serious adverse reaction to rifampicin the following recommendations were made:

1. The daily dose should not exceed 10mg per kg of body weight.

2. The concurrent use of other drugs capable of affecting the bone marrow (including methyldopa, tolbutamide and frusemide) and should be avoided if possible.

3. Careful note should be taken immediately of any symptoms of drug intolerance or hypersensitivity. The dose of rifampicin should be halved or ceased until all symptoms have disappeared and the dose then restored cautiously.

The incidence of purpura and/or thrombocytopenia fell from six cases during 1971–75 to one case (purpura without thrombocytopenia) during 1977–80.

The principal advances in chemotherapy in Australia during the 1980s have involved the widespread adoption of short-course chemotherapy and the selective use of fully supervised intermittent chemotherapy.

Maurice Joseph was an early proponent of short-course chemotherapy. In a letter to the National Tuberculosis Advisory Council dated 17.6.75 he wrote::

> I submit we are about to witness... the introduction of short course chemotherapy made possible by the discovery in 1967 of rifampicin, a drug which is of equal efficacy as isoniazid... all one has to be assured of is that it (short course chemotherapy) is at least equally effective and that relapse rates are acceptably low.

Dr Joseph concluded:

> One should not attempt to lay down rigid rules for the treatment of tuberculosis but guide lines should be clearly indicated. It has always seemed illogical to me that the length of treatment recommended should have no relationship to the severity of infection. Obviously the efficacy of the drugs must be related to the size of the inoculum ie. the extent of the disease and therefore the minimal lesion should not require treatment for nearly so long as an advanced cavitatory case.

> I suggest that we should revise our recommendations on the chemotherapy of tuberculosis and as a basis for discussion suggest that a standard recommended treatment should consist of streptomycin isoniazid and rifampicin daily for one month followed by daily isoniazid and rifampicin for a further eight months or for a period of six months from the time of sputum conversion.

The first recommendation towards shortening the standard two-year chemotherapy was made in the *Treatment of Tuberculosis* booklet (Fourth Edition 1977):

> Patients with active tuberculosis should usually continue treatment for 18 months unless rifampicin and isoniazid have been in use throughout in which case some physicians consider that 12 months of chemotherapy after bacterial conversion should be adequate.

However when this 4th Edition was reprinted in 1978, the following modification was inserted:

> Since the 4th Edition of this document in 1977, trials of daily chemotherapy of nine months duration have been reported including those of the British Thoracic and Tuberculosis Association. They describe satisfactory results ... following treatment of cases of pulmonary tuberculosis with three drugs for three months - rifampicin, isoniazid and either ethambutol or streptomycin - followed by rifampicin and isoniazid for six months.

This was unchanged in the Fifth Edition, 1980. It was only in the Sixth Edition (1982) that short-course chemotherapy of nine months duration was the general recommendation for pulmonary and extrapulmonary tuberculosis.

The other advance in chemotherapy over the past fifteen years has been the concept of fully supervised intermittent chemotherapy regimens. The results obtained from these regimens in Australia are the equal of those of the standard regimens. In practice these intermittent regimens are often used in easily recognisable groups such as recently arrived migrants or refugees with problems of communication, Aborigines in the more remote parts of Northern Australia, and in urban areas the alcoholic or drug dependent or otherwise "unreliable" patient.

These modifications of what was "standard chemotherapy" have gradually been accepted in Australia. The end result of these changes must always be the achievement of a 100 per cent cure-rate of tuberculosis using a safe and effective regimen which causes the least possible dislocation to the patient's life style and which effectively protects the public from infection.

Tuberculosis Experience, Australia

Bryan Gandevia

I graduated in 1948, by which time approximately 10 per cent of my year had developed symptoms of tuberculosis. Two of them, now distinguished practitioners in specialised fields, were saved, despite disseminated tuberculosis, by quite brief periods of streptomycin around 1948–1949. I was considered a candidate for tuberculosis because I had a flaming Mantoux reaction during my third year; I cannot recall my first-year reaction (tuberculin tests were, I think, compulsory for all of us). Despite the chemotherapeutic advances of the post-1948 period, my generation was acutely conscious of the significance of tuberculosis, both in children and adults. My interest in thoracic medicine was stimulated by an interest in asthma, fostered by a teacher at the Melbourne Hospital with whom I became closely associated (Dr H.J. Bolton) and by what seemed to me to be a specialty which required much further investigation of the environmental and occupational contributions. With John Bolton and Muriel Ross (then physiotherapist in charge of the Physiotherapy Department at the Melbourne Hospital) I did some research on asthma and some further studies in the allergy clinic, notably a study of antihistamines based on a latin square design, as far as I know for the first time used in medical research.

All this was done at a time when clinical research by clinicians was not regarded as a necessary step in one's education. When I was acting as assistant pathologist, I published a paper in the hospital's *Clinical Reports* on "Undiagnosed Pulmonary Tuberculosis", reporting several cases I had autopsied. In retrospect it was a rather tactless paper for a youngster with scarcely one foot on the ladder to write! I followed this up in the Division of Tuberculosis in the Department of Health in Victoria with a study of asthma in association with tuberculosis. I worked mostly at Gresswell

Sanatorium which was then in the charge of David Rosenthal, a dynamic little character who gave me the benefit of a vast experience precisely at the time when chemotherapy was slowly coming of age. He had a thorough knowledge of tuberculosis; few physicians were as well informed and few therapeutic regimens were as carefully and as effectively worked out as his. He had a very sound appreciation of the use of the three then available drugs, and I found many acknowledged experts overseas with a less critical approach to drug treatment (John Crofton was the most notable exception). He regarded artificial pneumothorax as no longer necessary, or very rarely so, some years, I think, ahead of conventional thinking overseas. Nonetheless, he taught me to induce a pneumothorax and of course maintaining them was still a routine procedure. At least partly under this influence, surgery was just beginning to become something of a last resort, although I suspect that in retrospect some unnecessary thoracoplasties were still being done, with resection becoming more common. The surgeons were chiefly Officer Brown and John Hayward. Altogether it was an extremely sound and disciplined training for a youngster about to go abroad.

At the Brompton Hospital I was house physician to James Livingstone, one of the most honest and conscientious clinicians I have ever seen in a hospital environment. He wrote his own notes in the hospital records and could be questioned on his findings at any time. He had re-instituted a vogue for plombage with Cleland (an Australian surgeon at the hospital) but I had the privilege of diagnosing the empyema in the last of those cases. It was successfully removed and Livingstone indicated the error that the operation had proved to be. He was also one of the last to abandon pneumoperitoneum and I induced one and maintained it for him in a case with a basal cavity, with what success I know not. At least I learned to use what I think was called a Maxwell box.

From the Brompton I went as registrar to Peter Stradling at Hammersmith Hospital. He ran a remarkable out-patient service with X-rays available on demand from general practitioners, thus providing his clinic with a vast amount of clinical material denied to the respiratory unit in the hospital which was then in the care of Charles Fletcher. We registrars read these X-rays and recalled those whom we were interested in for large films and clinical interview, an extremely educational process. We were also responsible for the out-patient management of tuberculous patients, including a large number of long-standing artificial pneumothoraces (I recall inducing none). I came to care for a ward full of patients with tuberculosis and other chronic chest diseases at the St Charles Hospital, which was a remarkable experience in relation particularly to non-tuberculous disease. Peter was an expert bronchoscopist but also very advanced in his chemotherapy, with a considerable experience of tuberculosis. He was almost obsessional in his approach and I greatly valued my time with him. Having one's own radiographic unit was a wonderful experience as one could obtain any kind of film one wanted, with any exposure in any position, on the spot and at the time, the only reservation being that one had to read them onself and then justify them at the clinic meeting each week. I was able to gain considerable experience in bronchography, which I did myself for the whole clinic, and Peter and I undertook various studies of observer variation in tomography and bronchography.

In 1956–57 when I became a Wunderly Scholar*, I wished to gain some understanding of respiratory physiology, and worked jointly at Hammersmith and Brompton Hospitals, with Charles Fletcher, Philip Hugh-Jones and John West at the former, and Francis Prime at the latter. This work had nothing to do with tuberculosis, although in later months when I travelled around England and Scotland to visit a variety of occupational health centres and occupations, including the coal and pottery industries, tuberculosis often came into consideration. Also at this time Scadding and Citron were studying tuberculin reactivity in sarcoidosis. I also managed to do lung-function tests on some of Guy Scadding's cases, and was particularly interested in two or three with widespread bronchial sarcoidosis. As a result I was able to diagnose a couple of cases in this country years later. I also saw some of his cases where there was some apparent relationship between sarcoidosis and tuberculosis, again leading to my being able to identify cases in my own unit years later. I think Scadding got a slightly biased view because cases of this kind were referred to him from all over the country, giving him the impression that the relationship was more frequent than it really was. Nonetheless, such cases did exist.

Just before I returned to Australia in 1957 I visited John Crofton's unit in Edinburgh. This dynamic man had welded together a number of disparate units to present a cohesive and rigid approach to tuberculosis control and treatment. He organised a devastating program for me, took me around personally to a multitude of clinical meetings, invariably introduced me as a specialist from Australia and equally invariably invited me to open the discussion on all the case presentations. It was a nerve-racking experience, especially as for a year or two I had done little or no teaching. There is no need to elaborate on his contribution to tuberculosis and he had a considerable influence on this country at a slightly later date. Blair Ritchie, Malcolm Schonnell and Brian Marks were amongst his trainees. As a physiologist I could not quite get the hang of his endobronchial pressure measurements but this was an odd diversion to which he was

---

* The Wunderly Travelling Scholarships are discussed in Ch. 11, and short biographies of all the Wunderly Scholars are given in the Appendix.

entitled! In, I think, 1962 he was guest Professor in New Zealand and I was invited as a sort of junior to him. We dined together the night before the course began. His first observation was "you must stop calling me Sir or they won't think that you're any good at all". He went on to indicate that I was to argue with him at every possible opportunity. We did so, a little to the amazement of the meeting, over several days, meeting each night to plot the program for the following day. It was again a tremendously stimulating experience. Years later he was chairing a session at an international asthma conference in England when he strongly opposed some point I made, and we argued quite fiercely for a few minutes. A senior English doctor later took me aside and apologised for the behaviour of the chairman, an observation which I conveyed to John, to our mutual amusement. I am sure he was an inspiration to those who worked closely with him and indeed he was to me. His book was moderately influential in this country; it was excellent on tuberculosis but perhaps a little dourly Scottish and dogmatic in some of the other sections. Perhaps one weakness was its failure to integrate the physiology with the clinical situation—they appeared separately so that the clinical application of the physiology was not obvious, a failing common to other textbooks in thoracic medicine.

Returning to Australia to a half-time appointment in occupational respiratory research in the University Department of Medicine at the Royal Melbourne Hospital in 1957, I was grateful when Alastair Campbell arranged for me to become a consultant to the Repatriation Hospital at Heidelberg, where I had at least some opportunity to retain some contact with tuberculosis. In those days an important consideration in general thoracic medicine was the breakdown of tuberculosis in patients given steroids; the ground rules were just becoming clear. Indeed, when steroids came out first, an allergist with severe asthma "cured" himself with cortisone but developed an acute tuberculous cavity! Occurring in a well-known member of the profession, the case received valuable widespread publicity in the tea rooms.

Just when I was faced with the difficulty of deciding between private consultant practice and the research I was so much enjoying—both had got out of control on a part-time basis—I was delighted to receive an invitation from Ralph Blacket to join him at the University of New South Wales and start a Department of Respiratory Medicine. Such a concept was obviously impossible in the Melbourne environment and although I was then offered a Readership in the University I could never have achieved the same independence as I was given in Sydney. I found the tuberculosis scene very different from Melbourne. There had not been the same unified approach and there had been no standardisation of treatment regimens. The various teaching hospitals were independent and the standards of treatment varied quite widely, being on average not as effective as in Melbourne. There was not the same concern about the emergence of resistant organisms, and such cases were not treated with the determination of a Crofton. There were exceptions, and the unit at Randwick was good. Bill Telleson was the young and enthusiastic physician there and although disappointed at not getting my job he collaborated well. We would like to have integrated my general unit at Prince Henry and the tuberculosis unit at Randwick but our efforts to do this were continually frustrated for one reason or another. Keith Harris was understandably cautious at losing control of the only metropolitan tuberculosis wards under his direct supervision. I did obtain beds there and I ran an out-patient clinic; this worked quite well while I supervised the beds personally. However, my interest in acquiring them was not for my own sake but rather because I wanted my senior registrars and thoracic trainees to gain the experience.

One major advantage throughout my time was the way in which out-patient clinics worked in what was a dedicated unit, which made them very efficient. For example, in all appropriate patients, we would have X-rays, ventilatory tests, skin tests, full blood examination and erythrocyte sedimentation rate performed before we saw the patient. Everything was under our control. The experienced nursing staff also knew the patients and their observations were often helpful. In later years when I had responsibility for the routine radiographs of follow-up cases, I found it invaluable experience for a senior registrar, once I had inducted him. I would then give him this responsibility, partly because I would have developed some faith in his ability, but also because I could trust the senior nursing staff to make sure that no radiographic changes were missed! In the early years there were quite interesting clinical meetings, once a week, with Harry Windsor, a dogmatic and forceful thoracic surgeon, Geoff McManis and Maurice Joseph attending from time to time. Bill Telleson was the only Randwick physician regularly to attend our meetings although John Murphy did so later and also Dr C.M. Mukerjee.

Following a lead from John Wright, who had started a chest surgical referral scheme at the Wollongong chest clinic, I began to accompany him down there and later we ran separate clinics once or twice a month. I enjoyed my association with that clinic partly because in the early years there was an enormous amount of untapped clinical material and there were no local physicians with specialised experience in modern respiratory medicine. I also appreciated the opportunity to see tuberculosis patients again. Another delight was the association with Sister Betty O'Brien, the archetype of the great tuberculosis nurse of the past—a good administrator, good with people, expert in tuberculosis and its treatment and thoroughly conversant with the public health aspects. I have been lucky to be associated with her successors and with others at Randwick of the same genre. I was most insistent on referring patients to their general practitioners, as far as possible, and in communicating with them. This was not a strong point of government clinics at the time, but the policy paid off handsomely in that we have continued to serve in a consultant way ever since, despite the appropriate and very necessary improvement in local services over the past twenty years. Keith Harris, I recall, kept an eye on chemotherapy there. In Sydney the doyen of tuberculosis specialists was Dr Cotter Harvey, a dedicated man, tall, lean and friendly. He must have exerted a considerable influence in the years before I came to Sydney but by the time I knew him his management of tuberculosis perhaps erred on the conservative side. While I agreed with Keith Harris that all patients with a positive sputum should be treated in hospitals, I would probably let them home earlier than he would have liked—this was a period of change. However, with the assistance of our nurses, our ambulant chemotherapy was possibly more determined and meticulous than in some of the other teaching hospitals. In recent years, Brian Jarvie in my unit began to insist upon supervised chemotherapy for all out-patient cases, and it was impressive that this was achieved with surprisingly little difficulty (I do not know if the policy continues). This procedure gave me a little more confidence in shortening the courses with the newer antibiotics, although with my memories of relapses from a bygone era I suppose I would always be asking for three months longer than some of my younger colleagues, or even than my enthusiastic and diligent literature surveyor, Dr Mukerjee.

The surgery at Randwick was done competently by Fred Ross who unfortunately lacked senior qualifications. This imposed problems in recognising him at the teaching hospitals and I gather there was a certain amount of conflict between the thoracic surgeons as a result. When he retired the work was done by our surgeons. Although they were also competent, one felt the lack of dedication to tuberculosis and perhaps the lack of experience in it, which was not the case when tuberculosis surgery was the main form of thoracic surgery. There is little doubt that pulmonary surgery has lost a lot from the development of cardiac surgery.

In the later years it was a pleasure to treat the delightful Vietnamese migrants, although I had comparatively little contact with them except in a remote supervisory capacity. I always enjoyed visiting them and appreciated their remarkable courtesy. They formed such a welcome contrast to those alcoholic, absconding and utterly unreliable characters concentrated at Randwick from time to time.

I guess I must record my first meeting with Gwyn Howells shortly after he became Commonwealth Director of Tuberculosis. He came to a meeting at Wollongong to consider equipment for the new wards. I asked only for a spirometer but he was disinclined to accept this, despite my indication that patients were now dying not of tuberculosis but of later respiratory failure. I replied, in some irritation, that the Commonwealth might care about patients with tuberculosis but it apparently didn't give a damn whether they returned to work or not. I am glad to report that we got along much better in subsequent years! The immediate problem was tactfully resolved by the donation of a spirometer from some other source, organised, I suspect, by the nursing staff.

Obviously,. there have been changes over the last twenty years in the mode of presentation of tuberculosis, in its treatment and in its public health aspects, not to mention the administrative side. Others can survey these issues with more experience than I. What has been interesting to observe is the evolution of today's respiratory physician from the old tuberculosis doctor. The former is lucky if he has had much exposure to tuberculosis, while the latter had a vast experience of a complex disease. There was a phase of conflict between these groups in the United States and England which I believe was less of a problem in Australia. Here tuberculosis was largely treated by full-time doctors not in competition with their colleagues, and not dealing with non-tuberculosis disease. Modern respiratory medicine and its exponents developed more or less *pari passu*; there was no real ground for conflict. Perhaps I am one of a small group who had a foot in both camps, at least for a time. The evolution is illustrated, perhaps paradoxically, by a review of the Wunderly Scholars' lifetime interests; I am not quite sure that Sir Harry wholly approved our deviation from "mainstream" of tuberculosis. Does anyone know?

A Physician's Overview of Tuberculosis 1940 - 1980

T. G. Paxon

At the time of my qualification (1939) tuberculosis was still rife in London's East End, yet I cannot recall any special emphasis being placed on the disease in teaching rounds (several others have made similar comments about the lack of teaching about tuberculosis in Australian teaching hospitals in the 1940s). The policy at the London Hospital was to transfer tuberculosis patients to the London Chest Hospital, or after its virtual destruction by bombing in 1941, to sanatoria outside London.

This lack of emphasis on tuberculosis was perhaps not surprising since tuberculosis was not considered an exciting clinical challenge especially to the young physician. This view was not helped by the presentation of the disease in Price's *Textbook of Medicine,* in 1944, which was hopelessly out of date. In the 1944 edition under the subheading "Climatic Treatment" the following were included:

> Residence by the sea at sea-level is undesirable... the climate of parts of Australia and New Zealand are admirably suited to this disease (p 1209)

My reaction to this some fifty years later is one of incredulity and anger. It was not the same with pathologists. I recall the interest with which Professor H.M. Turnbull, usually a very dour man, demonstrated a primary focus in a child's lung pointing out the tubercles along the lymphatics linking the focus with the hilar glands. At about the same time (1940) Arnold Rich at Baltmore's Johns Hopkins Hospital published *The Pathogenesis of Tuberculosis,* in my opinion one of the greatest medical texts of the first half of the 20th century and a work which clarified the subject in a way no other book has done.

I recall the period 1950–55 as years of revolutionary change in the treatment of tuberculosis. With chemotherapy and if necessary resectional surgery the cure became a relative certainty. The Australian tuberculosis program under the guidance of Sir Harry Wunderly applied these advances on a national scale.

These and other advances in tuberculosis during the 1950s gave impetus to research in various fields. The advances in the surgical treatment of tuberculosis under an umbrella of chemotherapy was associated with an appreciation of the segmental anatomy of the lung which in turn enabled surgeons to tackle other lung conditions and later cardiac surgery. It was tuberculosis which stimulated the whole science of epidemiology. The trials of various regimens of chemotherapy by the Medical Research Council set "Gold Standards" for trials of various drug therapies in other conditions. But it was probably in the field of immunology that research in tuberculosis produced remarkable advances in the whole understanding of the immune response. The study of delayed hypersensitivity evoked by the tubercle bacillus led to observations of macrophage behaviour in laboratory animals which in turn led to the discovery of the role of the T-lymphocyte and its ability to produce a range of chemical activators which are the basis of the cell-mediated immune system.

A significant recrudescence of tuberculosis in Australia may be unlikely. But the tubercle bacillus, this most ancient and persistent of organisms, will re-establish itself if given the chance.

CHAPTER 11

The Evolution of the National Tuberculosis Program

L.O. Goldsmith

The initial administrative interest in tuberculosis may be traced back to 1829 when the Royal College of Physicians in London, almost certainly responding to a request from the Colonial Office, sent a questionnaire seeking data on health matters in the colony to Governor Ralph Darling in Sydney.[1]

Public health services were slow to attract the attention of colonial governments and it was only between 1842–67 that local government legislation delegated some basic public health responsibilities to shires and municipalities in the various colonies. These bodies were inadequately funded and proved incapable of providing even the most rudimentary sanitary services.

Following the gold rushes of the 1850s, the populations of Melbourne and to a lesser extent Sydney rose dramatically, far outstripping municipal services such as pure water supplies and garbage disposal. At about this time tuberculosis became more common, due probably to the mass migration from Europe, England, California and China, stimulated by the stories of instant fortune on the goldfields of Bendigo and Ballarat. *The Victorian Year Book* of 1877 noted that "Phthisis resumed its place at the head of the causes of death—there were 1088 (deaths from phthisis) in that year." This Victorian report and others from New Zealand, Queensland and Western Australia all noted that an unduly high proportion of deaths from tuberculosis were in migrants from the United Kingdom seeking "the cure" in the Antipodes.

Central boards of health—forerunners of state departments of health—were established in all states by 1900. These boards varied in size from three to seven members with a chief medical officer, usually part-time, controlling a staff of health inspectors. The reports of these boards drew attention to the high tuberculosis mortality and this resulted in public health acts, including the compulsory notification of tuberculosis to the relevant authorities. South Australia was the first state to do so in 1899 and was followed by the other states within the following decade. As a consequence of notification, the medical officer of health or his deputy would despatch a health visitor to the home of the notified case, and in theory at least, examine the family contacts, and advise the patient and his or her family of basic hygiene and preventive measures including the disposal of sputum. Notification procedures and requirements varied from state to state; in most states only pulmonary tuberculosis was notifiable and the pressure applied to medical practitioners to notify cases was in general minimal. Only in Western Australia were doctors circularised twice-yearly, reminding them of their obligation to notify cases of tuberculosis and in addition offering a small fee for each notification. Tuberculosis carried a social stigma which severely affected employment and education and medical practitioners were in general reluctant to notify cases until the disease was obvious and far advanced.

In 1911 a national conference of chief health officers of the various states was convened by the Commonwealth in Melbourne to consider the most practical and effective methods of tuberculosis control. The Federal Director of Quarantine, Dr Perrin Norris, was chairman and the conference agreed to a series of recommendations including uniform compulsory notification of all forms of tuberculosis, free bacteriological examination of sputum in suspected cases and the more effective use of available sanatorium beds. These recommendations were pragmatic and achievable at a relatively modest cost, but the constitutional limitations of Federal power in health matters which were solely the responsibility of the states precluded any real progress. The states in general took refuge in the fact that while tuberculosis might be a serious problem in Australia, little more was being done in England or the United States where tuberculosis mortality was significantly higher.

The higher than expected rejection rate on medical grounds among volunteers for the Australian Imperial Force and the prevalence of tuberculosis in troops overseas in the first two years of the Great War came as a shock to politicians and the community and again focussed attention on tuberculosis. The Federal Government again assumed a leadership role despite constitutional limitations and an inter-departmental committee chaired by Dr J.H.L. Cumpston was convened in 1916 to investigate these health problems and make recommendations. The committee recommended the establishment of a Repatriation Commission to care for repatriated soldiers with disabilities including tuberculosis; initially this was possible only with the co-operation of the states who provided the sanatorium and hospital beds and were reimbursed by the Federal Government.

The Federal Department of Health with Cumpston as the Director-General was established in 1921. A Royal Commission on health was appointed by the Federal Government in 1925 and despite the constitutional limitations to its powers, the Federal Government was certainly playing a leadership role. The Royal Commission reported that the recommendations of the 1911 meeting of chief health officers in Melbourne had not been implemented due to apathy and a lack of financial resources. The recommendations of the 1911 meeting were reiterated and in addition the states were urged to appoint their own full-time Directors of Tuberculosis.

As a result Victoria appointed a well-qualified physician, Dr J. Bell Ferguson, and the Commonwealth created a Division of Tuberculosis within its own Department of Health, headed by Dr M.J. Holmes. Dr Holmes was actively encouraged by Dr Cumpston to formulate a national tuberculosis program which broke new ground with the notion of a special tuberculosis allowance to enable breadwinners to undergo treatment without impoverishing their dependents; this was undoubtedly inspired by the tuberculosis pension paid to ex-soldiers who developed tuberculosis after their discharge from the Services. The onset of the economic depression in late 1929 and the subsequent Premiers' plan under which all Australian governments pledged to reduce budget expenditure halted these promising efforts. The Division of Tuberculosis and the office of Director of Tuberculosis were abolished and the outbreak of World War II delayed any revival of the plan.

At the 1944 Ministers of Health conference the plan was resurrected and for the first time the Commonwealth government agreed to subsidise the states for maintenance costs of tuberculosis control facilities, assistance in capital costs for hospital beds and a food plan for families disadvantaged by tuberculosis. The Tuberculosis Act of 1945 gave formal expression to these proposals. This Act specified that:

> an amount... shall be payable in every year to each state upon the condition that the amount is applied by the state in making payments to or in respect of sufferers from tuberculosis or the dependents of such sufferers with the objects of :
>
> (a) encouraging such sufferers to refrain from working and to take treatment
>
> (b) minimising the spread of tuberculosis
>
> (c) promoting the better treatment of tuberculosis.

Thus the concept of a special tuberculosis allowance—a unique feature of the Australian Tuberculosis Campaign—was enshrined in legislation.

The allowance was too meagre to achieve its purpose and failure to achieve the co-operation of the states resulted in the Commonwealth making payments to the states which the latter refused to disburse to the tuberculosis sufferers. This led to undignified wrangling with some states, particularly Queensland. The Tuberculosis Act 1945 was a legislative and administrative failure; it was poorly drafted and insufficiently detailed. More importantly it highlighted the need to secure the enthusiastic co-operation of the states in view of the limited Commonwealth responsibility in the health field.

A constitutional amendment in 1946 broadened the Commonwealth powers in the health field to make laws about pharmaceutical, hospital and sickness benefits and medical and dental services. The Commonwealth also was able to use its powers under Section 96 of the Constitution to make grants to the states for health purposes. Dr Harry Wunderly was appointed consultant in tuberculosis to the Commonwealth and in 1947 Commonwealth Director of Tuberculosis in a reconstituted Division of Tuberculosis, Department of Health. He was determined to use the new Commonwealth powers to secure greater Commonwealth financial commitment, leadership and direction in the field of tuberculosis control. Like his predecessor Dr Holmes, he began by surveying every aspect of existing tuberculosis programs in the states and then in the United Kingdom, Europe, Canada and the United States.[2] He presented his report to Senator Niel McKenna, Minister of Health; the report made three key recommendations:

(a) A revised and more detailed Tuberculosis Act was essential, requiring action by the states on a standardised form of notification of tuberculosis and improvement in facilities for the treatment of tuberculosis patients.

(b) Full-time Directors of Tuberculosis should be appointed in all states.

(c) Extensive compulsory mass miniature radiography surveys (MMR) should be conducted in all states as the principal case-finding tool.

Senator McKenna took these recommendations to Cabinet and secured approval to meet State Ministers of Health in Melbourne in June 1948. At this meeting it was decided that the National Tuberculosis Campaign should be a joint Commonwealth/states undertaking with the states controlling policy through a National Tuberculosis Advisory Council and the Commonwealth controlling expenditure. The decisions of this conference were promptly encompassed in the Tuberculosis Act 1948. This was a far more detailed and wide-ranging Act; Section 5 detailed in five subsections the arrangements with the states "for the provision by the State subject to agreed conditions of services and facilities for the diagnosis, treatment and control of tuberculosis". The Commonwealth undertook to reimburse the states for capital and maintenance costs; the latter was restricted to "expenditure... not exceeding the amount by which that expenditure is in excess of the maintenance (during the base year 1947–48)". The 1948 Act conferred wide-ranging powers on the Director-General of Health, subject to the direction of the Minister:

(a) To take steps for the establishment or taking over the conduct of hospitals, sanatoria, laboratories, diagnostic centres, radiological and other units and clinics for the diagnosis, treatment and control of tuberculosis.

(b) To arrange for the provision of scholarships for post- graduate students of tuberculosis.

(c) To provide diagnostic and treatment facilities, rehabilitation units, health education and research facilities. Subsidies to

Universities were to be made available for research into tuberculosis.

The Act established the National Tuberculosis Advisory Council whose functions were to advise the Minister with respect to:

(1) Measures to be adopted in relation to prevention, diagnosis and control of tuberculosis.

(2) Provision of standards for equipment and apparatus in relation to the above.

(3) The standard of training of personnel engaged in the diagnosis, treatment and prevention of tuberculosis.

(4) The standards of hospitals and sanatoria used in the treatment of tuberculosis.

(5) The rehabilitation of patients.

By 1950 all the states had passed complementary legislation to enable the new Control Programme to begin; only the level of payment of the tuberculosis allowance remained to be agreed to. Before this could be achieved the Menzies Liberal Country Party Coalition assumed office following the December 1949 elections. The new Minister of Health, Dr Earle Page, was supportive of the program and immediately solved the impasse delaying the implementation of the tuberculosis allowance.

The Australian Tuberculosis Campaign

A.J. Proust

In 1947 the Commonwealth Government commissioned Dr H.W. Wunderly to investigate and report on tuberculosis control in Australia. Boag[3] describes it well:

> His appointment was no accident. An earlier sufferer of tuberculosis and a lucky pre-chemotherapy survivor, he had decided to do something to control the disease and enlisted the help of his wife Jeannie. Few if any parliamentary lobbyists can equal the success of the Wunderlys. How could a parliamentarian from the Prime Minister down, fail to listen to a quietly spoken expert doctor who lived with them in the Hotel Canberra and pleasantly repeated his simple message: "Tuberculosis can be controlled— give us the chance to do so".

Canberra was a small town of 16,100 people in 1947 and the Hotel Canberra was the focal point of Canberra society—many cabinet ministers lived there while Parliament sat, and senior public servants were constant visitors. The state Premiers and their advisers stayed there during Premiers' conferences and Loan Council meetings. Dr and Mrs Wunderly met them all; invitations to Mrs Wunderly's tea parties in the lounge of the hotel were eagerly sought after. At the same time the sincerity of the Wunderlys must have influenced those whom they met and entertained. Dr Wunderly had left an established consultant physician's practice in

Adelaide and Mrs Wunderly her beloved home and garden for an uncertain future in Canberra and the discomforts of life in the Hotel Canberra.

Wunderly was able to sum up his plan for the control of tuberculosis as follows [2]:

> The objectives of this plan are (1) prevention; (2) to discover every person suffering from tuberculosis—that is, case finding; (3) to isolate and care for every person in need of medical treatment; (4) to provide after- care and to rehabilitate every patient when this is possible; (5) to protect the patient and his or her dependents from economic distress.

Mass miniature radiography was the cornerstone of the case-finding program. It was compulsory from the outset in four states, voluntary in two. It took all Dr Wunderly's diplomatic and persuasive powers to bring the two reluctant states into line. Compulsory mass radiography on a national scale was the unique contribution Australia made in the field of tuberculosis control.

The National Tuberculosis Campaign was launched at what in retrospect was a propitious time. Tuberculosis mortality rates had been falling at first slowly and then more rapidly since 1900. The first effective chemotherapeutic agents against tuberculosis were undergoing clinical trials. Thoracic surgery was in its lusty infancy. Mass miniature radiography was becoming accepted and readily available. Australia was entering its "lucky country" phase of growth and prosperity and no problem seemed beyond solution. The post-war mass migration was just beginning and the campaign fitted in well with the concept of not only more migrants but more healthy migrants. Even the most conservative politicians supported the campaign which was based on free medical and hospital care for tuberculous patients largely at the hands of salaried medical staff.

The results were almost immediately impressive. The tuberculosis mortality rate fell 60 per cent in the six years 1949–54. In fact the results were so dramatic that chest hospitals built specifically for tuberculosis were never fully used as such; they were quickly and easily adapted for cardio- thoracic medicine and surgery.

There were many spin-offs from the campaign. Health education was given an enormous stimulus as health education in tuberculosis showed the way to secure the co-operation of all levels of government and all sections of the community. Without it, the compulsory mass X-ray surveys would not have been possible. Health education succeeded to a large degree in removing the fear and stigma of tuberculosis which had existed for centuries. The voluntary organisations broadened their horizons encompassing rehabilitation and sheltered workshops. The Association for the Prevention of Tuberculosis in Australia was formed and attracted leading chest physicians as active members. It affiliated with the International Union Against Tuberculosis (IUAT); a highly successful Eastern

Regional meeting of the IUAT was held in Sydney in 1972.

Sir Harry Wunderly retired in 1956 and was succeeded as Commonwealth Director of Tuberculosis by Dr Hilary Roche. Dr Roche reviewed the Australian Tuberculosis Campaign in the *Swiss Journal of Tuberculosis* (*Schweiz Z. Tuberk* 15.1.58) and an abridged version was published in the Department of Health's journal, *Health*, in June 1958:

> An outstanding feature of the campaign which makes it unique in the world is the payment of liberal allowances to tuberculous persons above the age of 16 years. This payment is regarded as an important public health measure since it enables patients to have adequate treatment which is completely free.

He highlighted the special responsibilities which the Commonwealth assumed with regard to the Aboriginal population and to the people of the Trust Territories of Papua New Guinea where the incidence of tuberculosis was directly related to their contact with Europeans. Both Australian Aborigines and the Papuans and New Guineans were highly susceptible to tuberculosis. BCG vaccination was used extensively in these populations.

He summed up the future after ten years of the campaign; tuberculosis still remained a formidable problem, the fall in tuberculosis mortality was not yet matched by a similar fall in notifications. The arrival of a million post-war migrants, already infected during the war years in Europe, would provide a steady source of new cases.

Dr Roche was Commonwealth Director of Tuberculosis 1956–60 and after retirement he continued as a physician in the Canberra chest clinic in the then Canberra Community Hospital until 1967. He was regarded by Marcus Faunce as an outstanding tuberculosis chest physician and was widely consulted by the small but growing medical community in Canberra.

Dr Alan King was appointed as Commonwealth Director of Tuberculosis in 1960. As Commonwealth Director of Tuberculosis he worked closely with the states, especially New South Wales and Queensland; Chermside Hospital (now Prince Charles Hospital) and the Brisbane Chest Clinic were built during his period as Commonwealth Director. He returned to Perth as Director of Medical Services, Department of Social Services in 1963.

Dr James Tremayne was appointed Commonwealth Director of Tuberculosis to succeed Dr King in 1963. He had been a resident medical officer at the Tasmanian sanatorium in Hobart under Dr Tommy Goddard and succeeded him as Director of Tuberculosis in Tasmania in 1951. As Commonwealth Director he travelled widely, visiting tuberculosis hospitals and chest clinics and was active in co-ordinating the work of the voluntary organisations. He died suddenly in 1965 while travelling to Sydney.

Dr Gwyn Howells, appointed Commonwealth Director of Tuberculosis in 1965, was the most innovative and effective of Sir Harry Wunderly's successors. He recognised that Australian physicians had acquired sufficient expertise to form expert committees which made recommendations on the microbiology of *M. tuberculosis*, the tuberculin test, and most importantly on the treatment of tuberculosis. The *Recommendations on Treatment* appeared in six editions from 1968 to 1982 and have been accepted in Australia, New Zealand and the South Pacific as a standard reference on chemotherapy. A more specialised and smaller publication, *Bacteriological Investigations of Mycobacteria* was first published in April 1967 and later renamed *Procedures for the Laboratory Diagnosis of Mycobacterial Infection.* The booklet, *The Tuberculin Test*, was first published in 1970 and led to a standardised Australian epidemiological tuberculin test.

Another successful innovation was the clinical tuberculosis conferences. The idea was to foster better communication between physicians, full-time and part-time, in the field of tuberculosis, both among themselves and also with nurses, microbiologists, social workers and administrators. Experts in related fields were invited; the effect was to raise confidence and self esteem among all these groups who hitherto had worked in relative isolation. Many excellent papers were presented, some of which were published in the *Medical Journal of Australia.*

Research projects were also undertaken; the Australian Tuberculin Survey and the Australian Rifampicin Trial were successfully completed with the medical staff of the Tuberculosis Division of the Commonwealth Department of Health co-ordinating the clinical work in the various hospitals and clinics in the states. In addition funds were made available to the Queensland Public Health Laboratory's Mycobacterial Section to investigate the epidemiology and pathogenicity of non-tuberculous mycobacteria; this work attracted international attention and the Queensland laboratory became a WHO Reference Laboratory for Australia and the neighbouring region.

Dr Howells also encouraged the adoption of proven advances from overseas, particularly fully supervised intermittent chemotherapy and the moves towards shorter regimens of chemotherapy. Concerted efforts were made to control tuberculosis among Aborigines in the Northern Territory; the notification rate in the Territory was for many years five- to ten-times higher than in the southern states. Regular visits by Dr Howells ensured that the recommendations of the National Tuberculosis Advisory Council were put into practice and physicians from various states made a series of visits to give support to the Director of Tuberculosis in the Territory. BCG vaccination in infancy of the Aboriginal population, fully supervised chemotherapy of both Aboriginal and white patients and mass miniature chest X-ray surveys, even in the least accessible areas of the Territory, were carried out despite problems of lack of electric power, the necessity of flying in radiographic equipment to rough airfields and the problems of identifying by name tribal Aborigines. Despite these efforts the notification rate in the Northern Territory remains at least five times the rate in Australia as a whole.

In September 1970, Dr Gwyn Howells reviewed the campaign in the journal *Tuberculosis*, published by the International Union Against Tuberculosis (IUAT).[4]

> The Australian tuberculosis campaign has registered massive successes. It has certain features that are unusual and when these are considered together, the whole campaign may well be considered unique... It was perhaps fortunate that the campaign, in being the product of fresh thought, did not suffer the disadvantages except in a minor degree, of an inappropriate and uncomfortable coupling to facilities and plans that already existed.

The campaign initially was based on the broadly accepted principles of public health but the individual approach to the patient was maintained. If a key to the success of the anti-tuberculosis enterprise is wanted, it might be in the word "legislation".[5]

> States and Commonwealth agreed to produce reasonably uniform legislation to cover compulsory notification of the disease by medical practitioners and compulsory examination where there was reasonable suspicion of disease and compulsory isolation of recalcitrant infectious patients. Later legislation to cover compulsory mass X-ray surveys was introduced.... The most significant thing about the legislation is how rarely its penalty clauses had to be invoked in the courts. The co-operation of the medical profession has been outstanding and failure to notify cases can now be said for practical purposes to be unknown.

The emergence of effective chemotherapy had fortunately coincided with the early development of the campaign.

> It has been an expensive Campaign... In capital expenditure on all new hospitals, clinics, X-ray and other machinery etc., the Commonwealth of Australia took over full responsibility subject to its own approval of its necessity. In maintenance, the Commonwealth Government took over all running costs for institutions and staff over and above that spent by the States in the financial year 1947–48.

The total cost until 1969 was about $238 million. Dr Howells continued:

> The Commonwealth role has been (after discussion) to define the principles, to co-ordinate and lead the campaign and to supply the finance. The role of the States has been the practical one of the field work and the integration of the tuberculosis services within the framework of the health services... Each State Director of Tuberculosis has as his brief the control of tuberculosis within his state...

Dr Howells then referred to the work of the voluntary anti-tuberculosis organisations:

> Various voluntary organisations have not only fully supported the campaign but have provided valuable activities of their own in the rehabiliation and educational fields as well as maintaining invaluable international connections. The most important of these is the Australian Tuberculosis and Chest Association. This ATCA organisation, whilst closely co-operating with governmental agencies, has remained at Federal level a purely voluntary one. It is a member of the International Union Against Tuberculosis. The State organisations affiliated with it have developed in different ways but four of them work in the field of rehabilitation. The most oustanding example is the massive Bedford Industries in South Australia which commenced in rehabilitating the tuberculous. Whilst it still gives priority to tuberculosis this activity provides only a small percentage of its work. It is now an organisation with an annual budget of $1,000,000 and nearly 600 patients per year pass through it. The Australian Tuberculosis and Chest Association has also contributed considerably to medical, patient and public education. State branches are continuously active in individual case problems and aid.

The post-war migration of people to Australia from Europe ran parallel to the tuberculosis campaign. Both began in 1948 and reached their peaks in the 1950s. It would have been

> folly to import active and possibly drug resistant disease into a population now largely tuberculin negative as far as natural infection goes...

wrote Dr Howells in 1970.

> With this in mind every potential migrant over 16 years of age has an X-ray of the chest in his own country and persons found to have active disease are excluded at least until treated. Despite this programme migrants still have at least double the prevalence of tuberculosis of the Australian-born. This applies particularly to extrapulmonary tuberculosis which is now almost entirely an imported disease. The main factor in the relatively high incidence of tuberculosis in migrants is the degree of tuberculinisation of the individual migrant; the undoubted stress involved in migration almost certainly plays a role in the reactivation of a long past infection.

The end of the campaign coincided with the massive intake of refugees from south-east Asia following the Vietnam War. As the last Commonwealth Director of Tuberculosis Dr D.B. Travers (1975–83) presided over the winding down of Commonwealth funding and responsibility for the control program. He encouraged and cajoled the states to assume again their responsibilities in this field of public health.

The publication of the national tuberculosis statistics continued until 1985. The medical and radiological screening of migrants and refugees, administered from Canberra until 1988 and then moved to Sydney, continues. Concern for the maintenance of standards led to a Commonwealth sponsored "Workshop on Migrant Health Screening", attended by representatives of all states and territories and the Department of Immigration, in Canberra in October 1988.

In his 1970 review of the National Tuberculosis Campaign, Dr Howells concluded:

> Few countries, these days, live in isolation and Australia will feel the impact of tuberculosis in terms of the efforts, the successes or failures of the countries around it and the countries from which it receives migrants and visitors. The migrant programme would appear likely to continue for many years yet and presumably it will continue to have the same effect on tuberculosis control as at present.

Those words are as true today (1988) as when they were written (1970). The significant difference is that in 1970 we had a fully operational national tuberculosis control program; Commonwealth funding of the program ceased on 31 December 1977 and the responsibility for tuberculosis control has now been returned to the states.

Dr J. H. L. Cumpston

*A. J. Proust and Robert Layland**

John Howard Leggett Cumpston was a great Australian pioneer in the field of public health and specifically tuberculosis. He was an epidemiologist and a forceful administrator who found his way through the minefield of Commonwealth-state relations in the early years of Federation when the states held the whip over the fledgling Commonwealth. Cumpston was appointed Commonwealth Director of Quarantine in 1913 at the age of 33 years; Quarantine was the only health power yielded by the states to the Commonwealth but even so the Commonwealth had to rely on state public health officers to act on its behalf. In 1921 Dr Cumpston was also appointed first Director-General of Public Health, remaining in both positions until his retirement in 1945.

During his tenure of office he established the Commonwealth Serum Laboratories, which produced tuberculin and later BCG vaccine, and the Commonwealth Health Laboratories, which were set up in regional centres throughout Australia and as far away as Rabaul in New Britain with the major aim of providing bacteriological services for the diagnosis of tuberculosis. The Institute of Health and the National Health and Medical Research Council were also established during his tenure of office.

---

* With acknowledgment to Dr Alan Cumpston, Canberra, ACT.

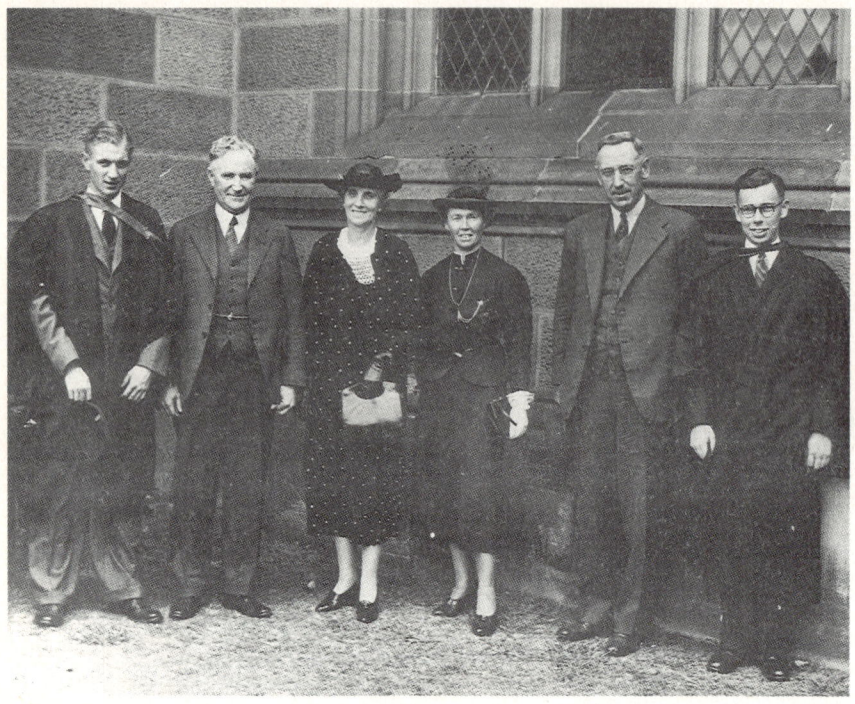

Outside the Great Hall of the University of Sydney in 1937. Left to right: Dr Ivan Page, Sir Earle and Lady Page, Mrs and Dr J.H.L. Cumpston and Dr Alan Cumpston.
(Photo courtesy of Dr A.G. Cumpston.)

John Cumpston was born in South Yarra, Melbourne, in 1880. He completed his education on scholarships at Wesley College and Queen's College, University of Melbourne. He graduated MB, BS in 1902 at the age of 22 and did his residency at the then Melbourne Hospital. Soon afterwards, he decided to devote his professional life to public health and preventive medicine taking full advantage of "the new bacteriology, the new pathology and the new epidemiology... the beacons indicating the new road to the prevention of disease on a national scale". In 1905 he sailed for Tokyo as a ship's surgeon and in Manila he contacted scientists of the Rockefeller Foundation who were working there in the control of smallpox and cholera, contacts which were later of benefit to Australia. In 1906, again as a ship's surgeon, he travelled to London, where he obtained the Diploma of Public Health, and in 1907 was awarded his MD. He visited the Pasteur Institute in Paris and Lille where he met Professor Albert Calmette who was even then working on BCG vaccine against tuberculosis. He returned to Australia in 1908 taking up the position of Medical Officer of Health in Perth.

In 1909, Cumpston wrote a paper on "Phthisis in Australia with more especial reference to Western Australia".* The tuberculosis mortality was declining in every state except Western Australia by the year 1890. This anomaly was attributed to the enormous increase in the state's population and migrants, mainly from the eastern states, particularly Victoria, who brought tuberculosis with them to the goldfields of Kalgoorlie.

Cumpston gave an exhaustive list of the possible factors associated with tuberculosis which if corrected could lead to its control: poverty, alcoholism and occupation, especially in those working in a dusty environment. The discovery of the tubercle bacillus by Koch led to suggestions such as tuberculin-testing of dairy herds and improved hygiene in dairies, to improve housing for the working classes, legal enactment of compulsory notification and isolation and treatment of infectious cases in sanatoria as possible effective control measures. He thought that public education was the most likely effective cause of the decline which had already taken place.[6]

> It may be fairly said that about this time (1860–80) there was a great awakening of intelligence among the lower classes—the classes chiefly affected by phthisis—and this awakening (through public education) brought with it a complete change in the social system.

As the social system was improved, the incidence of tuberculosis fell. No longer was there an apathetic acceptance of the dreadful toll of tuberculosis. Cumpston agreed that isolation of infected cases was also impor tant. But education in general and specifically about tuberculosis and its mode of transmission were vitally important in its prevention and control.

He concluded that:

> the principal preventive measure should be the immediate enactment of legal provisions for the strict prohibition of any phthisical patient from other shores landing at any port within the Commonwealth, should such a person land with the intention of becoming, even though only temporarily, a resident in Australia.

Thus Cumpston was among the first to think in terms of tuberculosis control; he was, of course, the first to achieve a position where he could influence governments along these lines.

In 1910 Cumpston was appointed Royal Commissioner to investigate the prevalence of miners' phthisis (fibrosis of the lungs) in the Kalgoorlie goldfields and if necessary make recommendations for control measures. He travelled extensively through the goldfields, examining miners, inspecting the underground mines and consulting local medical practitioners. There

---

* A copy of this paper was obtained through the courtesy of the Western Australian Archives.

was then no X-ray apparatus in Western Australia capable of taking chest X-rays on a mass scale.

Cumpston's report created quite a stir. He found that miners' phthisis was indeed a significant problem in the mining industry and that its prevalence was directly related to the presence of fine silica dust in the atmosphere of the mine. Where there was no dust there was no risk of miners' phthisis. Proper engineering practices to reduce dust and adequate ventilation to extract it where it did exist were recommended and later put in place. He also noted the association of tuberculosis with miner's phthisis.

Cumpston was to reflect on his experience in Western Australia and recognise that:

> apart from all other considerations, I was able to understand the attitude of State administration to the evolving Commonwealth.

This experience was put to good use in the years ahead.

Cumpston joined the fledgling Federal Quarantine Service in 1910 in Perth, transferred to Melbourne in 1911 and in the following year was Acting Director of the Service. He early asserted federal power when, in 1913, there was a smallpox epidemic in New South Wales.

Cumpston became concerned about the wider implications of infectious diseases, especially tuberculosis and venereal diseases. These had an impact on military manpower and invalid pensions which became obvious in the early days of the World War I. However, he was largely powerless to take preventive measures because of constitutional limitations. An inter-departmental committee of investigation was established in 1916, chaired by Cumpston, to investigate these problems and offer advice to the states, seeking a unity of purpose in the control of these and other health problems. This became Cumpston's hallmark; gather the facts, propose policies and relentlessly overcome apathy and opposition. The committee adopted recommendations which included a national system of oversight of industrial health problems (including miners' phthisis), legislation to control venereal diseases and Commonwealth financial assistance for laboratory diagnostic facilities and epidemiological research; these latter were aimed principally at tuberculosis control.

In 1918, faced with a world wide influenza epidemic and the return of over 300,000 troops from Europe, Cumpston again realised the limitations of his power as Director of Quarantine and he proposed the establishment of a Commonwealth Department of Health. This proposal was supported by the Commonwealth and the states as well as the medical profession, and the Rockefeller Foundation offered staff training and expertise. In February 1921 the Department was established and in March, Cumpston was appointed the first Director General of Health.

The important functions of the new department relevant to tuberculosis control included epidemiological research in morbidity and mortality, the establishment and control of diagnostic laboratories, the establishment of the Commonwealth Serum Laboratories (which produced tuberculin and later BCG vaccine) and health education of the public.

Laboratories were established at Bendigo, Townsville, Cairns, Toowoomba, Rockhampton, Darwin, Broome, Kalgoorlie, Port Pirie, Lismore and Launceston. When added to existing laboratories in capital and regional cities, Australia was to have in place a national network of microbiological laboratories ideal for incorporation into the National Tuberculosis Campaign 25 years hence. In Bendigo and Kalgoorlie, X-ray facilities were installed in or adjacent to the laboratories. Bendigo had the highest tuberculosis mortality rate among urban communities in Australia and it was chosen as the site of the epidemiological survey and a health educational campaign.

A Royal Commission into Public Health was established in 1924. The Commission sat throughout 1925 and among its recommendations was the establishment of the Federal Health Council which was the forerunner of the National Health and Medical Research Council. There were two recommendations with special relevance to tuberculosis; the first was that Commonwealth subsidies be provided for joint Commonwealth-state campaigns. This was to be the harbinger of the National Tuberculosis Campaign. The second recommendation was the creation of five new divisions in the Commonwealth Department of Health, tuberculosis, epidemiology, health education, maternal hygiene and child welfare.

The Federal Health Council comprised the State Directors of Public Health, representatives of the medical profession and leaders of the community appointed by the Minister. The chairman was the Commonwealth Director General of Health, Dr Cumpston. At its second meeting in 1928 the control of tuberculosis was discussed and comprehensive proposals adopted.

The transfer of the Department from Melbourne to Canberra must have been a blow to Cumpston's hopes. Melbourne, the seat of Australia's oldest medical school and until the turn of the century the largest Australian city, was the ideal place from which to orchestrate a national public health program. The Canberra offices of the Department, above the Blue Moon Cafe in Alinga Street, Civic Centre, could scarcely have been further removed from the medical establishment network of Melbourne, Sydney and Adelaide which Cumpston had striven so hard to cultivate.

The move to exile in Canberra was followed by a worsening of the economic depression. Health was an easy target for the "razor gangs" of the Cabinet and Public Service. Despite this Cumpston, now 50 years of age, retained his philosophy of public health. In the first *Annual Report of the Director General of Health* in 1930, he wrote:

> The community is gradually accepting responsibility for the
> health of its members within ever-widening limits; an evolution is
> in progress the end of which cannot be foretold.

He was beginning to see the realisation of his dream expressed in his
Phthisis in Australia (1909). He realised that community co-operation
through education was essential to attain his goals.

> No matter what legislative powers are conferred upon which au-
> thorities, without understanding and accord, efforts to improve
> the health of the people... cannot succeed.

As the depression persisted the functions of the Commonwealth and
states in the health field were reviewed in order to reduce expenditure and
eliminate duplication. The Commonwealth Department was at one time
under threat but survived with its activities drastically reduced. The
Health Council did not meet in 1932 and in 1936 it was reconstituted as the
National Health and Medical Research Council (NH&MRC). The Council,
which now became the major sponsor of medical research in Australia,
was a triumph for Cumpston, especially in the harsh economic climate of
1936.

The outbreak of World War II in 1939 must have severely curtailed any
long-term plans he had in mind; Cumpston was now 60 but was still able
to grasp the importance of a bold imaginative idea. It was to Cumpston
that Harry Wunderly turned in 1939 with his 35 mm mass radiographic
machine; Cumpston immediately referred it to an expert committee in
Melbourne who evaluated the idea and made positive recommendations
in less than two months.

Cumpston became involved in NH&MRC consideration of a national
insurance scheme under a Conservative Government (1939) and a plan to
socialise medical practice under a Labour Government (1945). He was
also involved with the groundwork for the successful referenda on health
and social welfare powers (1946).

Dr Cumpston retired in 1945. For over 35 years he had been a central
and often the dominating figure in public health in Australia. He laid the
groundwork for a national tuberculosis control program.

Sir Harry Wunderly

A.J. Proust *

Harry Wyatt Wunderly was born at Camberwell, Victoria, in 1892. Like
Cumpston he won a scholarship to Wesley College and then a University
Exhibition to the Faculty of Medicine, University of Melbourne and a

---

* With acknowledgement to E.W. Abrahams whose obituary of Sir Harry Wunderly was the source
of much of this section. Robert Layland was also helpful.

scholarship at Queen's College. He graduated in 1915. Wunderly developed pulmonary tuberculosis while at university, almost certainly following contact with his father who died of the disease. A long holiday in the country resulted in a remission and he lost little time from his studies. After graduation he joined a general practice at Mount Barker in the Adelaide Hills District and while there married Alice Barker, daughter of a well-known pastoral family.

Wunderly became an avid student of tuberculosis and began part-time practice in Adelaide as a consultant physician with a special interest in tuberculosis. This transition from general to consultant practice was interrupted by several relapses of his tuberculosis. His practice gradually centred around tuberculosis, the individual patient as well as the public health and preventive aspects.

Early in 1924, Wunderly submitted a report to the South Australian Government on his recent trip to England, Switzerland and Austria, pointing out the advances in prevention and treatment of tuberculosis. Two years after his report, Wunderly wrote about the various types of pulmonary tuberculosis, their diagnosis and treatment. As author, Wunderly gave no indication that he held any hospital affiliation, however by 1929, in an article with L.C.E. Lindon, Wunderly was described as an MD of the University of Melbourne and an Honorary Assistant Pathologist, the Adelaide Hospital. The subject of the article was "Advanced Pulmonary Tuberculosis Treated by Thoracoplasty" and described seven patients on whom a Wilms-Sauerbruch thoracoplasty was successfully performed. Six of the patients had unilateral cavities; a pneumothorax had been attempted without success. In these papers Wunderly showed he was an astute young physician, well qualified and experienced in tuberculosis, abreast with the latest overseas literature and well grounded in the pathology of tuberculosis. His interest was not limited to tuberculosis; in 1929 he wrote about the radiological picture of peptic ulcer and in 1937 he described two cases of giant-cell tumour of bone. By 1937 Wunderly had added Honorary Physician, Bedford Park Sanatorium, to his other hospital appointments.

In 1932 Wunderly wrote a lengthy monograph on Collapse Therapy in the Treatment of Pulmonary Tuberculosis. Of the 36 references quoted, all but one were from British, American, German or French journals. Wunderly summarised the essentials of the treatment, which were the improvement in the patient's general condition (by means of the sanatorium regimen) and the provision of rest for the affected part of the lung (by collapse therapy in selected cases). Tuberculin and gold therapy also had a role in treatment. The four accepted methods of collapse were artificial pneumothorax, thoracoplasty, extrapleural pneumolysis and avulsion of the phrenic nerve. Extrapleural pneumolysis consisted of the separation of part of the lung and its covering of pleura from the inner surface of the chest wall and filling the cavity with paraffin. Avulsion of the phrenic nerve paralysed the diaphragm which contracted and restricted lung

expansion on the affected side. He detailed the indications, contra-indica-
tions and complications of each method and indicated that great care was
taken to select the most effective method of collapse for the individual
patient.

By 1932 Wunderly was an established consultant:

> When going through my last hundred cases for the preparation of
> this paper, I was surprised to find that I had recommended some
> form of collapse therapy in fifty one. As this was so very different
> from the figures I had seen quoted, I then went through the previ-
> ous fifty cases and found that twenty five of the patients had been
> given similar advice... my patients were not exactly unselected
> because they came to me after some years of medical treatment
> had failed to give them relief...

In an address to the Australasian Medical Congress of 1937 he stressed
the importance of bovine tuberculosis as a source of infection among
infants though by this time bovine tuberculosis was relatively rare in
Australian dairy herds, compared with Great Britain and Europe.

Wunderly became an advocate of closer co-operation between governments and the great voluntary bodies which were entirely state-based.
The role of government was to legislate to provide control measures (such
as strict public health supervision of milk supplies), to improve the notification procedures and to provide funding to improve both public and
voluntary organisation facilities for treatment. He emphasised the importance of early diagnosis to reduce contagion and increase the chances of a
permanent remission; to this end he advocated mass tuberculin surveys of
whole communities. He also recommended the vaccination with BCG of
high-risk groups (such as nurses). He concluded his address:

> So government control must aim at stopping the spread of infec-
> tion, be it milk-borne or sputum-borne. It must hunt down the
> open case and either convert it to a closed case or prevent, by
> educative means, its spreading infection. Further it must seek out
> the early cases in the pre-clinical stage and take such measures as
> have been found to be effective to protect those who, with a
> negative tuberculin reaction, are compelled to be in contact with
> tuberculosis.

So more than a decade before its launching, Wunderly had enunciated the
logic and framework for a national tuberculosis campaign.

In 1940 Wunderly published the results of tuberculin surveys of young
women in Adelaide; the positive reactors were examined by photofluoroscopy in an effort to make a pre-symptom diagnosis and hence
institute treatment before the disease was well established. This survey
was similar to the landmark Prophett survey in Great Britain and certainly
the first to make some use of photofluoroscopy.

At the outbreak of World War II Wunderly immediately called for the
mass chest X-ray screening of recruits to the armed forces. He used his

access to the corridors of power to secure endorsement of this policy after the highly successful trial X- ray survey of the 6th Battalion, 6th Division of the Australian Imperial Force in December 1939. Subsequently all service personnel were radiologically examined on enlistment and again on discharge.

Despite their past history of tuberculosis both Dr and Mrs Wunderly were accepted into the armed forces early in the war. After a brief period as a Major in the RAAMC, Charters Towers, Wunderly was promoted Lieutenant Colonel in charge of an army sanatorium at Bonegilla in Victoria and was then transferred to the Army General Hospital, Heidelberg, in charge of the tuberculosis service and adviser on tuberculosis at Army Headquarters, Victoria Barracks. The armed service environment in which facilities for early diagnosis and adequate treatment of active cases were available, enabled Wunderly to refine and develop his notion of the requirements for a successful post-war national campaign.

Wunderly remained in the Army till 1947 when he was appointed the first Commonwealth Director of Tuberculosis by the Chifley Labor Government after the passage of the first Tuberculosis Act of 1946.

The timing of the Wunderly's arrival in Canberra was propitious. The Commonwealth had just achieved new powers in the health field through referendum and was willing to listen to Wunderly. He immediately began to compile a report on tuberculosis in Australia and overseas.

The report pointed to significant deficiencies in tuberculosis control in the various states. It noted shortages of beds and uneconomical use of available beds, medical and nursing staff shortages, unsatisfactory notification procedures, poor quality medical records and lack of co-ordination between the federal and state governments. Wunderly called for a comprehensive program to control tuberculosis with modern methods of detection, treatment, rehabilitation and prevention.

There were still many difficulties in implementing the scheme. Most of these problems were solved by Wunderly's diplomacy, determination and sheer hard work; the political lines of communication centered on their five years residence in the Hotel Canberra also solved many of these problems. Nothing highlighted their dedication more than this sojourn in Canberra, when both of them must have pined for their home in the Adelaide Hills.

At the same time Wunderly was helped enormously by the rapid progress in the diagnostic facilities, drug treatment and prevention of tuberculosis. The clinical trials of isoniazid, streptomycin and para-aminosalicylic acid (PAS) carried out by the Medical Research Council in the early 1950s in England and the Veterans Administration in America gave real hope that tuberculosis was curable. Resectional surgery, BCG vaccine and improved mass miniature radiograph machines were all making significant advances.

The combination of a well-funded national tuberculosis program with all these advances in diagnosis and treatment did not guarantee success. Some States were reluctant to adopt compulsory MMR, others remained suspicious of the Commonwealth's involvement in health matters. In 1950 in a letter to Cotter Harvey, Wunderly wrote:

> In the next few years I am determined to see action but the States must help... Tuberculosis should be and I thought it was, above politics.

Again he remarked to Cotter Harvey "I sometimes wonder whether this is a fight against tuberculosis or a fight about tuberculosis."

Dr Wunderly was actively aware of the need to have well- trained chest physicians playing a prominent clinical and teaching role in the tuberculosis control program. In this way the long-term goal of not only controlling tuberculosis but keeping it under control could be guaranteed. Dr and Mrs Wunderly established the Wunderly Travelling Scholarships within the Royal Australasian College of Physicians with a gift of £18,000. In making this gift Wunderly recalled the help he had received from scholarships as a student. The scholars were young physicians who travelled abroad, working usually at the Brompton Hospital in London and returned to take their place in teaching hospitals in Australia and New Zealand. They had an important impact on the emerging specialty of thoracic medicine.*

Sir Harry Wunderly retired in 1957, recognised in Australia as the "father of the National Tuberculosis Control Program" and by the World Health Organization as an expert in the field of tuberculosis control. He served on the WHO Expert Committee on Tuberculosis and advised the Malayan government on tuberculosis control. Of Wunderly's work with the World Health Organization (WHO) Dr H Mahler, later Director General of WHO wrote:

> with all his international authority as an outstanding clinician, combined with his unflinching courage, he moved into the international tuberculosis arena... Sir Harry succeeded in setting in motion the technical chain reaction that culminated in the eighth report of the WHO Expert Committee on Tuberculosis in 1964 in the preparation of which he was WHO's invaluable adviser. The resulting explosive Expert Committee Report was to become a monument of historical proportions in the fight against tuberculosis.

Wunderly continued to take a keen interest in the Australian control

---

* Short biographies of the Wunderly Scholars are given in the Appendix.

program In 1963 he wrote in the *Medical Journal of Australia:*

> there is no room for complacency when 3,500 new cases of tuberculosis were notified in 1961.

Dr Wunderly was knighted for his services to Australia in 1954.

Sir Harry Wunderly died suddenly in Canberra in April 1971, shortly after the death of his wife. Tributes were paid to him in the Medical Journal of Australia of 28 August 1971 by Dr Ellis Abrahams, who worked with Sir Harry in Canberra and later, as Director of Tuberculosis, in Queensland. Dr. Abrahams was a close colleague and friend of Sir Harry; he wrote a fine appreciation of Sir Harry and was joined by Dr H. Mahler, Assistant Director General of WHO (and later Director General) and Dr Cotter Harvey and others. Rarely if ever has the Journal published such lengthy tributes.

Dr William Cotter Burnell Harvey

H.P.B. Harvey

Cotter Harvey was born of Irish-German parents in 1897 in Grenfell, New South Wales, where his father Dr L W Harvey was in practice. Later the family moved to Manly where Dr Harvey established a flourishing general practice and young Cotter entered Sydney Grammar School. Following a minor accident, Dr Harvey coughed up some blood and pulmonary tuberculosis (the "Irish Disease" which had afflicted his family) was diagnosed. Dr Harvey semi-retired to a practice in the Blue Mountains while Cotter began his medical studies at the University of Sydney and St Paul's College. His father's condition deteriorated and finally the family except for Cotter travelled to Geneva, seeking the cure with tuberculin therapy. Dr Harvey had a massive haemoptysis and expired in the arms of his wife on the evening following his first injection of tuberculin. Cotter was at this time (1921) a resident medical officer at Royal Prince Alfred Hospital.

Cotter travelled to England, worked at the Brompton Hospital and was awarded the Tuberculosis Disease Diploma from the University of Wales. On his return to Australia Cotter was appointed to the staff of Royal North Shore Hospital in 1924 and to that of Royal Prince Alfred Hospital in 1925. He was to serve both hospitals as an honorary physician for 33 years. At Royal North Shore Hospital he worked tirelessly in the Wakehurst Block (1941) and the Thoracic Unit (1948). This unit became a trendsetter in Australia with Cotter Harvey as chief, Bruce White heading the second medical unit and Mick Susman as senior surgeon. Later, Gordon Bayliss and Geoff McManis (physicians) and Ian Monk (surgeon) joined the unit with Bruce Geddes as clinical superintendent.

At Royal Prince Alfred Hospital progress was less dramatic. The Thoracic Unit was established in 1945 when Cotter returned form World War II, and he committed himself entirely to the practice of thoracic medicine. The unit moved to the Page Chest Pavilion when the latter opened in 1955.

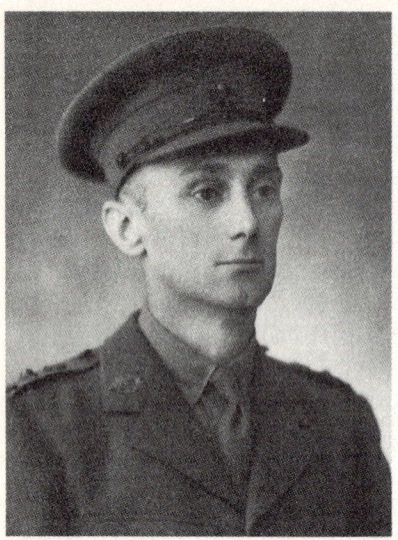

Lt Col W. Cotter Harvey in January 1941.
(Photo courtesy of the History of Medicine
Library, Royal Australasian College of
Physicians)

There Cotter Harvey headed a unit with Ted Rennie, Maurice Joseph and Geoff McDonald as physicians and John McMahon, Sandy Grant and Bruce Leckie as surgeons.

He worked extraordinarily long hours at both hospitals and at his own consulting rooms. He was at all times at the leading edge of advances in the treatment of tuberculosis and was one of the first to use streptomycin and isoniazid in Sydney. He also encouraged the surgeons to keep abreast of the advances in thoracoplasty and lobectomy in tuberculosis. He was an excellent teacher to both undergraduate and postgraduate students.

He enlisted without hesitation when World War II began, despite his age and family responsibilities. He was appointed head of the medical service in the 10th Australian General Hospital, and for four years he was a prisoner of war in Changi, Singapore. There he treated several cases of tuberculosis and administered artificial pneumothorax with an improvised apparatus.

Cotter Harvey returned to civilian life even more determined to win the big battles against tuberculosis and the other great killer, lung cancer, in which he became increasingly interested. He renewed his old friendship with Harry Wunderly and in the archives of the Royal Australasian College of Physicians Library are scores of letters to and from Wunderly, Darcy Cowan and others who in the euphoria of the early post-war period were determined to eradicate tuberculosis in Australia. Incidentally Cotter's chest X-ray, on his return to Australia, showed lung scars and active tuberculosis was suspected but finally disproved.

His enthusiasm and energy were boundless. He was a member of the New South Wales Medical Board 1940–67 and its president from 1956–67, the foundation president of the Association of Chest Physicians (1949) and later of the Laennec Society which laid the foundation of the Thoracic Society of Australia. D'Arcy Cowan of Adelaide in 1948 was instrumental in founding the Australian Tuberculosis Association with Cotter Harvey, Roy Mills and Harry Wunderly on the steering committee. This later became the National Association for the Prevention of Tuberculosis in Australia (NAPTA) of which Cotter was later president. He was to mobilise all these with other leaders in the fight to establish a national tuberculosis control program.

His interest in tuberculosis was truly international. He joined the precursor of the International Union Against Tuberculosis (IUAT) in 1920 and attended most post-war IUAT meetings. He was also a founder of the Eastern Region of the IUAT of which Australia was a member. In 1960 he was awarded the prestigious Philip Memorial Medal by the Chest and Heart Association of the United Kingdom. From 1949 to 1970 he was a member of the National Tuberculosis Advisory Council which supervised the national tuberculosis control program.

He was a man of immense energy. During the 1930s he would take his family on long journeys over indifferent roads to visit patients in sanatoria at Picton, Wentworth Falls, Springwood and Blackheath. No wonder his patients adored him. Their faces would light up at the mention of his name even 30 or more years after he had treated them. Basically an Irishman never known to shirk a fight, his battle against tuberculosis with its many victories (as well as the occasional wound) was the one he enjoyed most during his lifetime and for which he will be long remembered.

H.O. Lancaster

Oliver Lancaster was Professor of Medical Statistics at the University of Sydney for 30 years from 1959. He achieved international recognition for his publications on tuberculosis and cancer mortality.

He published his paper on "Tuberculosis Mortality in Australia 1908–1945" in 1950 (*MJA* 1950 1,665). He noted the problem posed by the priority traditionally given to tuberculosis as a cause of death over all other conditions save cancer and violence. This almost certainly exaggerated the tuberculosis death certification rate in the latter half of the 19th century and early decades of the 20th century.

Lancaster tabulated the crude tuberculosis mortality data according to age and sex and then calculated standardised mortality rates per million at risk. He then rearranged mortality rates "to give a presumed (tuberculosis) mortality experience of successive generations or cohorts". In doing this he was applying the work of W.H. Frost in the USA to Australian data.

Lancaster clearly demonstrated the continuing reduction in age and sex specific tuberculosis mortality first noted by Trivett. This fall occurred well before any possible influence of improved treatment techniques or public health measures with the exception of Dairy Supervision Acts of the 1880s. A comparison of tuberculosis mortality rates of 1908–10 with those of 1941–45 showed a 70 per cent decline in both sexes up to the age of 44 years. The fall in the female mortality rate outstripped that of the male. In males aged 65 years and over the fall was quite modest. In 1941–45 tuberculosis remained a significant cause of death in the 15 to 44 year age group, accounting for 14 per cent of male deaths and 16.3 per cent of female deaths. By 1941–45 the concentration of tuberculosis mortality in older males was well established.

The cohort or generation method of analysing age-specific tuberculosis mortality rates compared, for example, the rates of those born in 1901 with those born in 1931. In the USA Frost had applied this to tuberculosis mortality data and had demonstrated that the mortality rate at every age was lower as the cohort progressed in time. This decline gave the appearance that tuberculosis mortality was merely postponed from the earlier years of life to the later years. This was shown by Frost (and Lancaster) to be an artifact. The divergence in mortality between the sexes (the female rate falling significantly more than the male rate, especially in the older age groups) was also puzzling. Both sex cohorts had passed through high infection rates in early childhood. It was possible that prior to childbearing the natural selection pressure was greater in females in the early 1900s and resulted in a female genetic constitution with increased resistance to tuberculosis. There was evidence of increased resistance in females to most diseases in infancy and childhood. Another possible cause of the divergence between male and female tuberculosis mortality rates was the excess mortality in servicemen during and after the World War I. Male occupational hazards such as mining, excessive smoking and alcohol intake may also have been factors. These may have slowed the decline in male tuberculosis mortality.

The concentration of tuberculosis mortality in the older age groups, especially male, occurred because heavy tuberculosis infection was more common in the 1891 cohort for example compared with the 1921 cohort. As the heavily infected cohort grew older and survived longer due to increased longevity latent tuberculosis foci had greater chances of reactivation and caused death due to tuberculosis in the older age groups. The peak male tuberculosis mortality passed from the 30–49 year age group in 1901–05 to the 55 to 74 year age group in 1941– 45.

Lancaster charted the decline in tuberculosis mortality in Australia over nearly 70 years and predicted it would continue. The massive intake of migrants and refugees in the post-war period and again after the Vietnamese conflict slowed this decline only marginally. Without this influx of young people usually heavily infected with the tubercle bacillus in their own country, tuberculosis mortality in Australia would now be infinitesimal.

The Waxing and Waning of Tuberculosis in Australia 1788 to 1988

A.J. Proust

The Australian Aborigines were not infected with tuberculosis prior to European settlement at Sydney Cove in 1788. On the other hand the convicts and military and civilian personnel of the First and subsequent Fleets were heavily infected as they came from England which was experiencing the peak of a tuberculosis epidemic. Despite this tuberculosis was not a major cause of death in the infant colony.

Cunningham (1827) was the first of several medical observers who commented upon tuberculosis in New South Wales. The prevalence and natural course of the disease in the Antipodean climate became subjects of debate over then next 50 years.

The discovery of gold in Victoria in 1851 attracted an enormous number of prospectors and migrants, some with known tuberculosis and probably many more with unsuspected tuberculosis. As a result of this migration of mainly young people the birth rate soared in the middle 1850s, further skewing the age structure of the population towards the younger age groups which were highly susceptible to tuberculosis (and other infectious diseases). This combined with other factors (occupational and urban) resulted in a peak of tuberculosis mortality in Victoria and New South Wales in the 1880s. Queensland experienced a steeper peak in tuberculosis mortality at about the same time, due to the large scale importation of Kanaka labourers who were highly susceptible to tuberculosis; the other states maintained plateaux in their tuberculosis mortality rates at this time and then joined the larger states in a sustained fall which has continued up to the 1980s.

Most Australians, even those in the health professions, would be surprised at the numbers of people who have died of tuberculosis in Australia since 1850.

The Table of Mortality on the following page shows the tuberculosis mortality rate peaked in the decade 1881–90, fell rapidly in the first decade of the 20th century and thereafter more slowly to 1950. The advent of chemotherapy and other factors reduced the rate by a dramatic 70 per cent in the decade 1951–60 until by 1974 it had reached a minuscule one death per 100,000 population.

Morbidity in 1910

A careful review in South Australia in 1910 of tuberculosis notifications, death certifications and hospital and dispensary records concluded that on December 31, 1910 there were 457 persons with active pulmonary tuberculosis in the state, a point prevalence rate of 112 cases per 100,000 population.

As South Australia's tuberculosis mortality rate was similar to that of Australia's, one may assume there were about 5,000 cases in Australia's 4.4 million population. There were 3,094 deaths from pulmonary tuberculosis in Australia in 1914; assuming the total number of active cases of pulmonary tuberculosis was about 5,000, the case fatality rate was about 60 per cent. In Western Australia in 1914, 229 deaths were registered and 353 notifications received, a case fatality rate of 65 per cent.

Uniform criteria for notification of all forms of tuberculosis came into operation in Australia in 1950 and detailed Australian tuberculosis statistics were published by the Commonwealth Department of Health until 1985; these included notifications by sex and age group, deaths, details of bacteriology including drug sensitivity patterns, bovine tuberculosis, bacteriologically proven atypical mycobacterial disease, the case yield of mass miniature X-ray surveys, numbers of recipients of the tuberculosis allowance, capital and maintenance expenditure under the National Tuberculosis Control Program and beds available for tuberculosis patients.

Table of Estimated Mortality

Period	Mortality Rate per 100,000	Total Tuberculosis Deaths
1850–80	120	64,000
1881–90	150	47,000
1891–1900	120	45,000
1901–10	100	45,000
1911–20	75	36,000
1921–30	60	35,000
1931–40	42	28,000
1941–50	35	23,000
1951–60	10	8,000
1961–70	3	3,000
1971–80	1	1,200
1981–90	< 1	500
TOTAL		335,000

Explanatory notes:
1. Data prior to 1875 are generally unreliable. Registration of the cause of death was not universal and terminology (eg. phthisis, consumption) was not standardised.
2. Data from 1875 to 1909 are regarded as accurate particularly in New South Wales (Trivett, Coghlan), Victoria (Hayter) and Western Australia (Cumpston).
3. Data for the period 1908 to 1945 are from the published papers of H.O. Lancaster.
4. Data from 1948 to 1985 are from Australian Tuberculosis Statistics, Department of Health, Canberra and for the years 1986 and 1987 by courtesy of Dr Eddy Lo, Canberra.

Infection in the 1920s

The prevalence of infection in Australia as measured by skin sensitivity to tuberculin (using the Von Pirquet, Mantoux or Heaf tuberculin test) has been measured since the 1920s.

W.J. Penfold presented data to the 1923 Australasian Medical Congress which showed rates of infection in the cities of Melbourne, Sydney and Adelaide. In Melbourne, of 100 male and female medical students aged 18 to 27 years, 70 were tuberculin reactors. About 25 per cent of children aged 6 to 10 years and 50 per cent of adult hospital patients without any evidence of tuberculosis were positive reactors.

One must conclude that tuberculosis infection was common in adults and children in urban communities in Australia in the 1920s. It was however not as high as in industrial England where as late as 1930 90 per cent of children were tuberculin reactors.

The Death of the White Plague

In 1948 in Australia there was a happy coincidence of factors which was to spell the death knell of tuberculosis as a major public health problem. The decline in tuberculosis mortality, evident since 1900, continued up to 1945 with a marked shift of male mortality into the 60 years and over age group; the female mortality rate fell significantly across all age groups. The factors which were to result in a marked decline in tuberculosis mortality were

- The demonstrated efficiency of mass miniature radiography (MMR) as a reliable and cost-effective case-finding tool on a community-wide basis.
- The discovery of specific anti-tuberculosis drugs which were later proven capable of curing the disease.
- The national determination to tackle major problems was used to overcome political problems which had plagued tuberculosis programs in the past.

The result was that in the forty years from 1950 there were dramatic falls in tuberculosis infection, notification and mortality rates despite the entry of nearly 4 million migrants and refugees, most of whom came from countries with a much higher prevalence of tuberculosis than Australia's.

INFECTION RATES 1948–1980

In 1948 about 40 per cent of the white Australian adult population were infected with tuberculosis as manifested by a Mantoux reaction of 10 mm or more (Canberra and Queanbeyan Mantoux survey 1950). By the 1980s the adult population's infection rate was only 15 per cent.

In Australian-born schoolchildren aged 10 to 12 years the decline in infection was more dramatic; from 8 per cent in 1948 to less than 1 per cent in 1980 (ACT school tuberculin surveys).

In migrants and refugees from high prevalence countries (Asia, Central and South America) the prevalence of infection remains at about 50 per cent in adults.

MORBIDITY 1954–1986

Morbidity rates based upon compulsory notification of active cases of tuberculosis have fallen from a peak of 56 per 100,000 in 1954 when MMR was in full swing to 10 per 100,000 in 1974 and 6 per 100,000 in 1986.

The Australian tuberculosis notification rates are distorted because Australia unlike the UK, USA and Canada includes cases of atypical mycobacterial disease (AMD). These increase the notification rate by 7 to 10 per cent in Australia overall; in Queensland and Western Australia the increase is about 10 to 15 per cent. If AMD is discounted, the notification of tuberculosis has fallen to 5 cases per 100,000 in 1985–86.

Tuberculosis is now a disease of old age. In 1982 the notification rate according to age groups was:

0–19 years	1.5 cases per 100,000
20–24 years	6 cases per 100,000
45–64 years	12 cases per 100,000
65 and over	22 cases per 100,000

Not only has there been a reduction in notified cases of tuberculosis, there has been a significant reduction in the percentage of notified cases which are shown to be bacteriologically positive (and hence infectious).

The pool of infectious cases has been further reduced by the virtual elimination of "chronic positives", 71 cases of which were notified in 1969; with the introduction of rifampicin in 1969 this number was reduced to less than 10 in 1975.

This reduction in infectious tuberculosis has resulted in a generation of young Australians aged less than 20 years who have had virtually no contact with tuberculosis within Australia.

Mortality 1948– 1980

In 1948 the tuberculosis mortality rate in Australia was 28 deaths per 100,000; this fell to 5 (1959) to 1 (1974) and since then it has been less than one death per 100,000 per annum. Most of the deaths which do occur are in elderly people who die *with* tuberculosis rather than *from* tuberculosis.

If some form of tuberculosis control is maintained one may be reasonably confident that tuberculous infection, morbidity and mortality will remain acceptably low.

The Future of Tuberculosis Control in Australia

A .J. Proust and D.N.L.Seward

Tuberculosis like most infectious diseases in Australia is now responsible for only a negligible mortality and morbidity; improved living standards, public health legislation, the National Tuberculosis Campaign, BCG vaccination and modern chemotherapy have been jointly responsible.

Australia has however an active migration and refugee resettlement program mostly involving people already heavily infected with tuberculosis in their homeland. For this reason alone tuberculosis control is still relevant in Australia. Because there is usually a long latent period between infection and the development of overt active tuberculosis, migrants and refugees from countries of high tuberculosis prevalence will provide a trickle of tuberculosis during the remainder of their lifetime in Australia.

For more than 90 years the notification rate of active tuberculosis has been falling in the white Australian-born population. To maintain the present low incidence of tuberculosis in this population it is essential to keep a basic control structure in place; notification procedures, central case registers and registers of those at high risk of developing tuberculosis must be maintained. The teaching of tuberculosis to undergraduate and post-graduate students must continue and all large hospitals should have on the staff a designated physician with expertise in the management of tuberculosis and at least one graduate nurse knowledgeable in the public health aspects of the disease. There should be a large microbiological laboratory in each capital city which acts as the central reference laboratory for the full identification of mycobacteria including drug sensitivity testing in that state. There is also the need to have a small number of hospital beds for investigation and treatment of problem cases.

These control measures are now in place to varying degrees in the States and Territories of Australia. Despite these control measures however there will be during the 1990's about 350 cases each year among Australian-born whites, reflecting an estimated incidence rate of about 2.5 cases per 100,000. The impact of the acquired immune-deficiency syndrome (AIDS) on the incidence of tuberculosis in this population has so far been negligible in Australia.

The Australian Aboriginal population has a significantly higher tuberculosis notification rate than Australian-born whites. This applies in both the semi-tribal rural and the urban environments. About 25 to 40 cases may be expected in this population (estimated incidence 10 to 15 cases per 100,000) each year during the 1990s. Aboriginal health services should be constantly reminded of this; the most effective way of control is by the general application of BCG vaccination to infants soon after birth, repeated if indicated at the age of 10–12 years.

Migrants from the United Kingdom, Western Europe, North America and New Zealand are not significantly more likely to develop tuberculosis in Australia than the Australian-born white population; migrants from Central, Southern and Eastern Europe will have a higher incidence of tuberculosis after migration to Australia. The overall incidence of tuberculosis in these migrant groups is about 8 cases per 100,000 each year, about 200 notifications each year. This may fall steadily during the 1990s as migration from these countries diminishes. The long-established screening procedures to exclude active tuberculosis should remain in place.

The highest incidence of tuberculosis (about 80 cases per 100,000 each year) is to be found among migrants and refugees form high incidence countries (countries other than the United Kingdom, Europe, North America and New Zealand). This will result in about 350 notified cases annually, rising if the numbers admitted rise significantly or if screening procedures are not rigorously maintained.

The medical and nursing professions must remain aware of the possibility of tuberculosis in any person whatever his or her ethnic, social or cultural background. It is only with this constant awareness of tuberculosis that control can be maintained. This will lead to early diagnosis and effective treatment of the infectious case, identification by contact examination of those who have been infected and effective prevention of the disease by BCG vaccination.

Chapter 12

Migration of Consumptives to Australia

A.J. Proust

The migration of consumptives seeking "the cure" in Australia may be traced to the 1820s (Powell[1]). Most aspects of this subject in the 19th century have been covered in Chapter 2 ("The Long Sea Voyage and the Australian Climate").

From about 1830 Australia increasingly evoked among English people an image of an El Dorado, an Australian Felix, a rich country sparsely settled by healthy people of English stock; the climate was equable and disease was uncommon so much so that English medical practitioners thinking of migrating were warned they might have problems establishing a viable practice.

Prior to 1850 two myths about tuberculosis in Australia were established. The first was that tuberculosis was a rare or even unknown cause of death in the Australian-born population. This was stated categorically by Dr T.E. Dempster of the Indian Medical Service in Calcutta, who practised in Tasmania about 1835. The myth had been exploded by Dr McLeod of Sydney Hospital replying to a questionnaire about health and disease in the Colony in 1829. Most authorities agree that although tuberculosis was much less common than in England, it certainly occurred, especially in the younger age-groups.

The second myth was that "European phthisis is cured or relieved in the Australian climate" (Dr P. Cunningham 1827, later given great authority by Dr S. Dougan Bird in Melbourne in the 1860s). There is no doubt that some migrants with early disease or with chronic fibroid disease did do well in the climate, life-style and plentiful food in Australia. But many migrants arriving with pulmonary tuberculosis died within months of their arrival, especially in the second half of the 19th century.

In the 1860s the colonies began competing with one another for British migrants. Publicity in the British press emphasised the healthy life style in their particular colony; Victoria actually promoted the state as ideal for the consumptive migrant some of whom were given assisted passages. As Melbourne was the initial land fall, most migrants disembarked there and stayed in the city. Only a minority ventured to rural areas. Large-sale underground mining in Ballarat and Bendigo attracted large numbers of skilled miners from Wales.

Powell[1] summarises this episode in the history of migration to Australia:

> at no time were details kept of the actual number of consumptive immigrants who entered Victoria. Accurate diagnosis (of

the disease) was quite impossible and only the most cursory examination was ever required (prior to emigration). Had it not been for Thomson, Hayter and other sympathetic thinkers and for the opportunism of a crusading newspaper the chances are that the government of Victoria might have added the weight of its own successful promotional efforts to cast its net even wider among the consumptives of Europe.

The dramatic economic depression in Victoria in the 1890s caused the flow of migrants to almost dry up, to be revived only just prior to World War I.

1918 Onwards

L.J. O'Keefe and A.J. Proust

The newly established Federal Department of Health assumed the responsibility for the medical screening of migrants in 1921. The Director General of Health, Dr J.H.L. Cumpston was a highly experienced quarantine officer and he had chaired the inter-departmental committee of 1916 which investigated the principal causes of ill-health in the Australian community. One of its recommendations was that all intending migrants should undergo official medical inspection overseas and again on arrival in Australia.

Approximately 300,000 migrants arrived in the 1920s, the great majority from Britain and the remainder from Europe (Italy, Yugoslavia and Greece). The Great Depression of the 1930s halted migration although several thousand refugees from Central Europe arrived just prior to World War II.

Post World War II Immigration, 1947–1975

In 1946 an assisted passage scheme was announced by the Australian Government by which British emigrants would be brought to Australia. In July 1947 Mr A.A. Calwell, Minister for Immigration, signed an agreement in Geneva with the International Refugee Organisation for the resettlement in this country of refugees and displaced persons of whom a million or more remained in Western Europe, mainly in Germany and Austria. Thus was initiated the great post-war migration scheme which by 1981 had brought about four million people to Australia from about forty countries.

In order to ensure the good health of all prospective migrants, comprehensive health screening measures were introduced. Dr Harry Wunderly, Commonwealth Director of Tuberculosis, recognised that the prevalence of tuberculosis in many of the source countries was much higher than in Australia, particularly in a Europe still suffering the deprivations of six years of war. As the selection processes became established, Australian medical officers formed part of the migration teams. Applicants were physically examined and all persons sixteen years of age and over were required to undergo a chest X-ray examination. Doubtful films were referred to Australian radiologists stationed in central locations such as London, Athens and Rome. This same pattern was adopted when missions began to operate in places like Malta, Egypt, Turkey and the Lebanon.

Where there was radiological evidence of active disease or a recent history of such inadequately treated by Australian standards, the application for migration was rejected. Migrants with known but inactive tuberculosis who were accepted were required to sign an undertaking to report to the relevant state Director of Tuberculosis within a stated period after arrival in Australia.

Pulmonary tuberculosis accounted for a high proportion of rejections on medical grounds in Europe in the late 1940s and early 1950s. Mackay[2] found a rejection rate of thirty five per cent on account of tuberculosis in a series of 348 medical rejections between November 1948 and April 1949. On the whole the screening process was quite effective. Nevertheless, some persons with active tuberculosis did manage to escape the net. One of us (L.O'K), who served as a medical officer in Austria and Germany in the 1950s proffers the following reasons. Firstly, chest X-rays were performed under the direction of and reported on by local doctors employed by the host countries who were often not very experienced in radiology— for instance, Australian authorities had to circularise instruction on the technique of taking lordotic films. Secondly, facilities for examination were less than ideal, frequently being housed in makeshift quarters in barracks of displaced persons' camps. Thirdly, successful substitution by healthy friends or relatives did occur when the identification checks were not scrupulously observed; later, when O'Keefe was medical superintendent at Bonegilla Migrant Reception Centre in Victoria he recalls not infrequently seeing X-ray films from overseas which obviously were of different persons to those X-rayed on arrival. Fourthly, tuberculosis might develop or be reactivated during the interim between processing the application to migrate and his arrival in Australia, which could be six months or more. To minimise this intending migrants who had not left within twelve months of selection were required to have another chest X-ray. Finally the X-ray standards were occasionally relaxed on compassionate grounds.

For these reasons newly arrived migrants were examined in Reception Centres by miniature radiography. As a result at Bonegilla Reception Centre, two wards at the hospital were reserved for the treatment of arrivals with active tuberculosis. Later as the prevalence of pulmonary tuberculosis fell in newly arrived refugees, only high risk groups were examined radiographically as a routine on arrival at reception centres. Nevertheless it was a requirement that all new arrivals presumably free of tuberculosis present themselves within a month of arrival at their final destination in Australia. The special wards at Bonegilla were closed and those found to have active tuberculosis on entry were accommodated temporarily on chemotherapy pending transfer to a State sanatorium.

In 1963 F.G.B. Edwards, Director of Tuberculosis in Western Australia, reported that in that state[3] "the incidence of tuberculosis in persons born outside Australia (migrants) has been more than double that in the Australian born". Edwards divided the 1961 population census of Western Australia into the following categories.

Country or Region of Birth	Average Population (thousands) 1958 - 62	Average incidence of Tuberculosis per 100,000
United Kingdom	44.4	106
Italy	14.9	109
Other European	23.3	104
Other countries	8.1	126
Australian born	284.8	44.6

In Edwards's series of 1,130 notifications of tuberculosis in Western Australia during 1958–62, 494 (43.7 per cent) were in persons born outside Australia. The Working Party on Tuberculosis Services in Victoria (1982) reports that in 1974 the notifications per 100,000 population of Australian born of 6.4 was somewhat lower than in UK/European born (8.6) and considerably less than for those born in Greece (12.9), Italy (20.0) and Yugoslavia (26.3).

The 1970s saw an end to discrimination in immigration policy and the beginning of substantial Asian immigration. By 1986 Australia had taken more than 100,000 Indo-Chinese refugees as well as many migrants.

Dr Eddie Lo calculated that 48.6 per cent of notifications in Australia in 1986 were in persons born outside Australia. The highest notification rates were in Vietnamese-born (157 per 100,000), in those born in the Philippines (142 per 100,000) and in the Chinese born (72 per 100,000). The rate in the non-aboriginal Australian-born was 2.8 per 100,000 and in Australian Aborigines 11 per 100,000.

The rates of tuberculosis notifications in the Australian Capital Territory (ACT) were published in the *Australian Tuberculosis Newsletter* by A J Proust *et al* (No. 12 March 1990). The rate in the Australian-born was 2.2 per 100,000, in the European-born 8.5, and in those born in high incidence countries (those born in countries other than Europe, North America and New Zealand) 40 per 100,000. The authors noted that:

> The ACT has had since 1961 a higher proportion of its population born overseas than any state or territory except Western Australia.

During the period 1961–71 the overseas born component of the ACT population averaged 26.2 per cent compared with 18.5 per cent in the whole Australian population. The 1961 census revealed about 2.1 per cent of the ACT population was born in high incidence countries and this rose to 4 per cent in 1981.

The total notifications of tuberculosis in Australia during the period 1948–86 inclusive was 101,314 of whom at least 45,000 were in the overseas-born population. Seen in the context of four million migrants and refuges over the past 40 years and considering the urgency of the immediate post-war program and the humanitarian aspects involved in the intake of refugees from war-torn countries of Europe and Asia, it is believed that the medical screening processes have been effective in containing the problem to a level with which a prosperous nation such as Australia is well able to cope.

Dr Howells wrote:

> A study of this problem only reinforces the old principles of tuberculosis... the degree of infection in certain migrant groups is far higher and active tuberculosis derives from this infection.

He forecast in 1970 that Australia would feel the impact of tuberculosis in countries to the north folowing the entry of migrants and refuges from these countries.

Extrapulmonary Tuberculosis in Migrants

Stefan Csordas made some interesting observations on tuberculosis in migrants.[4] He reviewed 1,076 cases of extrapulmonary tuberculosis notified in Victoria 1961–71, comprising 13.5 per cent of all tuberculosis notifications; 50.3 per cent of patients with extrapulmonary tuberculosis were born outside Australia although the 1971 census showed that only 20.5 per cent of Victoria's population were migrants. The migrant population provided 75 per cent of all cases of tuberculosis of the female genital tract and 51 per cent of all cases of renal, bone and joint tuberculosis. Mainland European-born migrants comprised about 11.6 per cent of the Victorian population and they manifested 36.9 per cent of all cases of extrapulmonary tuberculosis. The Italian-born population comprised 4.4 per cent of the Victorian population yet provided half of all cases of tuberculosis of the female genital tract and about one-third of the renal, bone and joint tuberculosis.

Tuberculosis in Australian Troops in Two World Wars

L.J. O'Keefe

A total of 512,953 men volunteered for service overseas in the AIF during the Great War. A remarkably high number, 173,138, were rejected on medical grounds and of these only 1,359 were rejected because of tuberculosis.

Of the 339,815 passed for service, 343 died of tuberculosis overseas and 2,059 were repatriated with active tuberculosis. The problem of tuberculosis among servicemen became evident in 1915 when tubercular soldiers had to be evacuated from Gallipoli.

The unexpectedly large proportion (33.7 per cent) of volunteers rejected on medical grounds prompted the Federal Government to convene an inter-departmental committee chaired by Dr J.H.L. Cumpston to investigate the causes of ill-health in the Australian population. The wide-ranging investigations and recommendations of the committee led to the establishment by the Commonwealth of the Department of Repatriation (1918) and undoubtedly stimulated the government to create the Department of Health (1921). Both of these departments were involved with tuberculosis during the 1920s

According to Repatriation Department annual reports there were 1,820 ex-servicemen in 1920 with active tuberculosis, 487 of whom were in hospital. These included arrested cases suitable for light rural employment, advanced cases requiring hospice care and a growing number of early cases diagnosed only at or after discharge, for whom sanatorium care was required. The diagnosis of pulmonary tuberculosis was almost entirely clinical until the early 1920s. Chest X-ray examination and sputum examination for the tubercle bacilli are mentioned only briefly both in the official War History and the early annual reports of the Repatriation Department.

Pulmonary tuberculosis assumed much less importance in World War II. The reasons for this were two-fold; the incidence of tuberculosis gradually fell in the inter-war period and more importantly miniature chest radiography was used to screen all recruits from 1940 onwards, thus excluding those with minimal asymptomatic pulmonary tuberculosis who would otherwise have escaped detection. The introduction and successful application of MMR (mass miniature radiography) in the screening of Australian recruits in World War II is described in Chapter 7.

Walker in the Medical History of World War Two comments that MMR played an important role in the control of tuberculosis in the services. Walker reported that by the end of the war in 1945 the total number of service personnel notified and treated for tuberculosis while in the services was 1,500; the total of service men and women in the Australian Services during World War Two was 992,000. This represents a reduction of almost 80 per cent per 100,000 compared with World War I.

A comparison may be made between civilian notification rates 1914–18 and 1940–45 in Western Australia and notified and treated cases among service personnel in the two World Wars.

Average Notification Rates of Pulmonary Tuberculosis
per 100,000 Population

	1915-18	1940-45
Civilian Population Western Australia	140	44
Service Population Australia	143	25

The civilian notification rates in Western Australia were chosen because these rates are generally accepted as the most accurate in the early years when notification was introduced in Australia.

The conclusion to be drawn from this comparison is that MMR played a significant role in reducing the incidence of tuberculosis in Australian service personnel in World War Two.

A Tuberculosis Medical Officer in Stalag IV A 1942–45*

Alan King

I joined some twenty other medical officers mostly British but including two or three Australians and New Zealanders. I was at Lamsdorf from September 5th 1941 to the end of January 1942 when I volunteered as Medical Officer to Allied POW with tuberculosis, thinking that the living conditions and food would be an improvement. The tuberculosis hospital was at Konigswartha Stalag IV A about 100 miles south of Berlin. There were some hundreds of patients, mostly British, some Yugoslavs and a few French being treated mainly by French Army doctors; in addition there were several Yugoslav and one Polish doctor. The hospital was an old Home for the Blind with a barracks-type addition, housing about 100 patients in double-decker bunks. I was the only British Medical Officer here for some months; however as the French POWs with tuberculosis were repatriated together with their Army Medical Officers, they were replaced by British POWs who brought with them two English Medical Officers and four Australian Medical Officers who had been captured in Crete including my commanding officer Lt Colonel Le Souef, Captains Gallard and Mayrhofer also of my own unit and Captain Gerald Holt of the 2/5 AGH captured in Greece.

Although conditions were primitive in some ways, (one could hardly call Konigswartha a sanatorium—it was too crowded for that). I was soon taught a lot about tuberculosis by a French specialist physician Dr Maurice Blondeau. We had a fluoroscopic X-ray screen and were rationed to one

---

* Captain Alan King of the 2/7th Field Ambulance, AIF, was captured on Crete on 28 May 1941.

chest X-ray film (some on paper) every month or so. Thanks to Blondeau I was soon conversant with artificial pneumothorax which was induced in carefully selected patients. In turn I passed on this training to other newly arrived Medical Officers when Dr Blondeau was moved to another camp. Dr Blondeau also taught me how to perform "section de bride" or section of pleural adhesions.

We had all the usual accompaniments of a POW camp—barbed-wire fences and German guards and a senior German Army doctor, Hauptman Rindfleish, who had tuberculosis experience. We tried to secure better conditions (food and equipment) as patients increased in numbers. Some patients were very ill and the only treatment we could give was absolute bed rest. Those that died were given a decent burial with an Army-type funeral by the Germans.

At the beginning of March 1943 we moved to a standard German Army Hospital at Elsterhoist, still in Stalag IV A. Dr Blondeau was replaced by Dr Andre Chon, a young tuberculosis physician. There was a good X-ray room as well as a Theatre Block and Pharmacy. In September 1944 after a visit by a mixed German and Swiss commission, the first major repatriation of Allied tuberculosis POWs began and the Hospital was nearly emptied. Major Bert Palandri and Captain Frank Gallasch were the lucky Australian Medical Officers to accompany them back to England. Colonel Le Souef was transferred to another camp and Lt Colonel "Blue" Bull replaced him. However we soon filled up with patients again; we acquired patients via a network built up by Australian medical orderlies from the 2/5 AGH captured in Greece.

The Russian advance loomed from the East and we were regarded as "hostages" by the Germans who were resigned to inevitable defeat. February 18 1945 saw us, patients and staff, crowded into railway cattle trucks and shunted around Czechoslovakia and Eastern Germany. I remember one night vividly in the marshalling yards at Dresden (during the famous saturation raid). On February 24 1945 we arrived at a makeshift hospital in West Saxony—a polygot crowd of Russians, Italians, French and Americans—we even got the frost-bitten wounded from the Battle of Arnheim who had been force-marched through Germany in the snow for one week without any shelter. Fortunately we were freed by elements of General Patton's 4th Armoured Division of the American Third Army Corps and after about ten days cleaning up the sick and wounded, we were flown to England on May 12th 1945.

In England I was prevailed upon to continue my tuberculosis work in view of the number of cases being picked up on discharge in Australia. Russell Godby and I were promoted to Majors and given 6 months postgraduate training in the United Kingdom, Canada and the USA. Returning to Australia early in 1946 I took over as tuberculosis specialist at

Bonegilla, Victoria, from Colonel Harry Wunderly and later took my discharge in January 1947.

I completed two reports on my travels in the United Kingdom, Canada and USA: "The Present Trend of Treatment of Pulmonary Tuberculosis in England and Wales" (September 1945) and "The Problem of Tuberculosis in Canada and the USA" (February 1946). The latter included "Hospital Planning and Equipment" and it eventually became the basis for the planning of the Perth Chest Hospital (now Sir Charles Gardiner Hospital).

I joined the Health Department of Western Australian in 1947 but continued to work at the Repatriation Hospital in Perth for two days per week.

The Management of Tuberculosis in Ex-servicemen after World War I*

A.J. Proust and L.J. O'Keefe

The Department of Repatriation was established in 1918 just before the end of the Great War and rapidly became responsible for the treatment and rehabilitation of ex-service personnel with tuberculosis.

The initial steps were taken by the Defence Department. In 1916 Mont Park Mental Hospital and extensive sites at Bundoora and Janefield on the outskirts of Melbourne were taken over for the 14th Australian Auxiliary Hospital for Army recruits convalescing from illness. A further site at Gresswell was used for temporary tents for soldiers returning from overseas with tuberculosis and No. 1 Military Sanatorium was opened at Macleod in August 1916. At the same time Janefield was handed over to the Red Cross Society for a farm for the rehabilitation of ex-servicemen recovering from tuberculosis.

On 1 October 1920 the Defence Department handed over No. 1 Military Sanatorium to the Repatriation Department and this became known as the Macleod Repatriation Sanatorium. Initially there were about 130 beds available for tuberculosis patients. The first medical superintendent was Dr H.M. James who had served in the AIF in Egypt and France and had worked at the Red Cross Sanatorium, Wentworth Falls, NSW. He was also medical superintendent of Bundoora Convalescent Farm for non-tuberculosis chest patients (mainly suffering the effects of war gas) and medical officer to the Anzac Red Cross farm at Janefield for convalescent tuberculosis ex-servicemen. To complete this remarkable work-load Dr James was assistant medical officer for tuberculosis at the Royal Melbourne Hospital.

Those who developed tuberculosis during war service were entitled to

* Based on a history of the Victorian Division of the Repatriation Department by Dr A.H. Campbell.

a pension during treatment. This pension was only sixty shillings per fortnight and led to political agitation for an increase. A conference of ex-service organisations was held in Melbourne in September 1920 and proposals were put forward which were, after some delay, to become government policy. It was resolved that those being treated for tuberculosis in an institution for at least 6 months should receive a pension equal to those totally incapacitated, £8 per fortnight. This pension should be maintained for one year after discharge and should not be reduced below £4.4 a fortnight as an insurance agianst relapse. The conference also resolved that treatment should be directed by specialist medical officers.

Towards the end of 1924 the government established a Royal Commission of medical experts to enquire into the administration of the Repatriation Act. The Commission recommended and the government accepted that "a permanent pension in some degree should be paid to war-caused tuberculosis". The permanent pension was £4.4 per fortnight.

The Annual Report of the Repatriation Commission 1926–27 contained the results of a survey of tuberculosis mortality amongst ex-servicemen and soldiers in Victoria for the period 1916 to 1926. During this period there were 757 deaths from tuberculosis; for matched age-groups the tuberculosis mortality rate was 272 per 100.000 for ex-servicemen and soldiers compared with 300 per 100,000 for civilians. As the military mortality was very similar to the civilian mortality despite the fact that AIF recruits had been medically examined before enlistment, other factors were examined. Forty per cent of the soldiers with tuberculosis were found to have suffered severe war disabilities, including 15 per cent who had been severely gassed. These associated disabilities were probably responsible for the higher than expected tuberculosis mortality in the soldiers and ex-servicemen.

By 1929 with the passage of time it was becoming more difficult to prove that the onset of tuberculosis was associated with war service and increasing numbers of ex-servicemen with active tuberculosis were judged ineligible for the pension. In 1935 service pensions were introduced and ex-servicemen with tuberculosis were able to apply for this if they could not prove it was war-caused. In 1943 all cases of tuberculosis in service or ex-service personnel who had served in a theatre of war received the full tuberculosis pension benefits.

In 1945–46 the average daily number of tuberculosis patients in repatriation institutions was 675. The number peaked at 1,275 in 1951–52 but fell to 191 in 1967–68. In 1967 there were 11,890 ex-service personnel receiving a tuberculosis pension, the great majority of cases were inactive after treatment.

Tuberculosis in the New Zealand Expeditionary Force in World War II

Extracts from the Official History of New Zealand in the Second World War 1939–45, Chapter 16, by T. Duncan and M. Stout.

Tuberculosis did not constitute any great problem in 2 NZEF. At no time was the incidence high enough to cause any difficulty in management. The cases were, of course, segregated when diagnosed, and returned to New Zealand by the next hospital ship when the condition of the patient was considered to be satisfactory enough to stand the journey. The infectious diseases ward of the *Maunganui*, though small, was always able to accommodate all the tuberculosis cases. There were 115 cases of pulmonary tuberculosis invalided back to New Zealand from 2 NZEF during the war. More cases were discovered by routine X-ray at discharge, or became ill after return to civil life, than were diagnosed during their service with 2 NZEF.

In 1949, Dr D. Macdonald Wilson made a survey of pulmonary tuberculosis among New Zealand service personnel, embracing all the cases that had occurred in the ten-year period 1939–49 in the military population of 200,000 medically examined and passed fit for service, of whom about 134,000 served outside New Zealand. In the main this was a specially selected population, but, on the other hand, chest X-rays at discharge from the services, plus pension applications later, resulted in nearly all those developing tuberculosis being brought within the compass of the review. Up to 31 December 1949, 1,412 cases had applied for a pension, while there had been 8 deaths on service overseas and 30 among servicemen in New Zealand. Included were 193 cases of pleurisy with effusion. Approximately 37.5 per cent of the cases took ill on service, 42.5 per cent were diagnosed by routine X-ray (usually at discharge), and 20 per cent became ill after discharge from service.

It was found that whereas the Army and Air Force produced numbers roughly corresponding to their relative strengths, the Navy had almost double the number of cases on a comparative basis. This emphasised the fact that exposure to infection rather than the physical hardships of a campaign is the greater cause of tuberculosis in the services.

The importance of chest X-ray at enlistment was emphasised by the higher incidence among those army personnel of the first two echelons who were not X-rayed in 1939–40. The members of the Maori Battalion fortunately were nearly all X-rayed, so removing most of the potential sources of infection (16 per cent were rejected for chest conditions), and the Maoris in the services had an incidence of less than double the incidence for the whole group (13.5 against 7.4 per 1,000 over the ten years), whereas in the civil population the Maori rate is nearly five times that of Europeans.

By comparison with the annual civilian Maori rate of 23.5 per 1,000 the rate of 13.5 per 1,000 in Maoris who served overseas shows a marked reduction. (It has to be noted that on a comparative basis living conditions were much the same for Maoris and Europeans in the forces, but this was not so in civil life).

In prisoners of war the incidence was fairly high—over 17 per 1,000 over the period, but 84 of the 155 army POW cases had not been X-rayed on enlistment. Most of the prisoners of war were taken in the early campaigns and had entered the Army in 1939 and 1940 before the X-ray examinations were properly organised. Irrespective of prisoner-of-war privations, this group would have produced a higher incidence than the average. Of the total of 729 cases in the Army overseas, 222 were not X-rayed before going overseas. The First and Second Echelons, with 193 cases, produced an incidence of 14.3 per 1,000.

The annual incidence of new civilian cases in 1948 (the lowest on record at the date), was European 0.77 and Maori 3.6 per 1,000. The average annual incidence in returned service personnel for the years 1945 to 1949 was European 0.95 and Maori 1.73 per 1,000. It has be noted also that the service figures were swollen by the large number of cases brought to light by X-rays taken on discharge after return from overseas in 1945 and 1946.

Results of Treatment

All will agree that the best results of treatment should be obtained in the cases diagnosed early, for whom institutional treatment if required is available without delay, and who are relieved of financial worry should it be advisable for them to cease work. Except for prisoners of war, these two latter conditions existed for service personnel, and in over 40 per cent of cases the first condition was also present as they were diagnosed by routine X-ray before the patients were aware of any illness.

In the treatment of the 1,404 cases under review, some 300 required no treatment but were merely kept under observation at the chest clinics. On the other hand, in addition to inpatient observation in sanatorium or hospital required for the remaining cases, the following operative procedures were carried out:

- Thoracoscopy with pneumolysis or attempted pneumolysis, 33 cases.
- Artificial pneumothorax was induced in 316 cases.
- Pneumo-peritoneum was used in 22 cases.
- Phrenic crush or avulsion was carried out in 54 cases.
- Thoracoplasty was carried out in 27 cases.

Royal New Zealand Navy

Just before the outbreak of war, seven cases of tuberculosis were diagnosed in the crew of the cruiser *Achilles*. This was thought to be associated with overcrowding below decks and poor ventilation. From the end of 1940 chest radiography became part of the routine recruitment procedure. Of the 117 cases of active disease which occurred in male RNZN personnel during the period 1 September 1939 to 21 December 1946, the chest X-rays on recruitment were clear in 87.

Conclusion

From the survey it is difficult to compare the incidence of tuberculosis among service personnel with that of the civilian population, as the survey covered a closed group composed in the main of personnel of the age group in which the incidence of tuberculosis is the highest. Taking all factors into consideration, the incidence of tuberculosis in service personnel was much the same as for the civil population. Mass radiography reduced the spread of infection. Thus radiography, plus improved hygiene and the elimination of overcrowding, seems the best means of reducing the incidence of pulmonary tuberculosis in the military community.

Appendix

The Wunderly Scholars
Bryan Gandevia

Sixteen graduates from Australia and New Zealand were fortunate enough to benefit from the Scholarships provided by Sir Harry and Lady Wunderly over the decade 1948–58. Sir Harry's prime objective was to ensure that there were some Australian and New Zealand physicians with special expertise in tuberculosis, to the control of which he had himself made a major contribution. It is very much to his credit that although occasionally expressing a hint of concern that some later scholars were pursuing paths somewhat different form those he had envisaged, he continued his support, specifically declining invitations to contribute to the deliberations of the selection committee of the Royal Australasian College of Physicians.

Most of the scholars became teachers in the specialty of thoracic medicine; by the 1960s there were postgraduate units providing the specialised and concentrated training which the scholars had previously felt obliged to seek overseas. The generosity of the Wunderlys did more for thoracic medicine than Sir Harry could have anticipated.

The following biographies of the scholars are given in order of appointment.

Douglas Gauld

Douglas Gauld graduated with honours and the Exhibition in Medicine in 1939 at the University of Melbourne. After a year's residency at the Royal Melbourne Hospital, he joined the 2nd AIF, seeing service in Palestine, Syria and Egypt including Tobruk and El Alamein.

During his army service he was posted to the tuberculosis section of the Repatriation General Hospital, Heidelberg. Later he served with the 116th Australian General Hospital at Bonegilla, commanded by Lieut-Col Harry Wunderly where all the tuberculosis service patients were concentrated after 1944.

Awarded the first Wunderly Scholarship Gauld worked firstly at the King Edward VII Sanatorium at Midhurst with Dr (later Sir) Geoffrey Todd and then as house physician at the Brompton Hospital with Neville Oswald who at that time was developing his concept of chronic bronchitis and emphysema.

By the time of his return to Australia in 1951 chemotherapy and surgery were taking over the treatment of tuberculosis and the sanatorium system was beginning to wind down. At this time Gauld acquired the technique of bronchoscopy under the tuition of Ian McConchie which he continued on a sessional basis at the Repatriation General Hospital for the next twenty years.

In the early 1970s, with Alastair Campbell, fibreoptic bronchoscopy was introduced, perhaps for the first time in Australia, and it was associated with colour photography for teaching purposes at the weekly chest conferences.

From 1948 to 1978 Gauld was an honorary physician at the Prince Henry Hospital and subsequently a consultant physician; he was a consultant physician at the Repatriation General Hospital, Heidelberg; He was also a consultant at Heatherton Sanatorium from 1951 to 1978.

Stanley Wigley

Stan Wigley graduated MB BS, University of Melbourne, with honours and the Exhibition in Medicine in 1944. After a year at the Royal Melbourne Hospital he joined the Royal Australian Army Medical corps and served a period at Bonegilla, where Wunderly provided the stimulus to seek a career in tuberculosis. In 1947–48 he was a resident medical officer in the chest wing of the Repatriation General Hospital at Heidelberg.

Wigley was appointed a Wunderly Scholar in 1948 and worked as a house physician at the Brompton Hospital. He then took an unpaid job as a house surgeon to Sir Clement Price Thomas, and later took another unpaid research assistantship in the respiratory physiology laboratory at Hammersmith.

In London in 1950 Wigley again met Wunderly who suggested that he contact Dr E.V. Keogh, Director of Tuberculosis in Victoria. Keogh provided Wigley with a job with time off to act as associate physician to Clive Fitts at the Royal Melbourne Hospital. Over the next few years he conducted the Prahan and Central Chest Clinics and was medical superintendent at Greenvale Sanatorium.

In 1956 Wigley spent three months in New Guinea selecting cases for a tuberculosis surgical program to be carried out by C.J. Officer Brown and he combined this with a tuberculosis survey along the Sepik River. Attracted by the magnitude of the tuberculosis problem with its opportunities for treatment and control, he accepted an appointment as specialist medical officer with responsibility for the tuberculosis program. His achievements may be assessed from his publications which include papers on tuberculosis, leprosy, lung cancer and pneumonia. In 1973 with the coming of independence to Papua New Guinea he retired after training his Melanesian successor. Through an association with the World Health Organization he keeps in touch with trends in tuberculosis control; he also serves as co-ordinator of the Pain Clinic at the Prince of Wales Hospital, Sydney.

During his period in New Guinea Wigley acted several times as consultant to the South Pacific Commission and was twice a WHO Travelling Fellow, in 1961 to South-East Asia and in 1969 to Equatorial Africa.

A. Geoffrey McManis

Geoff McManis graduated from Sydney University in 1936. After resident appointments at St Vincent's Hospital, Sydney, and Newcastle Hospital (1936–39) he joined the RAAF, serving in the Middle East, Morotai and Borneo. In 1947 he was a medical officer in the chest wing of the Repatriation General Hospital, Concord, and at the end of the year went to England for post-graduate studies.

While at King Edward VII Sanatorium, Midhurst, McManis was awarded a Wunderly Scholarship which enabled him to take a post at the Brompton Hospital. Working at the Brompton and Midhurst was already a practice which almost all future Wunderly Scholars followed.

On his return to Sydney in 1950 McManis was appointed thoracic physician at St Vincent's Hospital and to the thoracic unit at Royal North Shore Hospital. From 1950 to 1956 he was medical officer-in-charge of the Eva Hordern Hospital for Pregnant Women with Tuberculosis. He was also consultant to the metropolitan mental hospitals and the Randwick Chest Hospital.

McManis's influence was felt more through his teaching than through his several publications although a paper on pregnancy and tuberculosis in 1953 was timely.

Malcolm Allen

Malcolm Allen graduated from the University of Melbourne in 1942. He was a diabetic and shortly after beginning his residency at the Royal Melbourne Hospital he was found to have pulmonary tuberculosis. He was admitted to the Austin Hospital under the care of Dr Hilary Roche who induced and maintained an artificial pneumothorax. After several months, Allen resumed his residency at the Royal Melbourne Hospital where he remained until 1945. He was then appointed registrar to the Thoracic Surgical Unit at the Alfred Hospital under C.J. Officer Brown; he became expert in the care of thoracic surgical patients.

In 1949 Allen was awarded a Wunderly Scholarship and worked at the London Chest Hospital and then at the Montana Sanatorium in Switzerland to which Dr Hilary Roche had returned after the war.

Allen returned to a part-time appointment as pulmonary function officer at the Alfred and Austin Hospitals in Melbourne, pioneering bronchospirometry in the pre-operative assessment of surgical patients. He was an accomplished bronchoscopist. He died after a car accident in June 1960. A modest and very likeable person, Malcolm was among the first thoracic physicians in Australia to interest himself in pulmonary function.

Bruce Geddes

Bruce Geddes graduated with credit from Sydney University in 1943. After a year's residency at Sydney Hospital he joined the AIF serving in the 2/13 Field Ambulance at Morotai and Borneo. He was with the 113 AGH at Concord until his discharge in 1946, and remained there in the chest wards until 1948. His next appointment was as registrar to the Thoracic Unit at Royal North Shore Hospital where he worked until 1950 when he was awarded a Wunderly Scholarship.

Early in 1951 he was appointed an assistant physician at the King Edward VII Sanatorium at Midhurst. With his fellow scholar Alec Priest, he spent some weeks in Scandinavia and visited the United States on the way back to Australia.

In 1953 he returned to Royal North Shore Hospital as a respiratory physician and played an active role in organising the Asian Pacific Conference on Tuberculosis held in Sydney in that year. In 1962 he became Director of the Thoracic Unit, retiring in 1984.

Bruce was an informed and delightful colleague whose experience and advice was always quietly and courteously available.

William Alec Priest

Alec Priest graduated in medicine from the University of Otago in 1933. After a year at Dunedin Hospital he moved to New Plymouth Hospital where he acquired a chest infection, presumably tuberculosis, which influenced his subsequent career. He recovered to work at Cashmere and Waipiata sanatoria. He was awarded a Wunderly Scholarship which he used to study lung disease overseas but details are unknown.

On his return to New Zealand he was appointed chest physician in Wanganui and he continued in this post till his death in 1973 at the age of 63. He conducted chest clinics over a wide area, gained the esteem of the Maori community and was active in lay anti-tuberculosis organisations.

Geoffrey Brinkman

Geoffrey Brinkman graduated in medicine in 1944 and was awarded his MD in 1952 at the University of New Zealand. After a year as house surgeon at Christchurch Hospital (1945) he went to London and worked at various hospitals including the London Chest Hospital (1946–48). He returned to New Zealand and was senior resident at Dunedin Hospital and later assistant director of Cashmere Sanatorium, Christchurch (1950–51). In 1952 he was awarded a Wunderly Scholarship in conjunction with a Fullbright Scholarship and worked at the Trudeau Sanatorium, Saranac, New York and Bellevue Hospital, New York and in pulmonary physiology at Johns Hopkins Hospital, Baltimore.

He was professor of medicine at Wayne State University School of

Medicine from 1968 until his return to Dunedin as professor of medicine, University of Otago. He was Dean of the Faculty from 1978 until his retirement in 1985.

Brinkman published some fifty papers mostly on the therapy of tuberculosis and its complications, clinical respiratory pathophysiology and some aspects of chronic bronchial disease.

Alastair Campbell

Alastair Campbell graduated in medicine in 1940 and was awarded the MD in 1961 at the University of Melbourne. After a year's residency at Prince Henry's Hospital, he joined the RAAF and served until 1946. Following his discharge he became a medical officer at the Repatriation General Hospital Heidelberg. He developed pulmonary tuberculosis but had returned to the chest service at Heidelberg when he was awarded a Wunderly Scholarship in 1952. In England he worked at Papworth and later at the Brompton. He then spent six months in the United States, primarily at the Veterans Administration Hospital, Sunmount, New York, when D'Esopo and Raleigh were establishing the value of long-term chemotherapy with the result that bed rest was no longer essential in the treatment of tuberculosis. Campbell attended a short course in respiratory function and visited the units of Amberson and Cournand in New York.

He returned to Australia to rejoin the Repatriation Department which was then the only organisation offering the practice of thoracic medicine as a separate specialty. From 1953 to 1955 he conducted the chest clinic at Caulfield, Melbourne, and from 1955–59 he was chest specialist at Greenslopes Repatriation Hospital, Brisbane. In 1959 he returned to Heidelberg as senior specialist and additionally consultant (chest diseases) at the central office of the Repatriation Department in 1964.

For many years he was a member of the National Tuberculosis Advisory Council and of the Council of the Victorian Tuberculosis Association.

Campbell's research interests reflect a continuing concern with changes in anti-tuberculosis chemotherapy and other clinical aspects of the management of tuberculosis. His interest in the development of a respiratory function laboratory was generally in advance of the thinking in most teaching hospitals.

Campbell also wrote a book, *John Batman and the Aborigines* (Kibble Books 1987) which was well received by critics .

H. Maynard Rennie

Maynard Rennie, commonly known as Ted, graduated from Sydney University in 1928 and from 1928 to 1930 he was a resident medical officer at Royal Prince Alfred Hospital. After post-graduate study in London he entered general practice in the Sydney suburb of Ashfield. In 1938 he was appointed honorary assistant physician at Royal Prince Alfred Hospital and became an honorary physician in 1956. About 1940 Rennie established a bronchoscopic unit and in 1946 he joined forces with Cotter Harvey to establish a thoracic unit at Royal Prince Alfred Hospital; Maurice Joseph also joined the unit at this time.

Rennie applied for a Wunderly Scholarship to extend his experience in thoracic diseases. He acquired some understanding of respiratory function studies in San Francisco, at the Mayo Clinic and by visiting Amberson, Cournand and Mitchell in New York. In England he visited the Brompton and Midhurst Hospitals.

From 1958 to 1964 Rennie was the senior honorary thoracic physician to Royal Prince Alfred Hospital, and from 1970 to 1972 he was the highly respected president of the Royal Australasian College of Physicians.

Philip Woodruff

Philip Woodruff graduated in medicine with honours from Melbourne University in 1936 (MD 1939). He was a resident at the Royal Melbourne Hospital 1937–38 and Medical Superintendent of the Mackay District Hospital, Queensland, 1939–1942. He spent the next four years in the Army and then became honorary physician to outpatients at the Prince Henry Hospital, Melbourne, from 1946 to 1950.

Wunderly sponsored him for a Rockefeller Fellowship which he spent in 1948–49 in the United States and Europe. On his return to Australia he was appointed Director of Tuberculosis in South Australia (1950–59) and in 1959 he became Director-General of Public Health (1959–78). From 1951 to 1969 he was a part-time lecturer at the Adelaide Medical School in tuberculosis, public health and preventive medicine.

The Wunderly Scholarship supplemented his previous overseas experience in Britain, Scandinavia and the United States.

Woodruff published papers on tuberculosis (especially epidemiology) on the control of communicable diseases and on human ecology. His book *Two Million South Australians* traced the health of the people of South Australia from the founding of the colony in 1836 to the early 1980s and is a reference book of lasting value.

H. Peter Harvey

Peter Harvey graduated in medicine at the University of Sydney in 1948. His resident years were spent at Royal Prince Alfred Hospital , from 1949 to 1951, in the last year as assistant clinical superintendent. In 1964 he was appointed honorary thoracic physician at Royal Prince Alfred Hospital.

Harvey spent his time as a Wunderly Scholar at the Brompton Hospital, Midhurst and Sully. He appreciated the concentration of experience and clinical material at these hospitals together with the clinical expertise of the post-graduate teachers.

Harvey now practices at Bathurst where he also owns a grazing property.

John Beveridge

John Beveridge graduated in medicine and was awarded the University Medal at Sydney in 1948. After a residency at Royal Prince Alfred Hospital he worked at the Royal Alexandra Hospital for Children, becoming its chief resident medical officer until 1955. In 1962 he was appointed foundation Professor of Paediatrics at the University of New South Wales. He played the major role in the development of the new Prince of Wales Children's Hospital. In 1977 he was a Sims Travelling Professor and also a WHO Consultant in paediatrics in Vietnam.

Beveridge was anxious to use his Wunderly Scholarship, awarded in 1956, to research respiratory disorders in childhood in the United Kingdom and at the Children's Medical Centre in Boston. He gained also special experience in cystic fibrosis.

Derek Meyers

Derek Meyers graduated in medicine from the University of Queensland in 1950. After a residency at the Brisbane General Hospital he worked at the Repatriation General Hospital, Heidelberg, from 1952 to 1954. He then became clinical supervisor at the Royal Melbourne Hospital (1955–56) and obtained his MD.

Meyers was awarded a Wunderly Scholarship in 1957 and worked at the Brompton Hospital and at Central Middlesex Hospital. He visited Sully and also Edinburgh hospitals where he was much influenced by John Crofton.

On his return to Australia he was appointed a visiting physician to the Princess Alexandra Hospital in Brisbane, an appointment he held until 1985 when he became a visiting physician to the Repatriation General Hospital at Greenslopes.

J.D. Sinclair

"Jack" Sinclair graduated in medicine at the University of New Zealand 1950 and was awarded his MD in 1955. He was medical registrar at Auckland Hospital and in 1956–57 he was research assistant at the Brompton Hospital in London. He was awarded a Wunderly Scholarship and continued his work in London with the Medical Research Council, and in respiratory physiology at the Post-Graduate Medical School. He then held a United States Public Health Service Fellowship at the Mayo Clinic.

Sinclair sought a Wunderly Scholarship to extend his clinical experience in thoracic medicine and he was particularly anxious to visit

Scandinavian chest units which by 1957 were studying gas exchange. He did some clinical work at Brompton Hospital and visited John Crofton's unit in Edinburgh.

He returned to New Zealand to become clinical physiologist at Green Lane Hospital in Auckland until 1966 when he accepted appointment as Scientific Secretary of the Medical Research Council of New Zealand. Since 1966 he has been Professor of Physiology at the School of Medicine in the University of Auckland. He was President of the New Zealand Thoracic Society from 1984 to 1986.

Sinclair has made fundamental contributions to cardio-respiratory physiology especially in recent years in relation to neurological control of breathing. His sixty odd papers include many studies in clinical respiratory physiology.

Sinclair's research experience in respiratory physiology led to a unique appointment as physician-in-charge of clinical physiology at Green Lane Hospital. It was his experience as a Wunderly Scholar which enabled him to communicate on an equal level with clinicians.

Bryan Gandevia

Bryan Gandevia graduated MB BS with honours in 1948 from the University of Melbourne, and obtained his MD in 1955. After a year at the Royal Melbourne Hospital he joined the RAAMC for military service in Japan and the Korean War. After his return in 1951 he held various appointments at the Royal Melbourne Hospital and the Tuberculosis Division of the Department of Health, he then went to England. After three months at the Wellcome Institute for the History of Medicine on a scholarship provided by the Victorian Branch of the British Medical Association, he became house physician at the Brompton Hospital and then chest clinic registrar at Hammersmith Hospital. Gandevia obtained a Wunderly Scholarship and spent the next eighteen months at the same two hospitals working on respiratory physiology and visiting centres in the United Kingdom concerned with occupational respiratory disorders.

He returned to Australia in 1957 and Dr E.V. Keogh organised a position in the Department of Health for him. This enabled Gandevia to work at the Royal Melbourne Hospital developing a respiratory laboratory on condition that he collaborated with the Division of Occupational Health in investigating occupational respiratory disorders.

In 1963 Gandevia was appointed Associate Professor in Medicine at the University of New South Wales and Chairman of the Department of Thoracic Medicine.

Since his resignation in 1985 Gandevia has practised as a consultant in occupational respiratory medicine. His other concerns have been mainly historical; he was the first president of the Australian Society for the

History of Medicine (1986–88) and he has been a member of the History of Medicine Library Committee of the Royal Australasian College of Physicians since 1963 and its chairman since 1983.

Gandevia's numerous publications relate to the clinical, allergic, radiological and physiological aspects of most forms of non-malignant respiratory disease with special reference to occupational disorders. His historical contributions have related mainly to Australian medicine with emphasis on occupational and respiratory medicine.

John Robert Read

John Read graduated in medicine with first-class honours and was awarded the Sydney University Medal in 1952.

Although his residency at Royal Prince Alfred Hospital was interrupted when he contracted pulmonary tuberculosis, he became registrar in thoracic medicine. In 1959 he obtained his MD for studies on the experimental production of pulmonary fibrosis in rats and was involved in respiratory physiology at Sydney University Department of Medicine.

As a Wunderly Scholar he worked mainly at the Post-Graduate Medical School at Hammersmith in London where the mass spectrometer was being introduced to physiological studies. Returning to the University of Sydney as senior lecturer in 1958, he became Associate Professor in 1962 and Professor of Medicine in 1966.

In 1967 John Read was a major contributor to a symposium on disorders of respiratory function in Melbourne (Campbell, Sinclair and Gandevia were other Wunderly scholars who contributed) and the resulting small published volume makes fascinating reading on the "State of the Art" in Australia at that time.

A grant from the Commonwealth Fund (New York) in 1964 allowed him to expand his concerns with medical education. His final contribution in the last months of his life was to prepare a functional brief for the new Westmead Hospital described as "one of the best, if not the best, ever produced for a teaching hospital".

Tragically he died when most of his colleagues expected the flowering and maturing of his contribution.

Conclusion

These biographical studies were based on material supported by the scholars in response to a questionnaire. For assistance in the biographies of deceased scholars, I am indebted to Julian Lee for J.R. Read, Alastair Campbell for M. Allen, J.D. Sinclair for A. Priest and A.G. McManis for B.L. Geddes. An evaluation of what the scholars achieved or wanted to achieve deserves deliberate historical study, perhaps better carried out in years to come.

References and Sources

Chapter One

References
1. RICH, A.R. *Pathogenesis of Tuberculosis*. C Thomas, Chicago. 1944 p.30.
2. BURNET, F.M. The Natural History of Tuberculosis. *Med J Aust*. 1948; 1, 57.
3. FRENCH, H. *The Index of Differential Diagnosis and Main Symptoms*. J Wright and Sons, Bristol. 3rd Edition, 1919, p288.
4. HOLMES, P.W. and FAULKS, L. Presentation of Pulmonary Tuberculosis. *Aust NZ J Med*. 1981, 11, 651.
5. ABRAHAMS, E.W. et al. Minor Epidemics of Tuberculosis. *Med J Aust*. 1967, 2, 1115.
6. HARRIS, K.W.H. Unpublished material 1973.

Source
International Nomenclature of Disease. Vol III. CIOMS and WHO. Geneva. 1979.

Chapter Two

References
1. GANDEVIA, B. and COBLEY, J. Mortality at Sydney Cove. 1788-92. *Aust NZ J Med* 1974, 4, 111.
2. O'BRIEN, E.M. *The Foundation of Australia*. Angus and Robertson, Sydney, 1950.
3. COWLISHAW, L. The First 50 Years of Medicine in Australia. *Aust NZ J Surg*. 1936-37, 6, 3.
4. ROYLE, H.G. The State of Health in New South Wales in the 1820s. *Med J Aust*. 1973, 1, 950.
5. THOMAS, B and GANDEVIA, B. Dr Francis Workman, Emigrant, and the History of Taking the Cure for Consumption in the Australian Climate. *Med J Aust*. 1959, 2, 1.
6. *Questionnaire on Health Matters addressed by the Royal College of Physicians to Governor Ralph Darling in New South Wales* 1829.
7. CUMPSTON, J.H.L. Quotation from Clutterbuck J.B. Port Phillip in 1849, London 1850. On page 55 in *Health and Disease in Australia*. AGPS Canberra 1989.
8 HAGGER, J. *Australian Colonial Medicine*. Rigby. Adelaide 1979, pp. 99-110.
9. BIRD, S.D. *On Australasian climates and their influence in the Prevention and Arrest of Pulmonary Consumption* Longmans London 1863.
10. GANDEVIA, B. Dr William Thomson and the history of the contagionist doctrine in Melbourne. *Med J Aust* 1953, 1, 398.
11. THOMSON, W. *Digest of the return ordered by the Legislative Council of all deaths from phthisis in Melbourne 1865-69 and the first half of 1870 etc.* Melbourne, Stillwell and Knight. 1871.
12. THOMSON, W. *On Phthisis and the supposed influence of climate*. Melbourne. Stillwell and Knight. 1870.
13. RICHARDSON, W.L. Notes on some of the diseases prevalent in Victoria, Australia. *Edin Med J* 1869, 14, 802.
14. HALL, E.S. On the epidemic diseases of Tasmania. *Trans. Epidemiol. Soc. Lond*. 1 863, 2, 69.
15. JOSKE, R.A. and JOSKE, E.J.P. Mortality pattern in Western Australia 1829-55. *Med J Aust* 1979, 1, 508.
16. MULLINS, George Lane. *Notes on Phthisis in New South Wales and other Australasian Colonies*. John Sands, Sydney. 1895.
17. TRIVETT, J.B. *Tuberculosis in New South Wales. A statistical analysis of the mortality from tubercular disease 1876 to 1908*. Govt Printer, Sydney. 1909.
18. *Victorian Year Book*. 1874 et seq. Govt Printer, Melbourne.
19. SUMMONS, W. *Report on the Ventilation of the Bendigo Mines*. Govt. Printer, Melbourne. 1906.
20............ *Miner's Phthisis: reports on an investigation at Bendigo into the prevalence, nature, causes and prevention of miners' phthisis*. Stillwell. Melbourne. 1907.
21. ROBERTSON, D.G. Inquiry into the prevalence of tuberculosis at Bendigo. Govt. Printer, Melbourne, 1920.

22. KERR, F.R. A Hundred Years Epidemic. *Health Bulletin,* 129-30, pages 3-16. Victorian Department of Health. Melbourne. 1965.

23........... Pneumoconiosis and Tuberculosis 1902-21. *Trans. Australasian Med. Cong.* (BMA) Suppl. Med J Aust. 1923, 273.

24. SMITH, F.B. Personal communication. 1990.

25. CUMPSTON, J.H.L. Edited by M.J. Lewis. *Health and Disease in Australia.* AGPS Canberra, 1898, p.163.

26. *Ibid.* p. 164-165.

27. Southgate IGP. Some aspects of tuberculosis in the New South Wales coalmining industry. *Med J Aust.* 1967, 2, 434.

28. Australian Archives. Canberra. personal search.

29. WUNDERLY, H.W. An investigation into the incidence of pulmonary tuberculosis in young women of Adelaide aged 15 to 30 years. *Med J Aust.* 1940, 2, 229.

30. WRYELL, Max. Personal communcation. 1988.

31. CLELAND, J.B. Tuberculosis lesions at autopsy in Adelaide 1925- 40. *Med J Aust* 1942, 1, 256.

Sources

BIRD, S.D. *Climate and Consumption.* Stillwell and Knight, Melbourne. 1870.

CLARK, C.M. *A short history of Australia.* Revised Illust. Edition Penguin Books Australia 1986.

CLELAND, J.B. Some early references to tuberculosis in Australia. *Med J Aust.* 1938, 1, 256.

COBLEY J. Medicine in the first 20 years of the Colony of New South Wales. *Med J Aust.* 1987, 2, 565.

CROWTHER, W.E.L. The Changing Scene in Medicine: Van Diemen's Land 1803- 1853. *Med J Aust.* 1938, 1, 340.

CUMMINS, C.J. The Colonial Medical Service.

(a)The General Hospital Sydney, 1788-1848. *Mod Med Aust* 1974, 17(1), 11.

(b)The administration of the convict hospitals of New South Wales. *Mod Med Aust.* 1974, 17(2), 11.

CUMPSTON, J.H.L. *An Analysis of the causes of invalidity in respect of claims under the Invalid Pensions Act 1910-1915.* Archival Collection, Dept of Health, Canberra. Phthisis was the largest single certified cause of invalidity - 16.4 per cent of all cases.

FORD, E. Medical Practice in early Sydney. *Med J Aust.* 1955, 2, 41.

CANDEVIA, B. Land Labour and Gold: The medical problems of Australia in the 19th Century. *Med J Aust.* 1960, 1, 753.

.... Medical History in an Australian environment. *Med J Aust.* 1967, 2, 941.

...........: Occupation and Disease in Australia since 1788. Part One. *Bull Post-grad Committee Med.* Univ. Syd. 1971. Vol 27, 8, 157.

GORDON, D. *Health Sickness and Society.* Univ. Queensland Press, St Lucia. 1976.

MULLINS, G. LANE *New South Wales as a health resort for British consumptives.* Sydney, J.A. Thompson, 1896.

NATHAN, C.V. Grim Times at the Sydney Infirmary. *Med J Aust.* 1968, 2, 688.

REPORT *Interim of the NSW Bd of Health Inquiry on the prevalance of miners phthisis and pneumoconiosis in certain industries.* Sydney Govt Printer, 1919.

REPORT *on an investigation of the pulmonary conditions of mine employees, Western Australia, 1925-26.* W.T. Nelson. Comm. Dept Health. Govt Printer, Canberra.

REPORT *of the Royal Commission on Miners' Lung Disease, Dec 1911.* Perth Govt Printer 1912.

THOMSON, W. *The Histochemistry and pathogeny of Tubercle.* Melbourne. Stillwell & Knight. 1876.

.... *The Germ theory of disease. Applied to eradicate phthisis from Victoria.* Melbourne. Sands and Dougall. 1882.

(NOTE: In these two publications Thomson postulated that the causal microorganism of tuberculosis was inhaled or ingested and was most likely present in the centre of the tubercle lesion; this was proven by Koch in 1882).

WOODRUFF, P. Revolutions in health in the Australian colonies. *Med J Aust.* 1987, 2, 572.

Chapter Three

References

1. GODDARD, T.H. The Control of Tuberculosis in Tasmania. *Med J Aust.* 1947, 1, 517.
2. JOSEPH, M.R. Chest Diseases in Australia. *Post Grad Med J* 1970, 46, 243.
3. McMANIS, A.G. The modern concept of pulmonary tuberculosis and pregnancy. *Med J Aust.* 1953, 2, 919.
4. FERGUSON, J. BELL and JAMES, H.M. Some observations on contact work in a tuberculosis bureau. *Med J Aust.* 1931, 2, 169.
5. HOLMES, M.J. Tuberculosis in Australia. *Med J Aust.* 1937, 2, 813.
6. JOSKE, R.A. and JOSKE, E.J.P. Mortality Patterns in Western Australia 1829-55. *Med J Aust.* 1979, 1, 508.
7. CUMPSTON, J.H.L. Edited by M.J. Lewis. *Health and Disease in Australia.* AGPS Canberra. 1989. p.163.
8. CLAYSON, Christopher. *Tuberculosis Control: The Beginning.* Unpublished material by courtesy of author. Edinburgh 1987.
9. CUSHING, Harvey. *Life of Sir William Osler.* OUP. London. 1940. p.536.

Chapter Four

References

1. WAKSMAN, S. *The Conquest of Tuberculosis.* Robert Hale. London. 1965.
2. BUTLIN, N.G. *Our Original Aggression.* George Allen & Unwin. Sydney. 1983.
3. MULVANEY, J and WHITE, J.P. *Australians to 1788.* Fairfax Syme Weldon, Sydney, 1987.
4. BARWICK, D. Changes in the Aboriginal Population of Victoria 1863- 1966. In: MULVANEY, D and GOLSON, J. *Aboriginal Man and Environment in Australia.* ANU Press, Canberra. 1971.
5. JENNINGS, H. In: *Aborigines. Report and Correspondence relative to the mortality amongst the Residents of the Aboriginal Stations of Victoria.* Govt. Printer, Melbourne. 1879.
6. MOODIE, P. *Aboriginal Health.* ANU press, Canberra, 1973.
7. COOK, C.E. Medicine and the Australian Aboriginal: A Century of contact in the Northern Territory. *Med J Aust.* 1966, 1, 559.
8. BASEDOW, H. Diseases of the Australian Aboriginal. *J Trop Med Hygiene.* 1932, 35, 209.
9. ARDEN, F. Tuberculosis at the Brisbane Children's Hospital: a ten year survey. *Med J Aust.* 1950, 2, 543.
10. KING, A., EDWARDS, G., GIBSON, P. A Survey of Australian Aborigines for pulmonary tuberculosis. *Med J Aust.* 1951, 2, 934.
11. ABRAHAMS, E.W. Tuberculosis in indigenous Australians. Med J Aust. 1975, 2, 23.
12. ANONYMOUS. Health in the Northern Territory, *Med J Aust.* 1964, 2, 799.
13 BATESON, E.M. Tuberculosis in the Australian Aboriginal: a radiological perspective. *Australasian Radiology.* 1986, 30, 63.
14. South Australia: *Report of the Aborigines Protection Board for the year 1958.* W.L. Hawes, Govt. Printer Adelaide, 1959.
15. CLELAND, J.B. Tuberculosis lesions at autopsy in Adelaide 1925- 40. *Med J Aust* 1942, 1, 256.
16. BREINL A. and HOLMES, M.J. Medical Report on the data collected during a journey through some districts of the Northern Territory.

Sources

MACKEN, F. Initial Comments on a tuberculosis case - finding survey among Australian Aborigines (State of Queensland) 1952. *Tubercle* (Edinburgh) 33, 376.
PENNY, M. THOMSON, N. A preliminary analysis of Aboriginal tuberculosis. *Aboriginal Health Information Bulletin* 1984, 8, 15.

Chapter Five

References

1. *Statistics of the Colony of New Zealand for the Year 1873*, Wellington, Registrar-General's Office, p.5.
2. Department of Public Health, Chief Health Officer *Annual Report 1901*, Appendices to the Journal of the House of Representatives (AJHR), H-31, p.1.
3. G. GORE GILLON, 'A Factor in Open-Air Treatment', read at annual meeting of the

New Zealand Branch of the British Medical Association, *New Zealand Medical Journal (NZMJ)*, 2, 5 (1901), p.1.

4. See G. R. SEARLE, The Quest for National Efficiency (Oxford, 1971).5.
   Department of Public Health, *Annual Report 1904*, p.ix.
6. SIR JOSEPH WARD, 'New Zealand's Attitude Towards Consumption from a Legislative Point of View', *NZMJ*, 3, 11 (1903), p.259.
7. See J. R. BIGNALL, Firmley: *The Biography of a Sanatorium* (London, 1979).
8. R. H. MAKGILL (Auckland District Health Officer), 'The Duty of the State in Regard to Tuberculosis', *NZMJ*, 19, 92 (1920), p.109.
9. See also BRIAN ABEL-SMITH, *The Hospitals* (London, 1964), pp. 36, 44, 45, 205.
10. Early twentieth-century British and American estimates placed morbidity at ten times mortality from tuberculosis.
11. Report by Dr POMARE, Department of Public Health, *Annual Report 1902*, p.65; ibid. 1903, p.72.
12. Quoted in Department of Health, Director General of Health, *Annual Report 1929*, p.2.
13. R. H. MAKGILL, NZMJ, 12, 92 (1920), p.102.
14. JAMES A. JENKINS, 'Thoracic Surgery', *NZMJ*, 28, 148 (1929), pp. 325-31; Jenkins, 'surgical Aspects of Pulmonary Tuberculosis', *NZMJ*, 31, 165 (1932), pp.315-27.
15. E. H. ROCHE AND A. H. G. ROCHE, *Green Lane Saga. Green Lane Hospital, Auckland: 1889-1982 and its development of cardiology and cardiothoracic and vascular surgery* (Auckland, 1983), p.16.
16. See for example, Editorial (J. O. Mercer), 'The surgery of Pulmonary Tuberculosis', *NZMJ*, 38, 205 (1939), pp.139-43.
17. *Prevention and Treatment of Pulmonary Tuberculosis in New Zealand.* Report of the Committee of Inquiry appointed by the Hon. Mr Young, Minister of Health', AJHR, H-31A, 1928, p.4' C. A. Taylor (Director of Tuberculosis, Department of Health), 'Notification of Tuberculosis in New Zealand', *NZMJ*, 42, 230 (1943), pp.151-4.
18. See also L. BRYDER, 'A wonderland of buttercups, clover and daisies: tuberculosis and open-air schools 1907-39', in R. Cooter (ed.), In *The Name of the Child. Health and Social Policy, 1880-1950*, London, 1991.
19. J. M. WOGAN (Department of Health, Division of Tuberculosis), 'Tuberculosis Control in New Zealand', *NZMJ*, 54, 301 (1955), p.246.
20. M. K. FINLAYSON & N. L. EDSON (from the Travis Laboratory, Medical School, University of Otago), 'Extra-Pulmonary Tuberculosis. Frequency of Infection with the Bovine Type of Tubercle Bacillus', *NZMJ*, 46, 253 (1947), pp.184-9. the Department of Public Health *Annual Report for 1906* estimated that 15 per cent of milk-cows were affected with tuberculosis.
21. H. B. TURBOTT, *Tuberculosis in the Maori, East Coast, New Zealand*, Wellington, 1935. See also Chapter by Wells.
22. J. M. WOGAN, *NZMJ*, 54, 301 (1955), p.250.
23. C. A. TAYLOR, *NZMJ*, 42, 230 (1943), p.151.
24. M. STRINGER BUCHLER (from the Department of Health), 'Pulmonary Tuberculosis in Wellington, A Radiological Investigation Among Office and Factory Workers and Secondary School Children', *NZMJ*, 43, 234 (1944), pp. 73-80.
25. J. M. WOGAN, *NZMJ*, 54, 301 (1955), p.245.
26. L.Bryder, 'BCG Vaccination', *Proceedings of First National Conference of the Australian Society of the History of Medicine 1989* (1991).
27. See NATALI ALLEN AND EVE BRISTER, 'Nurses with Tuberculosis: A Preliminary Study', *Women's Studies Journal*, 5, 2 (1989), pp.38-60.
28. Editorial, 'BCG Vaccination and New Zealand', *NZMJ*, 48, 265 (1949), p.261.
29. S. HICKLING (Preventive and Social Medicine Department, University of Otago), 'Tuberculosis in New Zealand, past, Present and Future', *NZMJ*, 62, 369 (1963), p.228.
30. J. M. WOGAN, NZMJ, 54, 301 (1955), p.244.31. Editorial, 'Streptomycin', *NZMJ*, 46, 253 (1947),pp.167-8.
32. Editorial, 'The Prevention of Tuberculosis', *NZMJ*, 73, 469 (1971), p.366.
33. A. R. KERR, secretary of the Thoracic Society of New Zealand, 'TB and Polynesians', Letter to the Editor, *NZMJ*, 76, 485 (1972), p.295.
34. J. B. MACKAY, 'Tuberculosis in Polynesians', Letter to the Editor, *NZMJ*, 76, 485 (1972), p.449.
35. Department of Health, Director General of Health, *Annual Report, 1983*, p.19.
36. THOMAS MCKEOWN, *The Modern Rise of Population* (London, 1976);

McKeown, *The Role of Medicine. Dream, Mirage and Nemesis?* (Oxford, 1979).

37. See for example, J. M. Wogan, *NZMJ*, 54, 301 (1955), p.255; J. W. Donovan, 'A Study of New Zealand Mortality; 5. Tuberculosis', *NZMJ*, 70 (1969), p.95.

38. J. J. COLLINS, 'The contribution of medical measures to the decline of mortality from respiratory tuberculosis: An age-period-cohort model', *Demography*, 19, 3 (1982), pp.409-427.

39. See also L. BRYDER, *Below the Magic Mountain. A Social History of Tuberculosis in Twentieth-century Britain* (Oxford, 1988); F. B. Smith, *The Retreat of Tuberculosis, 1850-1950* (London, 1988); Neil Macfarlan, 'Hospitals, Houses and Tuberculosis in Glasgow, 1911-51', *Social History of Medicine, 2*, 1 (1989), pp.59-86.

40. See also SIMON SZRETER, 'The importance of social intervention in Britain's mortality decline c.1850-1914: A re-interpretation of the role of public health', *Social History of Medicine*, 1, 1 (1988), pp.1-38.

41. J. J. COLLINS, *Demography* (1982), p.424.

Source

MACKAY, N.R. Tuberculosis in the Maori. A radiological investigation among Maoris of the North Island. *NZMJ*. 1933.

Chapter Six

References

1. WIGLEY, S. The first hundred years of tuberculosis in New Guinea. In: *The Melanesian Environment.* Editor J.H. Winslow. ANU Press, Canberra, 1977.

2. DOCKER, E.L. *The Blackbirders. The recruiting of South Sea labour for Queensland. 1863-1907.* Angus and Robertson, Sydney, 1970.

3. PARNABY, C.W. *Britain and the labour trade in the South West Pacific.* Durham Univ. Press. Durham, NC. 1964.

4. LAWES, W.G. Effects of the climate of New Guinea upon exotic races. *Aust. Med Gazette.* May 1877.

5. CLEMENTS, F.W. A tuberculosis survey of a Papuan Village. *Med J Aust.* 1936, 1, 253.

6. CILENTO, R. *Report of the International Pacific Conference.* Govt Printer Melbourne, 1926.

7. BACKHOUSE, T.C. Tuberculosis in Melanesian natives. A survey of autopsy findings from the pre-war era 1922-40. *Med J Aust.* 1956, 2, 62.

8. HEYDON, G.A.M. Tuberculin Schick and Dick reactions in Central New Guinea natives. *Med J Aust.* 1937, 2, 766.

9. NORTH, E.A. JAMIESON, D. Immunisation against tuberculosis in Australia and New Guinea. *Med J Aust* 1950, 2, 792.

10. WILSON, R.K. Chest Surgery in New Guinea. *PNG Med J.* 1957, 38, 117.

11. WIGLEY, S.C. Thoracic Surgery in Papua New Guinea. *PNG Med J.* 1971, 18, 3.

12. MYLIUS, L.E. and WIGLEY, S.C. The Squatter Settlements of Port Moresby and Tuberculosis. *PNG Med J .* 1971, 18, 3.

13. DOWNS, Ian. *The Australian Trusteeship of Papua New Guinea 1945- 75.* AGPS Canberra, 1980.

14. WIGLEY, S.C. *Report of the Goroka Conference on tuberculosis control in the Highlands region of the Territory of Papua New Guinea,* May 1961.

15. WARI, K. and WIGLEY, S.C. Defaulters and Absconders Proc. *8th Eastern Region, IUAT Conference* Sydney, October 1972.

Sources

WIGLEY, S.C. *Tuberculosis and New Guinea.* PHD Port Moresby, 1973.

DECKER, J.A. *Labour Problems in the Pacific Mandate* OUP London, 1940.

FARRELL, B.H. *Man in the Pacific Islands.* Ed. R.G. Ward. Clarendon Press, Oxford, 1972.

WIGLEY, S.C. BCG Vaccination in a tuberculosis-free community. A study of post-vaccination conversion reactions. *Proc. 8th Eastern Region, IUAT Conference* Sydney, October 1972.

Chapter Seven

References

1. ABRAHAMS, E.W. Clinical experiences with mycobacterium other than M. tuberculosis in Queensland. *Med J Aust.* 1965, 1, 787.
2. BLACKLOCK, Z.M., DAWSON, D.J., KANE, D.W., McEVOY, D. *Mycobacterium asiaticum* as a potential pulmonary pathogen. A clinicial and bacteriological review of five cases. *Am Rev Resp Dis.* 1983, 127, 241.
3. MacCALLUM, P., TOLHURST, J.C., BUCKLE, G., SISSON, H.A. A new mycobacterial infection in man. *J. Path Bact.* 1948, 60, 93.
4. KEERS, R.Y. *Pulmonary tuberculosis. A journey down the centuries.* Bailliere Tindall, London, 1978.
5. ROBERTSON, D.G. *Inquiry into the prevalence of tuberculosis at Bendigo.* Govt. Printer, Melb. 1920.
6. PINNER, M.G. *The incidence of tuberculosis infection.* Report of an epidemiological survey of the ACT and Queanbeyan. *Med J Aust.* 1950, 1, 717.
7. MILLS, R.M. The source of tuberculosis infection in patients of the Royal Alexandra Hospital for Children. *Med J Aust.* 1953, 2, 374.
8............ Tuberculosis infection and its source in primary school children. *Med J Aust.* 1953, 2, 530.
9............ Tuberculosis infection in children under the age of two years. *Australasian Annals Med.* 1953, 2, 195.
10. TRIVETT, J.B. *Tuberculosis in New South Wales; a statistical analysis of the mortality from tubercular disease 1876-1908.* Govt Printer, Sydney, 1909.
11. HOLMES, M.J. and ROBERTSON, W.A.N. *Bovine tuberculosis in man and animals in Australia.* Govt. Printer, Canberra, 1930.
12. WEBSTER, R. The Mathieson Memorial Lecture. Observations based on laboratory experience in tuberculosis. *Med J Aust.* 1947, 1, 605.
13............ Pulmonary tuberculosis; bacteriological examination supplementing routine thoracic radiography in the Australian Military Forces. *Med J Aust.* 1943, 2, 81.
14............ Tuberculosis in childhood; the incidence of bovine infection in Victoria. *Med J Aust.* 1932, 1, 315.
15............ Studies in tuberculosis. *Med J Aust.* 1947, 2, 49.
16. HEWLETT, H.M. Radiology; the past and the future. *Med J Aust.* 1938, 2, 109.
17. STEVENS, D.J. Evolution of x-ray equipment for tuberculosis case- finding programmes in Australia. *Med J Aust.* 1968, 2, 931.
18. WALKER, A.S. *Clinical Problems in War: Australia in the War 1939- 45.* Series 5 (Medical) Vol 1. Australian War Memorial Canberra 1952.
19. HARVEY W. COTTER. Tuberculosis as a problem for the States. *Med J Aust.* 1940, 2, 239.

Sources

ABRAHAMS, E.W. AND SILVERSTONE, H. Epidemiological evidence of the presence of non-tuberculous sensitivity to tuberculin in Queensland. *Tubercle* 1961, 42, 487.
ABRAHAMS, E.W. HARLAND, R.D. Sensitivity to avian and human tuberculin PPD in Brisbane school children. *Tubercle* 1967, 48, 79.
ABRAHAMS, E.W. Tuberculin sensitivity following BCG vaccination in Brisbane school children. *Tubercle* 1979, 60, 109.
Bacteriological investigations for Mycobacteria including drug sensitivity testing. Dept of Health, Canberra, 1967.
BEGG, A.C. The Father of Radiology in New Zealand. *NZ Med J.* 1975, 82, 1.
CARRUTHERS, K.J.M. Observer and Experimental Variations in Tuberculin Testing. *Tubercle* 1970, 51, 48.
.... *Tuberculin Testing in the Control of Tuberculosis in Western Australia.* M.D. Thesis, 1969 Univ. of WA.
.... Tuberculin Testing after BCG vaccination with freeze- dried vaccine. *Med J Aust.* 1959, 1, 1122.
.... and EDWARDS, F.G.B. Atypical Mycobacteria in Western Australia. *Am. Rev. Resp. Dis.* 1965. 91, 887.
.... Comparison of the Heaf and Mantoux tests using several tuberculins. *Tubercle* 1969, 50, 22.

EDDY, C.E. The Fiftieth Anniversary of the Discovery of X-rays. *Med J Aust.* 1946, 1, 138.
SWABY, L.J. *Bacteriological investigations for tuberculosis.* Unpublished paper. 1969.
  By courtesy of the author.

Chapter Eight

References

1. KEERS, R.Y. *Pulmonary tuberculosis; a journey down the centuries.* Bailliere Tindall, London. 1978.
2. O'CARRIGAN, CATHERINE. *Phthisis*, M.A. Thesis.
3. MULLINS, GEORGE LANE. *Notes on Phthisis in New South Wales and other Australasian Colonies.* John Sands, Sydney, 1895.
4. PEARN, J. Phthisis and philately. An account of the Consumptive Homes Stamps of New South Wales, *Med J Aust.* 1987, 2, 575.
5. Public Records Office of South Australia. Mr D. Benjamin State Archivist provided copies of the Annual Reports of the James Brown Trust 1906-14.
6. SPRINGTHORPE, J.W. *Progress Report on Koch's treatment of tubercular disease.* Stillwell & Co., Melbourne, 1891.
.... *Tuberculin as a diagnostic agent.* Stillwell & Co., Melbourne, 1894.
7. WILKINSON, W. Camac. *Treatment of Consumption.* McMillan & Co. Melbourne, 1908.
8. MORRIS, K.N. *A Tribute to a great man, Sir James Officer Brown.* Memorial, 1984.
9. BROWN, C.J. OFFICER. The Place of Surgery in the treatment of pulmonary tuberculosis. *Aust NZ J Surg.* 1945-46, 99, 117.

Sources

ALLEN, H.B. *Report on Professor Koch's remedy.* Melbourne, Govt Printer, 1891.
ELWELL, L.B. Some notes on treatment with tuberculin. Transactions Australasian Med Cong (BMA) *Med J Aust* Suppl. 1924. p33.
GILLIES, S AND McDONALD, C.G. Dispensaries and their value in the control of tuberculosis. Trans. Australasian Med Cong. (BMA) *Med J Aust.* Suppl. 1924, p.279.
GRIFFITHS F GUY Fibrosis of the tuberculosis lung produced by the injection of tuberculin. *Med J Aust.* 1909, 1, 309.
LATHAM, L.S. Artiifical pneumothorax in the treatment of pulmonary tuberculosis. *Med J Aust.* 1914, 1, 463.
REISSMAN, C. The nature of tuberculosis and its treatment by the physician. *Aust. Med Gaz.* 1908, 27, 6, 269.
MACLEAN, L.A. An account of the Queen Victoria Sanatorium at Thirlmere. *Med J Aust.* 1914, 1, 465.
ROCHE, H. Some observations of the treatment and prevention of tuberculosis.
.... Some clinical aspects of tuberculosis.
.... The tuberculous lung cavity and Monaldi's closed suction drainage. *Med J Aust.* 1945, 2, 293, 299, 307, respectively.
WILKINSON, W. CAMAC. The principles of immunity in tuberculosis and their value in diagnosis and treatment. *Med J Aust.* 1924, 1, 103.

Chapter Nine

Sources

GODBY, R. Chest Surgery in the Blue Mountains. *Med J. Aust.* 1953, 1, 774.
HAYWARD, J.H., THOMAS, G. GUILFOYLE, P. *Tuberculosis in the Repatriation Department*, 1964.
MONK, IAN Recent Experiences of Thoracic Surgery in New South Wales. *Med J Aust.* 1953, 2, 596.
TELLESON, W.G. The place of surgery in pulmonary tuberculosis. *Med J Aust.* 1965, 1, 785.
NICKS, ROWAN The Surgery of Pulmonary Tuberculosis. *NZ Med J.* 1953, 366.
.... Tracheal stenosis. *B.R.J.S.* 1954-55, 42, 267.
.... Surgeons All. *The Story of Cardiothoracic Surgery in Australia and New Zealand.* Hale and Iremonger, Sydney, 1984.
ROSS, F.W. Surgery for pulmonary tuberculosis over a ten year period at Randwick Chest Hospital. *Med J Aust.* 1970, 2, 982.

Chapter Ten

References

1. WAKSMAN, S. *The conquest of tuberculosis*. R Hale. London, 1965.
2. FERGUSON J BELL, BRISTOW, V.G. AND BULL, P.R. Streptomycin in tuberculosis. *Med J Aust*. 1949, 2, 192.
3. MUNRO FORD, R. Streptomycin in Pulmonary Tuberculosis: a review of six cases. *Med J Aust*. 1949, 2, 205.
4. PROUST, A.J. and BEACHAM, E.G. Isonicotinic acid hydrazide in the treatment of pulmonary tuberculosis; a preliminary report. *Bull. School Med. U. Maryland*, 1952, 37, 147.
5. PROUST, A.J. Correspondence. *Med J Aust*. 1953, 1, 622.
6. PROUST, A.J., BEACHAM, E.G. and ALLEN, H.S. isonicotinic acid hydrazide in the treatment of pulmonary tuberculosis. *Med J Aust*. 1953, 1, 179.
7. MUNRO FORD, R. Isonicotinic acid hydrazide in the treatment of pulmonary tuberculosis. *Med J Aust.*, 1953, 2, 366.
8. HEYWORTH, F. and NOBBS, N.S. A study of tuberculosis notifications in Queensland in 1958 with a 5 year follow-up. *Med J Aust*. 1968, 2, 926.
9. PROUST, A.J. The Australian Rifampicin Trial. *Med J Aust*. 1971, 2, 85.
10. PROUST, A.J. and EVANS, C.P.V. The Australian Rifampicin Trial. *Med J Aust*. 1972, 2, 861.
11 .O'CONNELL, J., CAMPBELL, A.H., VERUNS, A. Initial treatment of pulmonary tuberculosis with rifampicin. *Med J Aust*. 1973, 2, 881.

Chapter Eleven

References

1. GOLDSMITH, L.O. *Administrative aspects of tuberculosis control in Australia. Masters Thesis, Univ. Western Australia, 1969.* Copy provided by author.
2. WUNDERLY, H.W. *Tuberculosis Survey of British Isles, Western Europe, United States and Canada.* Dept Health Canberra, 1950.
3. BOAG, T.C. Community-wide chest x-ray surveys in Australia. *Med J Aust*. 1971, 2, 74.
4. HOWELLS, G. The Australian Tuberculosis Campaign. *Bull. Internat. Union Against Tuberculosis (IUAT)* 1970, 44, 147.
5. HOWELLS, G. Australia is Lucky. *Tuberculosis Quarterly Review*. IUAT. Sept. 1970. p.1.
6. CUMPSTON, J.H.L. *Phthisis in Australia with more especial reference to Western Australia.* Perth Govt. Printer, 1909.

Sources

CUMPSTON, J.H.L. Public Health in Australia. The First 42 years. *Med J Aust*. 1931, 1, 491.
.... The evolution of public health administration in Australia. *Med J Aust*. 1932, 1, 194.
.... Tuberculosis in Australia. *Med J Aust*. 1931, 2, 153.
.... Statistical review of tuberculosis in Australia. Trans Australasian Med. Cong (BMA) 1924. *Med J Aust*. Suppl. 237.
.... *Health and Disease in Australia.* Edited by M.J. Lewis. AGPS. Canberra, 1989.
LANCASTER H.O. Tuberculosis Mortality in Australia 1908-45. *Med J Aust*. 1950, 1, 655.

Chapter Twelve

References

1. POWELL, J.M. Medical promotion and the consumptive immigrant to Australia. *Geog. Review* 1973, 63, 449.
2. MACKAY, I.R. Medical selection of migrants from the displaced persons population of post-war Europe. *Med J Aust* 1953, 1, 369.
3. EDWARDS, F.G.B. Tuberculosis. Incidence in the non-Australian born. *Med J Aust*. 1963, 1, 501.
4. CSORDAS, S. *Extrapulmonary tuberculosis among migrants.* From the original paper forwarded by the author.

Sources

DR A.H. CAMPBELL provided reprints of his papers on the epidemiology of tuberculosis in ex-servicemen as well as a history of the Victorian Division of the Repatriation Department.

Glossary of Terms

Tuberculin. Koch's original tuberculin (called old tuberculin, O.T.) was prepared from cultures of tubercle bacilli grown in glycerol broth medium which were then sterilised by heat and filtered to remove the bacilli and associated debris. It was then concentrated to one-tenth its volume. Modern tuberculin is a purified protein derivative (PPD) of tuberculin prepared from the water-soluble fractions obtained from cultures of tubercle bacilli grown in a liquid synthetic medium.

Tuberculin Test. The tuberculin test is a diagnostic test of infection with *M. tuberculosis*. A person (or animal) is said to be tuberculin positive when a skin allergic reaction is elicited by the intracutaneous injection of a carefully measured volume of PPD tuberculin. The accepted standard test is the Mantoux test.

Tuberculosis. A usually chronic disease caused by *Mycobacterium tuberculosis* or rarely (in Australia) *M. bovis*. The lungs are the principal site of disease in about 80 per cent of cases.

Primary tuberculous infection. An initial infection of the lung and draining lymph nodes with *M. tuberculosis* in previously uninfected and tuberculin nonsensitive persons, usually children or young adults. In most cases there are no clinical symptoms and healing occurs; the infection may remain quiescent for many years and then reactivate to cause disease in the lungs or other organs of the body. Primary infection is recognized by a positive tuberculin test.

Progressive primary pulmonary tuberculosis. Occasionally primary tuberculous infection progresses to other areas of the lung to cause primary pulmonary tuberculosis; this progress depends upon the interaction between the resistance of the host and the size of the infection.

Miliary tuberculosis is an acute dissemination of tuberculosis via the blood or lymphatic vessels to the rest of the lungs and more distant organs including the meninges, liver, kidneys and bone marrow. It is a life-threatening condition especially in those with immune deficiencies.

Adult pulmonary tuberculosis. The most common and infectious form of tuberculosis which usually arises from a reactivation of a quiescent primary lesion. Most commonly the disease initially involves the upper lobe of the lung but there may be widespread involvement of one or both lungs. Diagnosis depends upon the demonstration of tubercle bacilli in the sputum, on smear or on culture. Persons who expel large numbers of tubercle bacilli by coughing or spitting are a grave risk to their close contacts, particularly children and young adults.

Extrapulmonary or non-pulmonary tuberculosis is disease affecting principally organs or tissues other than the lungs, most commonly lymph nodes in the neck, the kidneys and renal tract, the female reproductive tract and bone. The diagnosis is usually made by bacteriological or histological examination of fluid (such as urine) or biopsy tissue.

Aypical mycobacteria. A general term for mycobacteria other than *Mycobacterium tuberculosis*, *M. bovis*, (the cause of bovine tuberculosis) and *M. leprae* (the cause of Hansen's disease or leprosy). Atypical mycobacteria may cause disease in humans and the diagnosis depends on bacteriological examination.

Pneumothorax, artificial. The introduction of air into the pleural cavity to collapse the lung as a form of threatment.

Thorocoplasty. The surgical removal of part of the ribs to collapse the underlying diseased lung.

BCG (Bacille Calmette-Guerin).   A live vaccine against tuberculosis prepared from *M. bovis*. The bovine tubercle bacilli are attenuated so they do not cause disease but produce significant immunity

Chemotherapy.   The treatment of tuberculosis with chemical compounds or drugs. Anti-tuberculosis chemotherapy dates from 1947 with the demonstrated efficacy of streptomycin in human tuberculosis.

Haemoptysis. The spitting or coughing up of blood.

Mass Miniature Radiography.   Radiography using photography of the image of the chest on a fluorescent X-ray screen. The size of the film (35 to 100 mm) resulted in a much lower cost per film compared with standard chest X-rays.

Phthisis.   An obsolete term used to denote a wasting disease or consumption. Until the early 20th century it was generally applied to advanced pulmonary tuberculosis.

Miners' Phthisis.   An obsolete term used to denote pulmonary fibrosis occurring in underground miners exposed to the inhalation of quartz dust (silica). It was commonly complicated by pulmonary tuberculosis.

Sputum examination.   Microscopic examination of sputum to demonstrate acid-fast bacilli stained by the Ziehl-Neelsen method. Proof that these bacilli were tubercle bacilli depended on culture on special media, usually for 8 weeks.

Index of Names

Index of Subjects